T0262027

Encyclopedia of Diabetes: Diagnosis and Alternative Treatment of Type 1 Diabetes

Volume 09

Encyclopedia of Diabetes: Diagnosis and Alternative Treatment of Type 1 Diabetes Volume 09

Edited by **Rex Slavin, Windy Wise and Roy Marcus Cohn**

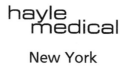

New York

Published by Hayle Medical,
30 West, 37th Street, Suite 612,
New York, NY 10018, USA
www.haylemedical.com

Encyclopedia of Diabetes: Diagnosis and Alternative Treatment of Type 1 Diabetes
Volume 09
Edited by Rex Slavin, Windy Wise and Roy Marcus Cohn

International Standard Book Number: 978-1-63241-151-8 (Hardback)

Contents

Preface

This book elucidates current developments in Type-1 Diabetes research across the world, focusing on distinct research fields significant to this disease. The areas covered are recognition & monitoring of diabetes mellitus and substitute treatments for diabetes. Top-notch investigators from across the world have contributed in this book. The book aims to elucidate understandable presentation of concepts on the basis of experiments and results from existing published reports as well as from research works of authors. The book will serve as a valuable source of reference for basic science and clinical investigators as well as for patients and their family.

Various studies have approached the subject by analyzing it with a single perspective, but the present book provides diverse methodologies and techniques to address this field. This book contains theories and applications needed for understanding the subject from different perspectives. The aim is to keep the readers informed about the progresses in the field; therefore, the contributions were carefully examined to compile novel researches by specialists from across the globe.

Indeed, the job of the editor is the most crucial and challenging in compiling all chapters into a single book. In the end, I would extend my sincere thanks to the chapter authors for their profound work. I am also thankful for the support provided by my family and colleagues during the compilation of this book.

Editor

Part 1

Identification and Monitoring
of Diabetes Mellitus

1

A Novel L-Arginine/L-Glutamine Coupling Hypothesis: Implications for Type 1 Diabetes

Paulo Ivo Homem de Bittencourt Jr.[1,2,3] and Philip Newsholme[4]

[1]*Department of Physiology, Institute of Basic Health Sciences,*
Federal University of Rio Grande do Sul
[2]*Federal University of Rio Grande do Sul School of*
Physical Education, Porto Alegre, RS
[3]*National Institute of Hormones and Women's Health*
[4]*School of Biomolecular and Biomedical Science and Institute for*
Sport and Health, UCD Dublin, Belfield, Dublin 4
[1,2,3]*Brazil*
[4]*Ireland*

1. Introduction

L-Arginine is synthesised *in vivo* from L-glutamine, L-glutamate, or L-proline via the intestinal-renal axis (**Fig. 1A**) in humans and most other mammals (Wu et al., 2009). In humans, plasma L-glutamine is the precursor of 80% of plasma L-citrulline while plasma L-citrulline, in turn, is the precursor of 10% of plasma L-arginine (van de Poll et al., 2007). Although the intestine consumes L-glutamine at a high rates, dependent on L-glutamine supply (and production from the skeletal muscle), approximately 13% of L-glutamine taken up by the intestine is converted to L-citrulline, so that quantitatively, L-glutamine is the major precursor for intestinal release of L-citrulline (van de Poll et al., 2007), which can be further converted to L-arginine. These observations highlight the importance of L-arginine/L-glutamine metabolic coupling, especially as L-arginine is one of the most potent secretagogues of insulin from the pancreatic beta cells (Palmer et al., 1976), whereas L-arginine deficiency is associated with insulinopenia and failure to secrete insulin in response to glucose (Spinas et al., 1999). L-Arginine is essential for metabolism and function of multiple body organs, with decreased plasma and cellular levels of L-arginine reported in type 2 diabetic subjects (Pieper & Dondlinger, 1997).

Since L-arginine is the precursor of nitric oxide (NO)[*], which serves as a key cell signalling molecule in pancreatic islet β-cells, restriction in the availability of L-arginine is likely to

---

[*] **Abbreviations used:** CAT, catalase; GSH, glutathione; GSSG, glutathione disulphide; GSPx, glutathione peroxidase; GSRd, glutathione disulphide reductase; HSP70, 70-kDa member of heat shock protein family; eHSP70, extracellular heat shock protein of 70 kDa; IFN-γ, interferon-γ; IκB, a member of the inhibitors of nuclear factor κB; IKK, inhibitor of κB kinase; IL-1β, interleukin-1β; IL1-ra, IL-1β receptor antagonist; iNOS, inducible nitric oxide synthase; NF-κB, a member of nuclear transcription factor κB; NO, nitric oxide free radical (•N=O); PPAR-γ, peroxisome proliferator activated receptor-γ; RNS, reactive nitrogen species; ROS, reactive oxygen species; SNOG, S-nitrosoglutathione; SOD,

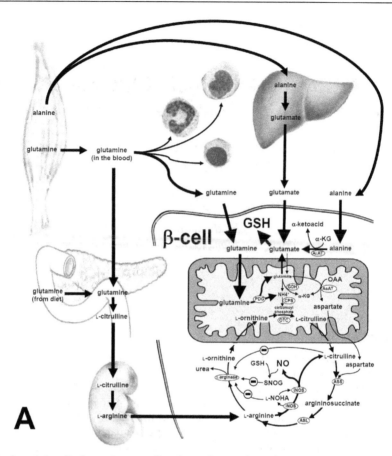

Fig. 1. The l-arginine/l-glutamine coupling hypothesis of insulin-secreting β-cells. (A) Pancreatic islet β-cells utilise l-arginine for the biosynthesis of NO and l-glutamate for GSH generation during secretagogue-stimulated insulin secretion. l-Arginine is provided to the pancreas by the intestinal-renal axis from l-glutamine, while l-glutamate is furnished by the liver mainly from muscle-derived alanine. In the β-cell, NH4+ may contribute to l-arginine biosynthesis, through the concerted action of carbamoyl phosphate synthetase I (CPS), ornithine transcarbamoylase (OTC), argininosuccinate synthetase (ASS) and argininosuccinate lyase (ASL) that eventually produces l-arginine. Skeletal muscle-derived l-glutamine is also substrate for the maintenance of GSH metabolism in β-cells, but rapidly-proliferating cells of the gut as well as immune cells compete with β-cell for the utilisation of l-glutamine. Hence, any minimal reduction in the supply of l-arginine to the pancreas may shift l-glutamate metabolism towards the synthesis of NO instead of GSH, thus leading to oxidative stress, inhibition of insulin secretion and eventually β-cell death. This is the case of undernourishment, cancer states, trauma, sepsis, major burns and low skeletal muscle

superoxide dismutase; TBARS, thiobarbituric acid-reactive substances; TNF-α, tumor necrosis factor-α; TNFR, TNF-α receptor; UCP, uncoupling protein-2.

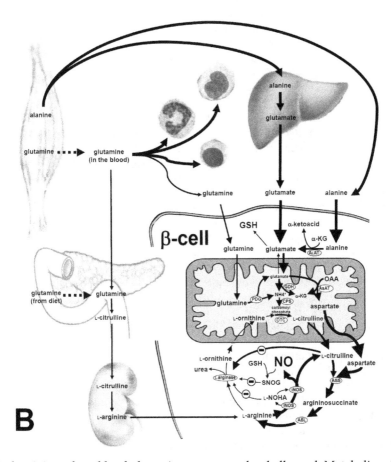

mechanical activity, where blood glutamine stores may be challenged. Metabolic acidosis, by increasing L-glutamine utilisation by the kidney, may also favour glutamine depletion unless enteral supplementation or enhanced physical activity takes place. This is also the case of psychological-stress motivated inflammatory reactions that may underlie by the activation of sympathetic-CRH-histamine system (**Fig. 3**), which ultimately leads to a Th1-centered immune response that augments glutamine utilisation. Therefore, L-glutamine imbalance, by virtue of deficiently supplying L-arginine to the pancreas, deviates β-cell glutamate metabolism from the synthesis of GSH to that of NO, leading to oxidative stress, impairment of insulin release and insulitis. This ongoing inflammation feeds forward NO metabolism, which enhances L-glutamine consumption thus perpetuating this cyclic condition that leads to type 1 diabetes mellitus (T1DM) **(B).** Physical exercise, on the other hand, may improve L-glutamine supply from the skeletal muscle and counteract Th1-mediated inflammation due to the production of type 2 cytokines, such as IL-6. Immunomodulatory action of exercise may also involve heat shock protein production and other anti-inflammatory mediators. Arrow widths indicate the intensity of the metabolic flux through each pathway.

contribute to derangements in the secretion and action of insulin (Newsholme et al., 2009a). Hypertension associated with diabetes is related with a decrease in levels of L-arginine (Spinas, 1999), as are inflammatory conditions characterised by release of L-arginase by activated macrophages (Murphy & Newsholme, 1998). While excessive NO production can trigger oxidative/nitrosative stress and is undoubtedly a key mechanism that results in β-cell death (Newsholme et al., 2009a; Spinas, 1999; Michalska et al., 2010), good evidence now suggests that lesser amounts of cellular NO, produced by the NF-κB-regulated inducible nitric oxide synthase (iNOS, EC 1.14.13.39), encoded by the *NOS-2* gene, serves as an important coupling factor in insulin secreting cells (Newsholme et al., 2009a; Spinas, 1999; Michalska et al., 2010). Recent data from the authors' laboratories has demonstrated that L-arginine is an important stimulator of β-cell glucose consumption and intermediary metabolism (M.S. Krause, N.H. McClenaghan, P.R. Flatt, P.I. Homem de Bittencourt Jr., C. Murphy & P. Newsholme, unpublished results). Such actions lead to increased insulin secretion, enhanced antioxidant and protective responses with greater functional integrity when challenged with pro-inflammatory cytokines. Given that insulin-secreting cells have very low expression levels of antioxidant enzymes, such as catalase (CAT) and glutathione peroxidase (GSPx), β-cells are particularly prone to chemical stress in the diabetogenic or inflammatory environment typical of type 1 and possibly type 2 diabetes (Newsholme et al., 2009a; Spinas, 1999). In fact, the pathogenesis of type 2 diabetes is now recognised to involve both innate and adaptive immunity, since type 2 diabetes is associated with low-grade systemic inflammation, infiltration of adipose tissue and pancreatic islets with $CD8^+$ T lymphocytes that precede invasion by inflammatory macrophages and activation of these cells resulting in pro-inflammatory cytokine secretion (Mandrup-Poulsen, 2010).

In this chapter, we discuss how the continued supply of L-arginine, physiologically provided by the metabolism of L-glutamine via the intestinal-renal axis and from active skeletal muscle (which will be enhanced during exercise) is essential for β-cell functional integrity and indeed for β-cell defence, which will be required to avoid/attenuate islet inflammation associated with the pathogenic mechanisms underlying type 1 and type 2 diabetes (**Fig. 1B**). L-arginine is therefore preserved for essential NO generation and stimulation of glucose metabolism, critical for insulin secretion. Additionally, the role of skeletal muscle (during exercise) on these metabolic processes is discussed.

2. Oxidative metabolism and oxidative stress in β-cells and type 1 diabetes

The intense aerobic metabolism, intrinsic to pancreatic β-cells, exposes these cells to the deleterious effects of high-turnover oxygen-based reactions. In fact, during secretagogue-stimulated insulin secretion, β-cells are associated with accelerated mitochondrial flux of electrons and, consequently, elevated tendency towards reactive oxygen species (ROS) production (Newsholme et al., 2007). However and notably, β-cells present a very low level of expression of antioxidant enzymes such as CAT and GSPx compared with other tissues and this reduced antioxidant activity is associated with significant increases in lipid hydroperoxides, conjugated dienes and protein carbonyls, which are markers for oxidative stress (Santini et al., 1997), so that β-cells are intrinsically prone to oxidative stress.

Moreover, a growing body of evidence indicates that, in the pre-diabetic condition, antioxidant status may be impaired (Rocie et al., 1997). Hence, the low antioxidant defence in certain individuals (even if transiently) may predispose to an enhanced oxidative stress and the eventual β-cell death that categorises the onset of type 1 and type 2 diabetes.

Oxidative stress has long been recognised to play an important role in the development of type 1 diabetes and its subsequent complications (Wierusz-Wysock et al., 1997) which are aggravated due to the low activities of oxygen free radical scavenging enzymes in islet β-cells, especially mitochondrial manganese-type superoxide dismutase (Mn-SOD; Asayama et al., 1986), glutathione peroxidase (GSPx; Malaisse et al., 1982; Mathews & Leiter, 1999) and glutathione disulphide (GSSG) reductase (GSRd; Mathews & Leiter, 1999). Also, the expression of mRNA encoding for several antioxidant enzymes, such as Mn-SOD, cytoplasmic copper-zinc type SOD (Cu/Zn-SOD), GSPx, and catalase (CAT), has been reported to be lower in islets of Langerhans compared with other mouse tissues (Lenzen et al., 1996). Additionally, the administration of antioxidants (nicotinamide, SOD, α-tocopherol, probucol and the 21-aminosteroid lazaroids), as well as oxygen free radical scavengers, have been used in vitro to protect islets from the cytotoxic effects of some pro-inflammatory cytokines (IL-1β, TNFα and INFγ), concurrently providing *in vivo* protection against the development of the autoimmune diabetes process (Nomikos et al., 1986). Conversely, studies on MnSOD and CAT transgenics have shown that protection of islets from oxidative stress does not alter cytokine toxicity (Chen et al., 2005), which indicates that, although related to each other, oxidative stress and cytokine-induced islet toxicity may use specific and diverse pathways to induce β-cell death.

An additional complication to this scenario is the fact that β-cells express mitochondrial uncoupling protein 2 (UCP2) which dissipates the coupling between electron transport from ATP formation favouring O_2- generation. Since O_2- anion is a powerful activator of UCP2, a positive feedback mechanism exists in that O2- generation enhances its own formation. This is particularly critical under prolonged hyperglycaemia, where UCP2 activity may be extremely high thus further depressing insulin secretion by β-cells (Newsholme et al., 2007). This situation is probably associated with the development of type 2 diabetes. Furthermore, the high-glucose, high fatty-acid environment created by either insulin-deficiency or insulin-resistance favours the expression of NAD(P)H oxidase with consequently enhanced ROS production and β-cell death (Morgan et al., 2007, Newsholme et al., 2009b).

Type 1 diabetic patients exhibit major defects in antioxidant protection compared with healthy, non-diabetic controls. A significant reduction in total antioxidant status in both plasma and serum samples from these patients is typically observed (Maxwell et al., 1997). Diabetic children show significant reduction in GSH and GSPx in erythrocytes, as well as in plasma α-tocopherol and β-carotene levels (Dominguez et al., 1998). Incubation of rat (Rabinovitch et al., 1992) and human (Rabinovitch et al., 1996) islet cells with a cytotoxic combination of cytokines (IL-1β, TNFα and IFNγ) has been reported as an inducing factor for lipid peroxidation (also known as lipoperoxidation). When individually administered, however, the same cytokines have been shown to inhibit insulin release without any increase in lipid peroxidation or cytodestructive effects in rat islets (Sumoski et al., 1989). Taken together, these findings suggest that cytokine-induced inhibition of insulin release may not be oxygen free radical-mediated, whereas the cytodestructive effects of cytokines on β-cells do appear to involve free radical-mediated events that induce the formation of toxic derivatives within the islets of Langerhans (Suarez-Pinz et al., 1996). This strongly suggests that type 1 cytokines interfere in β-cell metabolism at some point that is intimately related to insulin secretion. But where does reside this extreme sensitivity of β-cells to cytokine signals? The expression of iNOS, necessary for the synthesis of NO during insulin secretion, may provide an explanation.

NO has incontestably been shown to be a physiological regulator of insulin secretion in β-cells, in an elegant experimental protocol designed by Prof. Anne Marie Salapatek's group in Canada and reported in a seminal paper (Smukler et al., 2002). They have also reported that endogenous NO production can be stimulated by glucose, and that this stimulation can be blocked by NOS inhibition, whereas scavenging of NO specifically blocks insulin release stimulated by physiological intracellular concentrations of NO-donors (2 mM), but has no effect on the release stimulated by elevated K^+. It has also been reported that NO donation did not elicit a β-cell intracellular Ca^{2+} ($[Ca^{2+}]_i$) response alone, but was able to potentiate a glucose-induced $[Ca^{2+}]_i$ response. Since NO is a strong heme-reactant, it partially inhibits the mitochondrial respiratory chain by binding to cytochrome c and/or cytochrome oxidase. As a consequence, the mitochondrial membrane potential decreases and Ca^{2+} leaves the mitochondria. This is followed by restoration of the mitochondrial membrane potential and Ca^{2+} reuptake by mitochondria (Spinas, 1999). Therefore, overproduction of NO related to inflammatory stimuli may be related to cellular dysfunction but **not** normal levels of NO. As previously argued (Smukler et al., 2002), the precise level of NO is crucial in determining its resultant effect, with low levels being involved in physiological signalling and higher levels becoming cytotoxic (Moncada et al., 1991; Beck et al., 1999). Hence, the supraphysiological elevation of L-arginine, or the application of exogenous NO donors under the condition of already elevated NO, may result in excessive NO production, yielding cytotoxic effects (Smukler et al., 2002).

3. Nuclear factor κB-dependent L-arginine metabolism in β-cells

Pancreatic β-cells have to constantly express NF-κB-regulated iNOS in order to achieve appropriate amounts of NO produced from L-arginine. However, inflammatory cytokines, such as IL-1β and TNF-α, activate NF-κB in rodent and human islet cells (Eizirik & Mandrup-Poulsen, 2001). Contrarily, prevention of NF-κB activation protects pancreatic β-cells against cytokine-induced apoptosis (Giannoukakis et al., 2000; Heimberg et al., 2001). It is impressive that about 70 NF-κB–dependent genes have been currently identified in β-cells, including genes encoding for various inflammatory cytokines and iNOS (Darville & Eizirik, 1998). Remarkably, the expression of *ca.* 50% of the β-cell genes that may be modified after cytokine exposure is secondary to iNOS-mediated NO formation (Kutlu et al., 2003). It is of note that treatment of human, as well as rodent β-cells with purified IL-1β alone is not sufficient to induce apoptosis, but if IL-1β is combined with interferon-γ (IFNγ), β-cells undergo apoptosis after few days in culture (Eizirik & Mandrup-Pouls, 2001). This suggests that an intracellular IFNγ signal must synergise with IL-1β signalling pathways in order to trigger β-cell apoptosis. IFNγ binds to cell surface receptors and activates the Janus tyrosine kinases JAK1 and JAK2. These kinases phosphorylate and activate their downstream transcription factor STAT-1 (for signal transducers and activators of transcription), which dimerises and translocates to the nucleus where binding to γ-activated sites on target genes occurs (Eizirik & Mandrup-Pouls, 2001). STAT-1 mediates the potentiating effect of IFNγ on IL-1β-induced iNOS expression (Darville & Eizirik, 1998). Because excessive activation of JAK/STAT signalling may lead to cell death, STAT transcriptional activity is regulated by multiple negative feedback mechanisms. These include dephosphorylation of JAK and cytokine receptors by cytoplasmic protein-tyrosine phosphatases SHPs (for Src homology 2 domain phosphatases), and inhibition of JAK enzymic activities by the suppressors of cytokine signalling (SOCS) family. Upregulation of either SOCS-1 or SOCS-3 protects β-cells against cytokine-induced cell death in vitro and in vivo (Karlsen et al., 2001; Flodstrom et al., 2003). SOCS-3 also protects insulin-producing cells against IL-1β–mediated apoptosis via NF-κB inhibition (Karlsen et al., 2004). Evidence indicates that the fate of β-cells, after cytokine exposure, depends on the duration and severity of perturbation of key β-cell gene networks.

Besides its activation by cytokines, NF-κB is also a potential target for reactive oxygen/nitrogen species (ROS/RNS). It is noteworthy that NF-κB was the first redox-sensitive eukaryotic transcription factor shown to respond directly to oxidative stress in many types of cells (Dröge, 2002), while its activation leads to the expression of at least a hundred of inducible proteins directly involved in inflammation, such as cyclooxygenase-2 (COX-2), iNOS, TNFα and IL-1β (Moynagh, 2005). Therefore, NF-κB is, at the same time, both a target and an inducer of inflammation and inflammation-induced oxidative stress. In resting (unstimulated) cells, NF-κB dimeric complexes are predominantly found in the cytosol where they are associated with members of the inhibitory IκB family (Moynagh, 2005), so that NF-κB gene products are entirely inducible proteins whose activation is dictated by specific stimuli that activate IκB kinase (IKK) complexes. These stimuli include high intracellular GSSG levels and oxidative stress *per se* (Dröge, 2002). IKKs, in turn, phosphorylate IκB proteins directing them to proteasome-mediated degradation, which sets NF-κB dimers free to bind to DNA in the nucleus.

NF-κB activation is responsible for both initiation and amplification of immune and inflammatory responses in all cells. Actually, NF-κB activation is *sine qua non* for the control of immune and inflammatory responses (Baldwin, 1996; Nakamura et al., 1997; Winyard et al., 1997), and since inflammatory factors, such as pro-inflammatory cytokines, chemokines, adhesion molecules, colony-stimulating factors and inflammatory enzymes, are NF-κB-dependent gene products, dysregulation or aberrant activation of NF-κB could initiate inappropriate autoimmune and inflammatory responses. Conversely, inhibition of NF-κB activation has been argued as a potential therapeutic approach in several immune and inflammatory-related diseases (Chen et al., 1999). This is why cyclopentenone prostaglandins (cp-PGs), which are powerful inhibitors of NF-κB activation (Rossi et al., 2000), are now considered to be the physiological mediators of the "**resolution of inflammation**" (Piva et al., 2005), whereas cp-PG-based pharmacological approaches, *e.g.* LipoCardium technology, which is a liposome contained cp-PG-based formulation specifically directed towards atherosclerotic lesions in arterial walls (Homem de Bittencourt et al., 2007; Gutierrez et al., 2008) have proved to be powerful anti-atherosclerotic strategies (Piva et al., 2005; Ianaro et al., 2003; Homem de Bittencourt Jr., 2007).

Finally, considering that all the known forms of inflammation finish with the formation of naturally-occurring anti-inflammatory agents (e.g. cp-PGs, IL-10), an important question remains as to how does β-cell not resolve inflammation by triggering such responses? A fault in the expression of the anti-inflammatory heat shock proteins may give a clue to this question.

4. Heat shock protein pathways

Heat shock proteins (HSPs) have been found to play a fundamental role in the recovery from multiple stress conditions and to offer protection from subsequent insults (De Maio,

2011). The function of HSPs during stress goes beyond their intracellular localization and chaperone role as they have been detected outside cells activating signaling pathways. Extracellular HSPs are likely to act as indicators of the stress conditions, priming other cells, particularly of the immune system, to avoid the propagation of the insult (see De Maio, 2011 for review). As we shall present below, the delicate balance between the "danger signalling" extracellular HSPs and its intracellular counterparts may dictate pancreatic β-cell response to cytokines and, eventually, the precipitation of diabetes. By regulating L-arginine consumption through iNOS, and, consequently, NO generation, intracellular HSP response (or its deficiency) may unravel unpredicted facets of both type 1 and type 2 diabetes.

Heat shock proteins (HSPs) are a set of highly conserved polypeptides in both eukaryotic and prokaryotic organisms. They are categorised in families according to their molecular sises and include HSP110, HSP100, HSP90, HSP70, HSP60 HSP30 and HSP10 subclasses. By far, the most studied (due to its evident high expression in mammalian cells under stress conditions) and conserved is the 70-kDa family (HSP70), which comprises a number of related proteins whose molecular weights range from 66 to 78 kDa. HSP70 isoforms are encoded by a multigene family consisting presently of, at least, 13 distinct genes in humans so far studied (Kampinga et al., 2009; Henderson, 2010). Human HSP70 is 73% identical to *Drosophila* HSP70 and 47% identical to *E. coli* DnaK (the *E. coli* orthologue of eukaryotic HSP70) while, surprisingly, the nucleotide sequences of the human and *Drosophila* genes are 72% identical and human and *E. coli* genes are 50% identical (Hunt & Morimoto, 1985). HSP70s function as molecular chaperones that facilitate protein transport, prevent protein aggregation during folding, and protect newly synthesised polypeptide chains against misfolding and protein denaturation (Henderson, 2010). While the constitutive form is expressed in a wide variety of cell types at basal levels (being only moderately inducible), the so-called inducible HSP70 forms (which are barely detectable under non-stressful conditions) could be promptly synthesised under a condition of "homeostatic stress", this being any "homeostasis threatening" condition, such as heat, glucose deprivation, lack of growth factors and so forth. Traditionally, research groups indistinctly use HSP70 as a unified term for both inducible (72 kDa, HSP72 encoded by the *HSPA1A* human gene) and constitutive (73 kDa, HSP73 or HSC70, for heat shock cognate protein, encoded by the human *HSPA8* gene whose product differs from *HSPA1A* protein by only 2 amino acids, Kampinga et al., 2009; Tavaria et al., 1996; Arya et al., 2007; Tavaria et al., 1995). However, HSP70 is the preferable form to be used only when one refers to the inducible HSP72 protein encoded by *HSPA1A* gene (Heck et al., 2011).

Many different events can induce HSP expression, among them are environmental, pathological and physiological factors, such as heavy metal exposure, UV radiation, amino acid analogues, bacterial or viral infection, inflammation, cyclo-oxygenase inhibitors (including acetylsalicylic acid), oxidative stress, cytostatic drugs, growth factors, cell differentiation and tissue development, which strongly activate the main eukaryotic heat shock transcription factor, HSF-1, leading to HSP70 expression (Lindquist & Craig, 1988). Physical exercise, even at single low-intensity bouts (Silveira et al., 2007), is able to induce HSP70 expression in different cell types leading to augmented plasma HSP70 concentrations (see Heck et al., 2011 for review). In our hands, rats submitted to swimming sessions of as short as 20 min (2-4% body weight overload, a mild exercise) demonstrate increased HSP72 (mRNA and protein) in circulating monocytes and lymphocytes and in lymph node lymphocytes and peritoneal macrophages, which is paralleled by a rise in plasma HSP70 levels immediately after the exercise (C.M. Schöler, S.P. Scomazzon, P. Renck Nunes, T.G. Heck, P.I. Homem de Bittencourt Jr., unpublished work).

4.1 Intracellular hsp70

Aside the now classical molecular chaperone action, the most remarkable intracellular effect of HSP70s is the inhibition of NF-κB activation, which has profound implications for immunity, inflammation, cell survival and apoptosis. Indeed, HSP70 blocks NF-κB activation at different levels, by inhibiting the phosphorylation of the inhibitor of κB (IκBs), by directly binding to IκB kinase-γ (IKKγ) thus inhibiting tumour necrosis factor-α (TNFα)-induced apoptosis (Ran et al., 2004). In fact, the supposition that HSP70 might act intracellularly as a suppressor of NF-κB pathways has been raised after a number of discoveries in which HSP70 was intentionally induced, such as the suppression of astroglial iNOS expression paralleled by decreased NF-κB activation (Feinstein et al., 1996) and the protection of rat hepatocytes from TNFα-induced apoptosis by treating cells with the NO-donor S-Nitroso-N-acetylpenicillamine (SNAP), which reacts with intracellular glutathione (GSH) molecules generating S-nitrosoglutathione (SNOG) that induces HSP70, and, consequently, HSP70 expression (Kim et al., 1997).

HSP70 confers protection against sepsis-related circulatory mortality via the inhibition of iNOS gene expression in the rostral ventrolateral medulla through the prevention of NF-κB activation, inhibition of IκB kinase activation and consequent inhibition of IκB degradation (Chan et al., 2004). This is corroborated by the finding that HSP72 assembles with hepatocyte NF-κB/IκB complex in the cytosol thus impeding further transcription of NF-κB-depending TNF-α and NOS-2 genes that would worsen sepsis in rats (Chen et al., 2005). This may also be unequivocally demonstrated by treating cells or tissues with HSP70 antisense oligonucleotides that completely reverses the beneficial NF-κB-inhibiting effect of heat shock and inducible HSP70 expression (see, for instance, Kim et al., 1997; Chan et al., 2004). Hence, HSP70 is anti-inflammatory per se, when intracellularly located, which also explains why cyclopentenone prostaglandins (cp-PGs) are powerful anti-inflammatory autacoids (Rossi et al., 2000; Homem de Bittencourt & Curi, 2001; Beere, 2004; Gutierrez et al., 2008).

Another striking effect of HSP70 is the inhibition of apoptosis, which occurs via many intracellular downstream pathways (e.g. JNK, NF-κB and Akt) that are both directly and indirectly blocked by HSP70, besides the inhibition of Bcl-2 release from mitochondria (Beere, 2004). Therefore, intracellularly activated HSP70s are cytoprotective and anti-inflammatory by avoiding protein denaturation and excessive NF-κB activation which may be damaging to the cells.

It is strikingly noteworthy that L-glutamine attenuates TNF-α release and enhances HSP72 expression in human peripheral blood mononuclear cells (Wischmeyer et al., 2003). In fact, L-glutamine induces HSP70 expression via O-glycosylation and phosphorylation of HSF-1 and Sp1 (Singleton, K.D. & Wischmeyer, P.E., 2008) in a process that is mediated, at least partially, by the increase in the flux through the hexosamine biosynthetic pathway (Hamiel et al., 2009). Also, it has been shown that a single dose of L-glutamine relieve renal ischaemia-reperfusion injury in rats in 24 h by a mechanism associated with enhanced HSP70 expression (Zhang et al., 2009).

4.2 Extracellular hsp70

HSP70s may also be found in the circulation and its presence is associated to oxidative stress. While healthy people usually have low plasma levels of HSP70, the association of increased blood concentrations of such proteins with illness and disease progression has been hypothesised. In this way, oxidative stress, inflammation, cardiovascular disorders and pulmonary fibrosis have been directly correlated with HSP70 concentration in the bloodstream (Ogawa et al., 2008). On the other hand, L-glutamine supplementation, which rises circulating HSP70 levels in critically ill patients, is associated with lower hospital treatment period (Ziegler et al., 2005). Therefore, these studies may suggest that elevation of HSP70 levels could be an important immunoinflammatory response against physiological disorders or disease.

Inasmuch as HSP70s exist in the extracellular space, molecular interactions with cell surface receptors may occur and signalling pathways could be triggered in many cell types, whereas there are a variety of receptors to HSP70 binding, amplifying the possible targets to these extracellular molecules (Calderwood et al., 2007a, 2007b). However, the function of circulating HSP70 is incompletely understood yet. HSP70s are released towards the extracellular space by special mechanisms that include pumping across cell membranes through the highly conserved ABC cassette transport proteins. Recent studies have demonstrated that exosomes provide the major pathway for the vesicular secretory release of HSP70s and that heat stress strikingly enhances the amount of HSP70 secreted per vesicle, but does not influence the efficiency of stress-induced rate of HSP70 release and the number of exosomes neither (Sun et al., 2005; Lancaster & Febbraio, 2005; Multhoff, 2007). A similar profile was observed in our hands (T.G. Heck; P. Renck Nunes; S.P. Scomazzon & P.I. Homem de Bittencourt Jr., manuscript in preparation), in which lymph node lymphocytes from exercised rats submitted to a further (other than the exercise bouts) challenge (heat shock) presented an HSP70 accumulation into the culture medium that is dependent on previous exercise load. Apparently, systemic extracellular HSP70 (eHSP70) could arise from many tissues and different cell types and this may involve distinct mechanisms of release (including necrosis) and a large variety of inducing factors (Mambula et al., 2007). Finally, HSP72 is clearly the major component of the secreted eHSP70 found in the circulation, although recent evidence suggests that other forms may also be released into the blood, as recently pointed out by De Maio (2011). eHSP70 has been shown to bind to type 2 and 4 toll-like receptors (TLR2 and TLR4) on the surface of antigen-presenting cells (APCs) similarly to lipopolysaccharides (LPS), inducing the production of the pro-inflammatory cytokines IL-1β and TNF-α, as well as NO (a product with prominent anti-microbial activity), in an NF-κB-dependent fashion (Ao et al., 2009; Asea, 2003; Asea, 2008).

Taken together, the above findings suggest that the body must attain a precise equilibrium between pro-inflammatory eHSP70 and anti-inflammatory intracellular HSP70 production in order to avoid chronic non-resolved inflammations, such as those observed in sepsis and during the onset of type 1 diabetes. However, why such a balance is not achieved in these illnesses is a matter of intense study.

4.3 Heat shock proteins and exercise

As recently reviewed (Heck et al., 2011), physical exercise and its inherent physiological alterations induce HSP70 expression in many tissues and cell types, not only in the muscle cells. The breakdown of cell homeostasis produced by modifications in temperature, pH, ion concentrations, oxygen partial pressure, glycogen/glucose availability, and ATP depletion are among the factors that activate HSP70 synthesis during exercise (Noble et al., 2008). Rise in core and muscle temperature during exercise seems an obvious way to induce HSP70. However, while skeletal muscle sustains HSP70 expression in the absence of heat stimulus, the heart is not able to do the same, thus suggesting that the mechanisms of HSP70 protein synthesis are specifically driven in each tissue (Harris & Starnes, 2001; Skidmore et al., 2005; Morton et al., 2007; Staib et al., 2007) and that augmented temperature is insufficient to elicit HSP70 synthesis during exercise. Moreover, the susceptibility of tissues to be stressed by the environmental changes elicited by exercise varies enormously and other protective pathways may be activated in the heart, as we have shown for MRP/GS-X pump ATPases whose expression seems to prevent HSP70 expression in the cardiac muscle after exercise bouts (Krause et al., 2007). In spite of free radicals may be produced under normal conditions, a burst in reactive oxygen species does occur during exercise (Fisher-Wellman & Bloomer, 2009). Besides enzymatic and non-enzymatic antioxidant apparatus, studies in both animal models and humans implicate HSP70s as a complementary protection against oxidative damage (Smolka et al., 2000; Silmar et al., 2007; Hamilton et al., 2003), particularly because HSP70s may recover oxidatively denatured proteins. After an acute exercise session, skeletal muscle (Hernando & Manso, 1997), cardiac muscle (Locke et al., 1995) and other tissues, such as the liver (Gonzalez & Manso, 2004; Kregel & Moseley, 1996), have shown a state of oxidative stress, concomitantly to high concentrations of intracellular HSP70 (Salo et al., 1991). Even though oxidative stress is a strong factor to induce HSP70s in response to exercise, free radical production is not the only pathway involved in this process, since sexual hormones and adrenergic stimuli may modulate HSP70 response (Parro & Noble, 1999; Paroo et al., 2002a, 2002b; Paroo et al., 1999) and circulating monocytes from acutely exercised rats do not show appreciable changes in erythrocyte glutathione disulphide (GSSG) to glutathione (GSH) ratio (an index of intracellular redox status) and plasma thiobarbituric acid-reactive substances (TBARS), even in a state of high-profile synthesis of hydrogen peroxide (Silveira et al., 2007).

More recently, however, it has been demonstrated the presence of HSP70s in the circulation in response to exercise (Walsh et al., 2001). Since exercise is able to induce high concentrations of HSP70s in both muscle and plasma, the most obvious hypothesis was, primarily, that skeletal muscle should be the releaser of HSP70 during exercise. However, further studies have revealed that this is not the case, at all. Postural muscles express high levels of HSP70s under basal conditions, which has led to the belief in a preventive role for these proteins against muscle damage through the stabilization of ionic channels (Tupling et al., 2007), as well as myotube development (Kayani et al., 2008). HSP70s were also believed to be an important way to preserve low twitch (oxidative) muscle phenotype after frequent activation, as in physical training (Kelly et al., 1996; Murlasits et al., 2006). Preservation of intracellular muscular function during different exercises, venous-arterial HSP70 differences in different territories (Febbraio et al., 2002a), and the lack of evidence supporting the proposition that the muscle could be the major source of circulatory eHSP70 precluded the 'muscle hypothesis' and suggested that other tissues/cells should be responsible for the increase of eHSP70 in the circulation. Once HSP70 protein release from the muscle to the extracellular fluid could eventually happen by lysis process, and considering that the lysis of muscle fibre occurs only under severe cellular stress condition, the presence of eHSP70 during moderate exercise, as we normally employ, was found to be unfeasible. Though it had been shown that both the intensity and duration of exercise have effects in plasma eHSP70 (Fehrenbach et al., 2005) and muscle (Milne & Noble, 2002) HSP70 immunocontents, this rise in circulating levels of eHSP70 precedes, however, any gene or protein expression of HSP70 in skeletal muscle (Febbraio et al., 2002b), which is another strong argument against the 'muscle hypothesis'. As stated above, other tissues synthesise HSP70s during physiological challenges to the homeostasis, as in an acute physical exercise bout. In this way, after treadmill exercise protocol, the rat liver has been found to enhance the expression of HSP70s (Gonzalez & Manso, 2004). Moreover, and finally, in a human study featuring leg and hepatosplanchnic venous-arterial eHSP70 difference in response to exercise it was unequivocally demonstrated that the contracting muscle does not contribute to eHSP70 circulating levels, while hepatosplanchnic viscera release eHSP70 from undetectable levels at rest to 5.2 pg/min after 120 min of exercise (Febbraio et al., 2002a). Additional studies have shown that oral glucose administration may exclusively reduce HSP70 release from the liver without any effect on muscle glycogen content or intracellular expression of HSP70 (Febbraio et al., 2004). Taken together, these results suggest that other cells may release eHSP70 during exercise, as verified during an experiment that analysed cerebral venous-arterial HSP70 difference (Lancaster et al., 2004). Although the liver seems to participate in this process, the nature of eHSP70-releasing cell(s) during exercise remains to be established.

4.4 HSP70 and glucose/insulin status

Intracellular HSP70 expression produces a clear anti-inflammatory effect by knocking down the expression of pro-inflammatory NF-κB-dependent pathways. However, the activation of HSP70 pathways produces a much more delicate effect. Accordingly, in obese insulin-resistant mice, chronic heat shock treatment has been shown to dramatically reduce insulin resistance by HSP72-specific prevention of c-Jun N-terminal Kinase (JNK) phsophorylation, an effect which is also observed in high-fat fed HSP72$^{+/+}$ transgenic mice (Chung et al., 2008). Also, elevated expression of HSP70 has also been found in circulating mononuclear cells from type 2 diabetic patients (Yabunaka et al., 1995), which, as discussed above, is a immunoinflammatory disease as well. On the other hand, in rat islets, L-glutamine, which is an activator of HSF-1, was shown to attenuate ischaemic injury through the induction of HSP70 (Jang et al., 2008). Moreover, the well known inhibitory effect of IL-1β and TNF-α (alone or combined) on insulin secretion may be completely prevented by a 1-h heat shock (42°C) pre-treatment of both human and rat islets (Scarim et al., 1998). These authors have also shown that the protective effects of heat shock on islet metabolic function are associated with the inhibition of IL-1β- and TNFα-stimulated NF-κB nuclear localization and the consequent iNOS expression. Conversely, NO was found to be one of the triggers of HSP70 expression in human islets (Scarim et al., 1998), which is similar to that previously encountered by Kim et al. (1997), who described a protective effect of NO (via the formation of SNOG that induces HSP70) in rat hepatocytes against TNFα-induced apoptosis. Moreover, J-type cyclopentenone prostaglandins (cp-PGs), which are the most powerful anti-inflammatory substances ever known (see Gutierrez et al., 2008 for review) and natural ligands of peroxisome-proliferator activated receptor-γ (PPAR-γ; Forman et al., 1995; Kliewer et al., 1995), are the strongest inducers of HSP70 expression and consequent NF-κB blockade, a pattern that is shared with synthetic antidiabetic thiazolidinediones (TZDs), such as rosiglitazone, pioglitazone, troglitazone, and ciglitazone (see Zingarelli & Cook, 2005, for review).

The above observations point out again to the importance of poised L-arginine-dependent NO production by β-cells in order to achieve an optimum of HSP70 expression, which may, in turn, allow iNOS expression (needed to NO-assisted insulin secretion) but not at exaggerated ratios that culminate with β-cell death and failure in insulin secretion. In fact, physical exercise, which may also present an anti-inflammatory effect by virtue of its ability to induce the expression of HSP70, is inversely associated with L-arginine utilisation by β-cell iNOS (Atalay et al., 2004). Furthermore, a dramatic scenario does exist in that the susceptibility to oxidative damage to β-cells in type 1 diabetes is associated to the impairment of HSP70-induced cytoprotection, while endurance training may offset some of the adverse effects of diabetes by upregulating tissue HSP70 expression (Atalay et al., 2004). Indeed, in many, if not all, severe inflammatory manifestations of acute nature, such as sepsis or insulitis, the stage of HSP70-based "resolution of inflammation" is simply not seen at all. For instance, in the serum of septic patients with highly oxidative profile (whose prognosis is death), it is observed 30-fold increase in serum HSP70 (eHSP70) compared with control subjects (Gelain et al., 2011), whereas the amount of intracellular HSP70 expressed in the cells of such subjects is, as a rule, lower that that expected. Corroborating this proposition, the expression of HSP70 by pancreatic islets from diabetes-prone BB rats has been found to be lower than that in diabetic-resistant LEW rats of same age and, in the diabetes-prone BB rats, HSP70 expression has shown to be much lower in young as compared to adult animals (Wachlin et al., 2002). Since intracellular HSP70 functions as a potent anti-inflammatory cellular tool due to the impairment over NF-κB downstream pathways, a deficient HSP70 may threaten β-cell survival (see Hooper & Hooper, 2005, for review).

Results from our group have also shown that, besides a reduction in peripheral insulin resistance, heat shock treatment (which also enhances HSP70 export towards the plasma) may impair insulin action under hypoglycaemic conditions in the rat model (M.S. Ludwig.; V.C. Mingueti; P. Renck Nunes; T.G. Heck; R.B. Bazotte & Homem de Bittencourt, P.I. Jr., manuscript in preparation) so that HSP70 balance seems to be crucial for glucose-insulin homeostasis. Now, we are currently evaluating the possibility that exercise may stimulate Th2-based immune response and protect β-cells from pro-inflammatory cytokine pathways through HSP70 induction, which, ultimately, may prevent type 1 diabetes. Since **a)** L-glutamine is a major precursor of L-arginine, which is capital for β-cell survival, **b)** L-arginine-dependent moderate NO synthesis induces HSP70 and **c)** physical exercise is able of directly inducing HSP70 and of enhancing L-glutamine production by the skeletal muscle, both exercise and/or L-glutamine supplementation are argued as preventive agents against the installation of type 1 diabetes by re-establishing the HSP70 equilibrium between the intra and extracellular spaces, as previously hypothesised (Krause & Homem de Bittencourt, 2008).

5. Participation of L-arginine/L-glutamine coupling in diabetes

From the above discussion, it seems clear that the development of diabetes is not simply a question of cytokine imbalance culminating in a redox disruption and consequent oxidative stress that disrupts or kills β-cells. This, in fact, raises another question: is beta cell susceptibility to stress solely a question of compromised antioxidant defence? If this were the case, it would appear preposterous that such a sophisticated cell remains prone to endogenously-generated NO-mediated self-destruction. The intricate metabolism of L-arginine in β-cells may unravel some important points in this regard.

In β-cells, pro-inflammatory cytokines induce the production of NO, synthesised from L-arginine, via a reaction catalysed by iNOS, whose functionality depends on NF-κB-driven gene transcription and *de novo* enzyme synthesis. iNOS also utilises NADPH and O_2 as co-substrates (**Fig. 1A**) and, physiologically, L-arginine is the limiting substrate for NO production. In addition to this, pancreatic β-cells express another L-arginine-metabolising enzyme, *i.e.* L-arginase (L-arginine amidinohydrolase, EC 3.5.3.1), which allows for the completion of urea production through the formation of L-ornithine and urea from L-arginine (Cunningham et al., 1997). Physiologic levels of L-arginase gene expression and activity have been measured in rat β-cells and the insulin-secreting cell line RINm5F (Cunningham et al., 1997; Malaisse et al., 1989; Cardozo et al., 2001; Rieneck et el., 2000). β-Cells express both the cytosolic (L-arginase I) and the mitochondrial (L-arginase II) isoforms of the enzyme. Therefore, under certain circumstances, a true competition may occur in that the activity of iNOS relative to L-arginase dictates either NO or urea production in the pancreas (compare **Fig. 1A and 1B**). Consequently, L-arginase may impair NO production by limiting the availability of L-arginine for iNOS catalysis (Wu & Morris, 1998; Boucher et al., 1999; Mori & Gotoh, 2000). This notion is supported by the finding that inhibition of L-arginase results in enhanced NO synthesis in cytokine-activated cells (Chang et al., 1998; Tenu et al., 1999).

It has been demonstrated that cytokine-elicited co-induction of both NO (iNOS) and urea (argininosuccinate synthetase and argininosuccinate lyase) metabolic pathways occurs in many cell types (Nussler et al., 1994; Hattori et al., 1994; Nagasaki et al., 1996), including β-cells (Flodstrom et al., 1995), *in vitro* as well as *in vivo*. L-Arginase activity may be increased in peritoneal macrophages after exposure to LPS (Currie, 1978), while wound and peritoneal macrophages convert L-arginine to L-citrulline and L-ornithine at comparable rates, indicating that both iNOS and L-arginase pathways are functional (Granger et al., 1990). In clonal β-cells, IL-1β increases L-arginase activity with concomitant increase in NO production (Cunningham et al., 1997), which suggests a kind of coordinated regulation of L-arginase and iNOS in these cells.

There is also evidence for a reciprocal regulation of NOS and L-arginase during immune responses via the antagonistic effects of cytokines released from Th1 and Th2 lymphocytes. While L-arginase activity may be induced by the "anti-inflammatory" Th2 cytokines IL-4, IL-6, IL-10, and IL-13 (Modolell et al., 1995; Waddington et al., 1998; Munder et al., 1999; Wei et al., 2000), the Th1-derived "pro-inflammatory" cytokine IFNγ increases iNOS expression and activity, both alone and in synergy with other pro-inflammatory cytokines, such as IL-1β and TNFα (Gill et al., 1996). Reciprocal effects of Th1- and Th2-derived cytokines on L-arginase and iNOS activities have also been shown by the treatment of murine macrophages with cytokines (Modolell et al., 1995; Corraliza et al., 1995), and by co-culturing murine macrophages with Th1 and Th2 T-cell clones (Munder et al., 1998). In mouse bone marrow-derived macrophages, iNOS and L-arginase activities are regulated reciprocally by Th1 and Th2 cytokines, a strategy that guarantees a precise and efficient production of NO (Modolell et al., 1995).

Because of the above statements, a Th1/Th2 lymphocyte dichotomy has been proposed to play a central role in the pathogenesis of type 1 diabetes (Rabinovitch & Suarez-Pinzon, 1998), whereas evidence suggests that the progression of the disease correlates with a Th1-type immune response (Currie, 1978; Granger et al., 1990; Simmons et al., 1996). Increased generation of NO following cytokine-elicited iNOS induction during insulitis may contribute to β-cell destruction (Modolell et al., 1995; Morris et al., 1998). Therefore, competition between L-arginase and iNOS may be particularly important in protecting β-cells against the establishment of type 1 diabetes.

That macrophages exposed to LPS and IFNγ increase iNOS expression and NO production is well known. A novel clue for the understanding of NO-mediated β-cell damage is that

N^G-hydroxy-L-arginine (L-NOHA), an intermediate in the biosynthesis of NO, is a potent competitive inhibitor of L-arginase I (Boucher et al., 1994; Daghigh et al., 1994). Indeed, substantial amounts of this metabolite are released by LPS-treated rat alveolar macrophages (Hecker et al., 1995), while inhibition of L-arginase by L-NOHA may ensure sufficient availability of L-arginine for high-output production of NO in activated cells. L-Citrulline, the co-product of iNOS catalysis, and S-nitrosoglutathione (SNOG), an adduct produced by the reaction of NO with GSH, are also inhibitors of L-arginase in many cell types (Daghigh et al., 1994; Knowles & Moncada, 1994), including β-cells (Cunningham et al., 1997). Hence, intermediates of NO synthesis, as well as NO itself, precisely coordinate a maximum of flux through iNOS in insulin-producing pancreatic cells (**Fig. 1**). Conversely, dexamethasone and dibutyryl cAMP block both iNOS and L-arginase expression, which is paralleled by a strong decrease of NO production (Gotoh & Mori, 1999). Additionally, macrophages treated with LPS and IFNγ undergo NO-dependent apoptosis, which may be prevented by L-arginase DNA plasmid transfection (Gotoh & Mori, 1999). In such cells, L-arginase I and II seem to play a role in determining the route(s) for NO-elicited outcomes.

Competition between L-arginase and iNOS has also been found in activated murine macrophages incubated with another L-arginase inhibitor, nor-L-NOHA (Tenu et al., 1999). Contrarily, L-arginase induction by the type 2 cytokines IL-4 or IL-13 has been shown to inhibit macrophage NO synthesis due to increased L-arginine utilisation by L-arginase (Rutschman et al., 2001). Similar results have been obtained by using different cell types (Gotoh & Mori, 1999; Hecker et al., 1995). In β-cells, both L-arginase I, the major isoform expressed in rodent pancreas, and L-arginase II, the main human isoform, seem to reciprocally regulate iNOS-dependent NO production under physiological L-arginine concentrations (Wu & Morris, 1998; Stickings et al., 2002; Castillo et al., 1993), which suggests that islet L-arginase may be able to compete with iNOS *in vivo*, where L-arginine ranges at non-saturating concentrations for both enzymes. This fact may be of relevance for β-cells during Th1-driven insulitis, since L-arginine concentrations are likely to be reduced at sites of inflammation due to the release of soluble L-arginase from infiltrating macrophages (Albina et al., 1990). Corroborating this proposition is the fact that IL-1β-induction of NO synthesis in RINm5F insulin secreting β-like cells is accompanied by a reduced flux of L-arginine through L-arginase, an effect that appears to be mediated by L-NOHA (Cunningham et al., 1997). Hence, it is likely that, following immune cell-elicited NO production via iNOS, L-NOHA inhibits islet L-arginase activity to some degree *in vivo*, which may be strongly exacerbated by the pro-inflammatory cytokine IL-1β that inhibits L-arginase expression in β-cells (Cardozo et al., 2001; Rieneck et al., 2000). In fact, a remarkable reduction in L-arginase expression has been recently observed during insulitis in the NOD mouse model of type 1 diabetes (Rothe et al., 2002).

In the β-cell, NH_4^+ may contribute to L-arginine biosynthesis, through the concerted action of carbamoyl phosphate synthetase I, ornithine transcarbamoylase, argininosuccinate synthetase and argininosuccinate lyase that produce L-arginine (**Fig. 1B**). L-Glutamate is also believed to amplify glucose-induced insulin secretion in a K_{ATP} channel-independent way (Brennan et al., 2003). However, L-glutamate is, at the same time, an obligatory substrate for GSH synthesis, which, in turn, enhances the ATP/ADP ratio by optomising mitochondrial function and scavenges ROS/RNS leading to insulin secretion. L-alanine, may replenish the β-cell L-glutamate pool via an L-alanine aminotransferase-catalysed reaction. This explains why L-alanine is cytoprotective to β-cells against cytokine-induced apoptosis (Cunningham et al., 2005), *i.e.*, under cytokine-stimulated NO production,

L-alanine may provide L-glutamate for GSH synthesis thus avoiding oxidative stress and NO-induced apoptosis.

Since, as discussed above, β-cells have poor NADPH-dependent GSSG reductase (GSRd) activity, necessary to regenerate GSH from GSSG in situations of oxidative stress, and NADPH production from the hexose monophosphate shunt is limited because β-cell glycolytic activity is committed to mitochondrial ATP production during glucose-stimulated insulin release, *de novo* GSH biosynthesis from L-glutamate becomes crucial for insulin release and avoidance of β-cell death. Hence, it is easy to envisage that any metabolic disequilibrium in providing L-arginine for NO-assisted insulin secretion, during secretagogue-stimulated insulin release, forces β-cell metabolism to utilise L-glutamine-derived L-glutamate to synthesise GSH, thus ensuring little L-glutamate can undergo oxidative deamination via glutamate dehydrogenase (GDH) in these conditions. The kidney is considered to be the physiological producer of L-arginine since it is the only organ known to take up L-citrulline released from the metabolism of L-glutamine in the gut and release L-arginine into the blood (**Fig. 1 and 2**), although other tissues strongly express argininosuccinate synthetase and lyase but without any net delivery to the circulation (Vermeulen et al., 2007). In fasted humans, the contribution of L-glutamine via L-citrulline to the *de novo* synthesis of L-arginine is about 65% in neonates, where the gut is the major source of systemic L-arginine, even though some residual production in the adult gut could be accounted for by L-arginine release as well (Vermeulen et al., 2007). A minor part of circulating L-arginine may also be provided by the enterocyte metabolism of proline, as stated in the Introduction. Consequently, if, by any chance, the flux through the coupled L-glutamine/L-arginine pathway between intestine and kidney is reduced or lost, then the knock on consequences for NO synthesis are severe (**Fig. 1**). L-Glutamate, however, is a unique source of GSH in β-cells, so that a disruption or hypofunctionality of intestinal-renal L-glutamine/L-arginine axis, would promptly decrease GSH synthesis thus reducing insulin release, leading to oxidative stress and β-cell death. On the other hand, L-glutamine which is a major and immediate L-glutamate precursor, is also a primary nutrient for the maintenance of immune cell function (Curi et al., 1999; Newsholme et al., 2003; Pithon-Curi et al., 2004). Hence, we believe that an immune response triggered by an immune or chemical challenge in a redox-sensitive subject (in which the expression/activity of antioxidant and GSH enzymes is low) might decrease the availability of L-glutamine for GSH generation in β-cells, leading to oxidative stress (**Fig. 1B**). Analogously, it seems likely that other situations, in which the circulating L-glutamine pool is severely endangered (Curi et al., 1999; Newsholme et al., 1987; Lagranha et al., 2008), such as in undernourishment, strenuous-exercise or cancer cachexia-associated muscle loss, chronic inflammatory diseases (including obesity), severe metabolic acidosis, major burns, polytrauma and bacteremia, should result in β-cell dysfunction.

L-Glutamine deficiency can occur during periods of critical illness. In patients with catabolic diseases, plasma and muscle L-glutamine levels are dramatically reduced, which correlates with the poor prognosis and high degree of protein catabolism in those patients. For instance, in patients with major burn injury, plasma L-glutamine concentration is lower than 50% of that in normal controls and it remains low for at least 21 days after the injury (Parry-Billings et al., 1990). Conversely, in LPS-endotoxemic rats, a single dose of L-glutamine, which is known to induce anti-inflammation via HSP70 expression (Wischmeyer et al., 2003; Singleton, K.D. & Wischmeyer, P.E., 2008; Hamiel et al., 2009; Zhang et al., 2009) has been shown to attenuate the release of TNFα and IL-1β and to be associated with a significant decrease in mortality due to the attenuation of pro-inflammatory type 1 cytokines (Wischmeyer et al., 2001), whereas L-arginine-enriched diet limits plasma and muscle L-glutamine depletion in head-injured rats (Moinard et al., 2006). Remarkably, however, **predominately Th1** (but not Th2) cell responses require the presence of optimal concentrations of L-glutamine (Chang et al., 1999). Since β-cell death that accompanies the onset of type 1 diabetes is an essentially Th1-elicited cytotoxic challenge, it is not unreasonable to suppose that the specific recruitment of Th1 cells may greatly enhance L-glutamine and L-arginine utilisation leading to an L-arginine deficit, which causes a reduction of insulin release and redox imbalance.

The positive actions of L-arginine on viability, antioxidant status and insulin secretion are likely to reflect, in large part, the importance of GSH and the glutathione disulphide (GSSG) reductase systems as the main lines of antioxidant defence in β-cells which are characterised by low levels of CAT and GSPx. In order to adequately provide GSH, β-cells may either regenerate GSH from GSSG via a GSSG reductase-catalysed reaction or synthesise it, *de novo*, through the concerted action of γ-glutamylcysteine synthetase (γ-GCS) and GSH synthetase, which are ATP-consuming enzymes (see **Fig.** 2 for metabolic schemes). Regeneration of GSH from GSSG, which utilises NADPH as a co-factor but does not require ATP, is metabolically less expensive than the *de novo* synthesis from the constituent amino acids (L-glutamate, L-cysteine and L-glycine). However, unlike the majority of cell types, pentose phosphate shunt activity is relatively low in β-cells (Dröge, 2002), which is exacerbated by the high flux of glucose directed towards ATP production (Spinas, 1999). Therefore, β-cell NADPH must be obtained from the cytosolic malic enzyme (**Fig. 2B**), capable of converting malate to pyruvate with the concomitant production of NADPH from $NADP^+$ (MacDonald, 1995). *De novo* GSH synthesis, on the other hand, is completely dependent on the supply of L-glutamate, not only because this amino acid is a constituent of the GSH molecule, but also because L-glutamate acts as an amino acid donor in the synthesis of serine, which can subsequently, be converted to L-glycine, via a reaction requiring tetrahydrofolate.

We have found that L-arginine significantly increased glucose consumption in β-cells, while decreasing lactate formation, regardless the presence or not of pro-inflammatory cytokines, (unpublished results, also see **Fig. 2B**). This may suggest that L-arginine is able to divert glucose from mitochondrial CO_2 production towards the formation of NADPH via the cytosolic malic enzyme so requiring that glucose-derived malate is transported from the mitochondrial matrix to the cytosol. Indeed, we believe that, in the presence of L-arginine, L-glutamate can be generated from both L-arginine and glucose (via 2-oxoglutarate formation and transamination) and is subsequently utilised for GSH synthesis (please, compare **Fig. 2B and 2C**). L-Arginine addition enhances the conversion of AMPK into its active phosphorylated form, thus favoring fatty acid oxidation and ATP synthesis while glucose metabolism is supporting malate formation and L-glutamate formation for NADPH and GSH generation respectively. This requirement, however, results in a reduction in stimulus-secretion coupling and the associated insulin release.

We have also observed that NOS-2 expression is stimulated by the cytokine cocktail (which enhances iNOS activity) but NO synthesis was not enhanced by changing L-arginine in the culture medium. This suggests that iNOS is saturated with L-arginine which, in turn, results in elevated urea production. This shunt in L-arginine metabolism efficiently preserves β-cell redox status by favoring the production of GSH in conditions which generate excessive levels of NO (**Fig. 2C and 2D**).

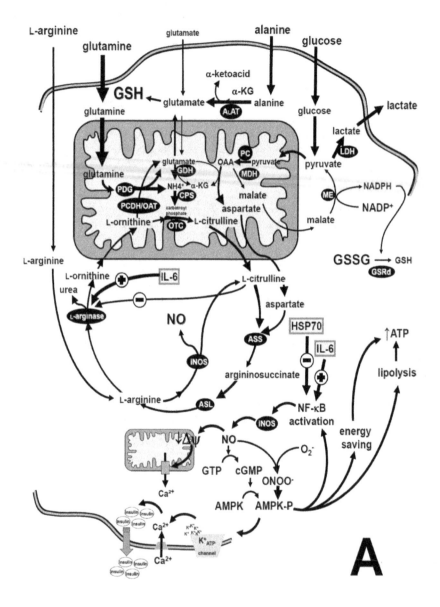

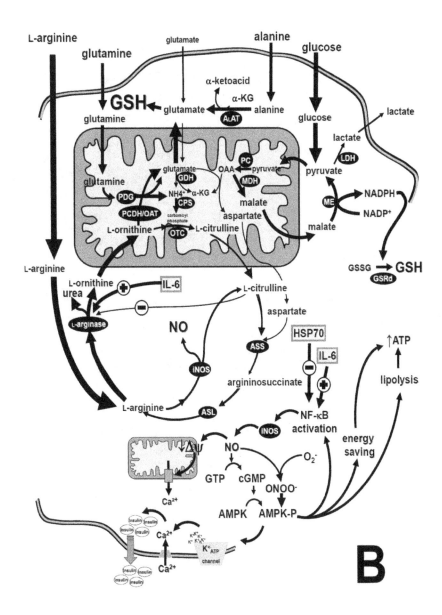

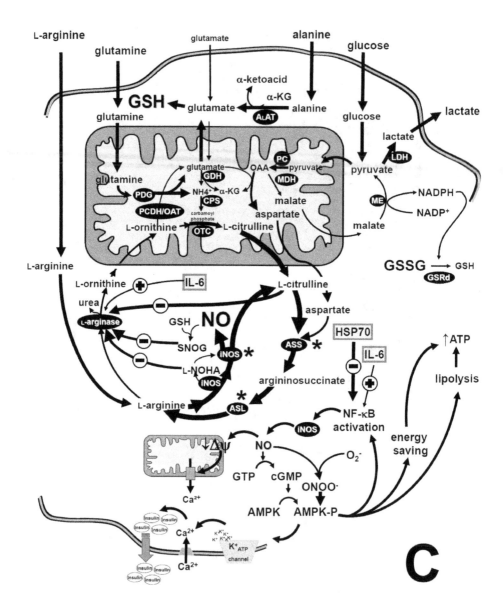

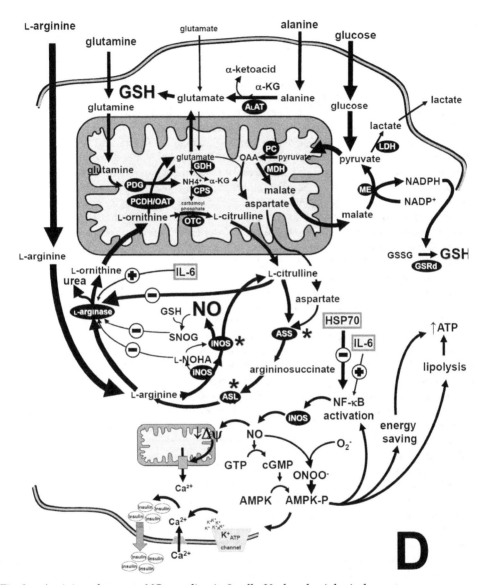

Fig. 2. L-Arginine-glutamate-NO coupling in β-cells. Under physiological secretagogue-mediated insulin release, both NO and GSH are obligatory intermediates. Accordingly, β-cells have an intricate iNOS-cantered machinery to produce NO, which potentiates insulin secretion physiologically. At the same time, insulin-secreting pancreatic cells utilise glutamate-derived GSH in order to maintain redox status needed to allow hormonal secretion and to avoid a possible NO-mediated cytotoxicity. L-Arginine derived from the kidney is the physiological substrate for the NF-κB-dependent iNOS-catalyzed NO production in β-cells. Under insufficient L-arginine supply, however, the high throughput of NO for β-cells may be attained

by the concerted action of phosphate-dependent glutaminase (PDG), glutamate dehydrogenase (GDH), aspartate aminotransferase (not shown), carbamoylphosphate synthetase I (CPS), ornithine transcarbamoylase (OTC), argininosuccinate synthetase (ASS) and argininosuccinate lyase (ASL), which, dramatically enhances the flux of L-glutamate towards NO production. In the presence of an inflammatory NF-κB-centered cytokine insult, multiple negative feedback systems act in β-cells in order to warrant L-arginine entry in iNOS metabolic pathway (lower part of the figure). This is achieved mainly due to the inhibition of L-arginase activity by L-citrulline, N^G-hydroxy- L-arginine (L-NOHA, an intermediate in NO synthesis) and S-nitrosoglutathione (SNOG), which is formed during NO biosynthesis. On the other hand, β-cells have to synthesize GSH from L-glutamate, L-cysteine and L-glycine, once regeneration of GSH from glutathione disulphide (GSSG) via NADPH-dependent GSSG reductase is relatively low in β-cells because of the high flux of glucose towards ATP production that empty pentose-phosphate shunt impairing NADPH production. In turn, *de novo* GSH synthesis is mainly dependent on liver-emanated supply of glutamate, which is not enough to allow for the enormous flux towards γ-glutamylcysteine synthetase (glutamate-cysteine ligase) and GSH synthetase in the GSH biosynthetic pathway. Therefore, muscle-derived L-alanine and L-glutamine constitute the principal sources of L-glutamate for GSH synthesis. Because of this, any reduction in L-arginine supply to β-cells accounts for a rapid shift in L-glutamate metabolism from GSH synthesis towards NO production. For instance, during Th1-elicited immune responses, the concerted enhancement of NF-κB-mediated (*) expression of ASS, ASL and iNOS dramatically boosts NO production from L-glutamate. If this rise in NO production is not accompanied by an enhanced L-arginine supply to β-cells, NO becomes very cytotoxic. Type 2 cytokines, such as interleukin-6 (IL-6) may alleviate NO toxicity by enhancing L-arginase expression that diverts L-arginine to the formation of L-ornithine and urea. At the same time, intracellular expression of the 70-kDa family of heat shock proteins (HSP70), which blocks a surplus activation of NF-κB-dependent genes, is cytoprotective because it warrants an equilibrium for NO production via NF-κB-dependent iNOS expression thus avoiding NO cytotoxic effects. Results from the present work reveal a novel as yet unpredicted facet of L-arginine metabolism in that an increase in its plasma concentrations (**from A to B**) could drift GSH metabolism from its original main source, via L-glutamine metabolism, towards the production of L-glutamate via the left side of the β-cell urea cycle, by the consecutive action of L-arginase, pyrroline-5-carboxylate dehydrogenase (PCDH), ornithine aminotransferase (OAT), γ-glutamylcysteine synthetase (not shown) and GSH synthetase (not shown). Under inflammatory stimuli (**C and D**), enhancement of L-arginine concentration may alleviate the excessive flux through iNOS by limiting L-arginine availability due to its conversion into GSH. Concomitantly, elevation of L-arginine levels are thought to deviate glucose mitochondrial metabolism towards its cytosolic utilisation as a NADPH precursor via malic enzyme (ME). This favors the regeneration of more GSH molecules from GSSG under oxidative stress conditions. L-Arginine may also stimulate AMPK activation which modulates closure of K_{ATP} channels and insulin secretion. NO is also capable of activating AMPK. However, in a high L-arginine environment, the excessive activation of AMPK may stimulate lipolysis and energy saving at the expense of insulin secretion. Since physical exercise stimulates L-glutamine flux towards L-arginine production, peaks IL-6 secretion by the stretching skeletal muscle and induces HSP70 expression throughout the body tissues, exercise continues to be the cheapest and most efficient way of preventing type-1 diabetes onset. Arrow widths indicate the intensity of the metabolic flux through each pathway.

L-Arginase is normally associated with a K_m value for L-arginine that is much higher than that of iNOS but a greater V_{max} value compared with iNOS (Mori, 2007), so that the V_{max}/K_m ratios of both enzymes are close to each other and thus these enzymes may be expected to compete for L-arginine equally in β-cells. In our hands, iNOS seemed to be saturated in β-cells, regardless of the presence of inflammatory cytokines, so that β-cell urea production is able to furnish L-ornithine and thus L-glutamate for GSH synthesis in appropriate conditions. Moreover, L-arginine may protect β-cells via the induction of haem oxygenase (HO-1) expression (data not shown). HO activity is an important detoxifying enzyme, due to its ability to scavenge haem groups thus providing redox protection (Abraham & Kappas, 2008). However, it is plausible that HO expression in β-cells in response to L-arginine may also play a metabolic role, since one of its direct products, carbon monoxide (CO), has recently been reported to induce insulin secretion and to improve *in vivo* function of β-cells after transplant (Abraham & Kappas, 2008). Moreover, the long-lasting expression of this enzyme has been shown to delay the progression of type 1 diabetes in NOD mice (Li et al., 2007). Hence, L-arginine can be recognised as an antioxidant in its own right, being comparable with known antioxidant stimuli, such as phytochemical supplements (Velmurugan et al., 2009).

Furthermore, and interestingly, chronic hyperlactataemia, in which high plasma levels of lactate block intestinal proline oxidase activity leading to severe hypocitrullinaemia and hypoargininaemia (Dillon et al., 1999), has been described as an independent risk factor for diabetes development, with lactate being an important factor for maintaining insulin resistance (DiGirolamo et al., 1992; Lovejoy et al., 1992). Conversely, L-arginine supplementation to critical care patients did induce L-glutamine rise in the plasma (Loï et al., 2009), which may be related to the fact the L-arginine supplementation spares plasma glutamine pools.

In synthesis, L-arginine derived from the kidney (**Fig. 1**) is the physiological substrate for the NF-κB-dependent iNOS-catalysed NO production in β-cells. Under **insufficient** L-arginine supply, however, the high throughput of NO for β-cells may be attained by the concerted action of phosphate-dependent glutaminase (GDP), glutamate dehydrogenase (GDH), aspartate aminotransferase (AsAT), carbamoylphosphate synthetase (CPS), ornithine transcarbamoylase (OTC), argininosuccinate synthetase (ASS) and argininosuccinate lyase (ASL), which, dramatically enhances the flux of glutamate towards NO production. Multiple negative feedback systems act in β-cells in order to warrant L-arginine entry in iNOS metabolic pathway. This is achieved mainly due to the inhibition of L-arginase activity by L-citrulline, N^G-hydroxy-L-arginine (L-NOHA, an intermediate in NO synthesis) and S-nitrosoglutathione (SNOG), which is formed during NO biosynthesis. On the other hand, β-cells have to synthesise GSH from L-glutamate, L-cysteine and L-glycine, because regeneration of GSH from GSSG via NADPH-dependent GSSG reductase is relatively low in β-cells because of the high flux of glucose towards ATP production that empty pentose-phosphate shunt, the major NADPH-producing system. In turn, *de novo* GSH synthesis is mainly dependent on liver-derived supply of glutamate, which is not enough to allow for the enormous flux towards γ-glutamylcysteine synthetase and GSH synthetase in the GSH biosynthetic pathway. Therefore, muscle-derived L-alanine and L-glutamine constitute the principal sources of L-glutamate for GSH synthesis in order to spare β-cell L-arginine stores. In fact, previous reports from our laboratory have highlighted the importance of L-glutamine and L-alanine for GSH generation, insulin secretion and protection against pro-inflammatory cytokines (Brennan et al., 2003; Brennan et a., 2002; Cunninham et al., 2005). Because of this, **any reduction** in L-arginine supply to β-cells accounts for a rapid shift in L-glutamate metabolism from GSH synthesis towards NO production. For instance, during Th1-elicited immune responses (*e.g.* as **in Fig. 2C and 2D**), the concerted enhancement of nuclear factor NF-κB-mediated expression of ASS, ASL and iNOS dramatically boosts NO production from L-glutamate. If this rise in NO production is not accompanied by an enhanced L-arginine supply to β-cells, NO becomes very cytotoxic. Type 2 cytokines (T2-CK) may alleviate NO toxicity by enhancing L-arginase expression that deviates L-arginine to the formation of L-ornithine and urea.

6. Psychological stress and the role peripheral sympathetic nervous system-histamine-CRH axis activation in type 1 diabetes

It has long been recognised that stressful situations are closely related to the onset of type 1 diabetes. In fact, many stressful conditions that are associated with immune system imbalances, including psychological ones, are associated with the incidence of type 1 diabetes (Soltesz, 2003; Dahlquist, 2006). Indeed, it has recently been shown that stressful life events and psychological dysfunctions dramatically augment the likelihood of the incidence of type 1 diabetes in children and adolescents (Sipetic et al., 2007). These include parents' job-related changes or lost job, severe accidents, hospitalization or death of a close friend, quarrels between parents, war, near-drowning in a pool, falling down, being an unhurt participant of an accident, conflicts with parents/teacher/neighbours, to be lost in town, physical attack, failure in competition, penalty, examination, death of pet, presence of lightning strike, loss of housing accommodation and learning problems.

As a general rule, stress is considered as immunosuppressive. Surprisingly, however, a growing body of evidence strongly suggests that acute stress serves as a pro-inflammatory stimulus via the production of corticotropin-releasing hormone (CRH) by peripheral sympathetic nerve terminals (Elenkov et al., 1999). CRH stimulates lymphocyte proliferation (McGillis et al., 1989; Jessop et al., 1997) and secretion of IL-1β and IL-2 by mononuclear cells isolated from the peripheral blood of healthy subjects (Singh & Leu, 1990). Peripheral CRH exerts a pro-inflammatory effect in autoimmune diseases with a selective increase in Th1-type responses, which is mediated by an NF-κB-dependent pathway (Benou et al., 2005). Additionally, it is possible that, upon a stressful situation, peripherally delivered CRH activates mast cells that secrete histamine, which acts via H1 receptors to induce local inflammation (Elenkov et al., 1999). In fact, diabetes is associated with increased basal hypothalamus-pituitary-adrenal (HPA) activity and impaired stress responsiveness (Chan et al., 2005). Therefore, psychological stress may selectively activate Th1 lymphocytes that mediate type-1 cytokine-induced iNOS expression, exacerbated NO production and β-cell cytotoxicity. Enhanced Th1 activity, in turn, increases L-glutamine utilisation with the consequent shift of L-glutamate metabolism from GSH biosynthesis towards NO production, as discussed above (Fig. 2 and 3).

Taken together, these findings suggest that psychological stress may have a dual and cross-potentiating role in determining the onset of type 1 diabetes: an immunoinflammatory (Fig. 3) and a metabolic one (Fig. 2C and 2D). Arguing in proof of such a hypothesis is the observation that orally administered L-arginine supplementation significantly improves patient status in a series of different pathological conditions associated with immune dysfunctions, including in pre-term neonates (Wu et al., 2004), without increasing urea

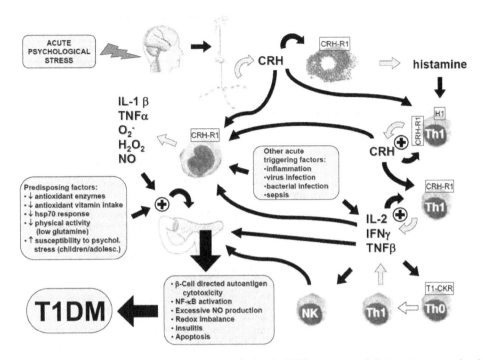

Fig. 3. Psychological stress and autoimmune diabetes. Different stressful situations may lead to the activation of sympathetic-corticotropin-releasing hormone (CRH)-histamine axis that triggers a Th1-specific immunoinflammatory response. Peripheral sympathetic nerve-derived CRH released under acute psychological stressful situations is capable of stimulating mast cells and Th1 lymphocytes, which arm an immunoinflammatory response. Auto-reactive Th1 cell subset and its cytokine products (type 1 cytokines, T1-CK) raised against islet β-cell antigen(s) mediate the activation of macrophages and Th1 lymphocytes, favouring insulitis. Additionally, other predisposing factors may also exacerbate β-cell injury and the onset of type 1 diabetes mellitus (T1DM).

levels (Wilmore, 2004). Curiously, intraperitoneal L-arginine injection, where the physiological coupling of L-glutamine/L-arginine through the intestinal-renal axis is bypassed, does **not** improve diabetes in animal models. On the contrary, it seems to worsen it (Mohan & Das, 1998), while **oral** administration of L-arginine to alloxan-treated rats restores blood glucose and insulin levels (Vasilijevic et al., 2007). Oral L-arginine administration has also been shown to improve, but not completely, peripheral and hepatic insulin sensitivity in type 2 diabetes (Piatti et al., 2001), where oxidative stress (Carvalho-Filho et al., 2005; Oliveira et al., 2003; Hirabara et al., 2006) and NO overproduction (Newsholme et al., 2007; Carvalho-Filho et al., 2005) are also involved. If this is so, nutritional management of L-glutamine and/or L-arginine, **enterally** administered in order to allow for the physiological re-establishment of L-glutamine/L-arginine homeostasis (Vermeulen et al., 2007), may rescue β-cell redox balance in ongoing type 1 diabetes. Additionally, skeletal muscle is a major site for L-glutamine synthesis in the human body and contains over 90% of the whole-body L-glutamine pool. Quantitative studies in humans

(Newsholme et al., 2003) have demonstrated that, in the postabsorptive state, 60% of the amino acids released comprise L-alanine plus L-glutamine (**Fig. 1A**). Therefore, moderate physical exercise, which is known to accelerate the rate of L-glutamine delivery into the circulation, may be of value in protecting L-glutamine/L-arginine metabolic coupling between the gut and β-cells.

7. Influence of regular physical exercise in L-arginine/L-glutamine coupling in β-cells

During physical exercise sessions, pro-inflammatory cytokine production is downregulated and anti-inflammatory cytokines, such as IL-1 receptor antagonist (IL-1ra), IL-10 and IL-6, are upregulated (Drenth et al., 1995; Nieman & Pedersen, 1999; Rohde et al., 1997). In this sense, IL-6 seems to play a capital role during exercise-induced changes in immune function. In fact, the level of circulating IL-6 has been shown to increase dramatically (up to 100-fold) in response to exercise (Pedersen & Hoffman-Goetz, 2000; Febbraio et al., 2002; Pedersen & Steensberg, 2002; Pedersen et al., 2001). Most studies have also reported that exercise, *per se*, does not increase plasma levels of TNFα, although some have shown that strenuous, prolonged exercise, such as marathon running, results in a small increase in the plasma concentration of TNFα (Pedersen et al., 1998; Suzuki et al., 2000). This long-term effect of exercise may be ascribed to the anti-inflammatory response elicited by an acute bout of exercise, which is partly mediated by muscle-derived IL-6.

Physiological concentrations of IL-6 stimulate the appearance, in the circulation, of the anti-inflammatory cytokines IL-1ra and IL-10, and inhibit the production of the pro-inflammatory cytokine TNFα. Hence, exercise-induced IL-6 release downregulates pro-inflammatory cytokine production while increasing anti-inflammatory cytokine production and action, which may induce a very strong anti-inflammatory cytokine response. The main modulator of these responses is likely to be the appearance of IL-6 in the circulation. Since IL-6 strongly downregulates NF-κB activation, we believe that moderate exercise-induced IL-6 production may suppress NF-κB-dependent iNOS while stimulating L-arginase activity/expression with a consequent decrease in NO-dependent β-cell death upon Th1-driven β-cell assault. Therefore, besides any possible beneficial effect that moderate exercise may have on L-glutamine/L-arginine coupling that is responsible for the maintenance of β-cell redox homeostasis and insulin secreting capacity (see above), mild physical exercise may shut off pro-inflammatory cytokine machinery, which gives rise to an additional protection against the development of type 1 diabetes.

Even though the effects of IL-6 on β-cells remains a matter of debate and controversies (Wadt et al., 1998), it has been found that IL-6 hinders the development of type 1 diabetes in different mouse models (Campbell et al., 1994; DiCosmo et al., 1994). Moreover, IL-6 has proven to be effective in protecting insulin-secreting MIN6 cells and freshly isolated pancreatic islets against Th1-derived cytokine (IL-1β, TNFα and IFNγ)-induced apoptosis while improving cellular viability and insulin secretion (Choi et al., 2004). Altogether, the above propositions support an important protective effect of exercise-dependent muscle-derived IL-6 on β-cells against the development of diabetes. Moreover, exercise-induced HSP70 expression in non-muscular cells may have a critical influence in maintaining an anti-inflammatory status, as discussed above. However, exercise-induced HSP70 in pancreatic β-cells has never been addressed. Therefore, we are currently evaluating the effects of acute and chronic (training) exercise sessions (swimming) on HSP70 pathways and L-glutamine/L-arginine coupling enzymes in animal pancreatic islets and isolated β-cells.

8. Conclusion

Continued supply of L-arginine, physiologically provided by the metabolism of L-glutamine via the intestinal-renal axis and from skeletal muscle, which is enhanced during exercise, is essential for β-cell functional integrity and, indeed, for β-cell defence. The dysregulation of immune system function, characteristic of Th1-elicited β-cell toxicity and impaired insulin secretion, which accompany the onset of type 1 diabetes, may be triggered when an individual faces a strong **psychological stress** that determines an enhanced L-glutamine utilisation by Th1 lymphocytes. The oxidative stress that takes place upon reduced intracellular GSH levels allows for the activation of NF-κB, which, in turn, positively feeds back on iNOS expression and activity, thus perpetuating the inflammatory process within β-cells where **excess** NO is harmful. Defective HSP70 induction in response to physiological levels of intraislet NO may also be involved in the pathogenesis of type 1 diabetes. Physical exercise, on the other hand, is capable of inducing a huge production and release of IL-6, which is a key anti-inflammatory mediator that suppresses NF-κB-dependent responses. Moreover, exercise-elicited activation of HSP70 biochemical pathways completely blocks NF-κB activation, impedes apoptosis and is cytoprotective due to HSP70 chaperone activity, which protects against protein denaturation. HSP70 induction is also associated with enhanced Th2 cell activity over Th1. Metabolically, exercise may restore L-glutamine supply thus normalizing pancreatic production of NO from kidney-derived L-arginine, and not from L-glutamate which is necessary for GSH synthesis and antioxidant defence. Thus the enormous changes in human life style, compared with that of our 3-4 million-old ancestors, could be related with our current inability in maintaining healthy β-cells. As previously argued (Krause & Homem de Bittencourt, 2008), we advocate that present-day levels of physical activity and dietary patterns (Simopoulos, 2006; Wisloff et al., 2005) seem to have changed much faster than the time needed to allow evolutionary metabolic changes. In other words, our metabolism evolved to fit a level of physical activity and availability of a variety of food supplies different from those of nowadays (favouring energy conservation and storage). As a corollary, unless humans enhance their pattern of physical activity, diabetes will become more and more of a risk factor in the population. Therefore, the notion that β-cells are solely bystanders of oxidative stress-mediated cell toxicity because their antioxidant defences fail in managing physiological stress is an unfortunate misconception. Since the L-glutamine/L-arginine duet may influence β-cell function and survival, the knowledge of physiologically adequate levels and fluxes of both amino acids may serve as a predictor of β-cell susceptibility to dysfunction or death in diabetes. Additionally, although the possibility of pharmacologically exploiting Th1/Th2 duality relative to L-arginine metabolism may open new avenues for diabetes therapeutics, physical exercise is still the cheapest and easiest physiological measure to avoid the onset and/or worsening of diabetes. In summary, if the prevention of diabetes is dependent on HSP70 expression and both restoration of adequate L-arginine supply to β-cells and blockage of NF-κB overstimulation, moderate physical exercise is presented as the most convenient solution for these two lacunes.

9. Acknowledgements

We thank UCD School of Biomolecular and Biomedical Science, Science Foundation Ireland and the National Council for Scientific and Technological Development (CNPq), Brazil, for their support of this work.

10. References

Abraham, N.G. & Kappas, A (2008). Pharmacological and clinical aspects of heme oxygenase. *Pharmacological Reviews*, Vol. 60, pp. 79-127

Albina, J.E.; Mills, C.D.; Henry, W.L. & Caldwell, M.D. (1990). Temporal expression of different pathways of L-arginine metabolism in healing wounds. *Journal of Immunology*, Vol. 144, pp. 3877-3880

Ao, L.; Zou, N.; Cleveland, J.C., Jr.; Fullerton, D.A. & Meng, X. (2009). Myocardial TLR4 is a determinant of neutrophil infiltration after global myocardial ischemia: mediating KC and MCP-1 expression induced by extracellular HSC70. *American Journal of Physiology. Heart and Circulatory Physiology*, Vol. 297, N° 1, pp. H21–H28

Arya, R.; Mallik, M. & Lakhotia, S.C. (2007). Heat shock genes – integrating cell survival and death. *Journal of Biosciences*, Vol. 32, N° 3, pp. 595–610

Asayama, K.; Kooy. N;W. & Burr, I.M. (1986). Effect of vitamin E deficiency and selenium deficiency on insulin secretory reserve and free radical scavenging systems in islets: decrease of islet manganosuperoxide dismutase. *Journal Laboratory and Clinical Medicine*, Vol. 107, pp. 459-464

Asea, A. (2003). Chaperokine-induced signal transduction pathways. *Exercise Immunology Review*, Vol. 9, pp. 25–33

Asea, A. (2008). Heat shock proteins and toll-like receptors. *Handbook of Experimental Pharmacology*, Vol. 183, pp. 111–127

Atalay, M.; Oksala, N.K.; Laaksonen, D.E.; Khanna, S.; Nakao, C.; Lappalainen, J.; Roy, S.; Hanninen, O. & Sen, C.K. (2004). Exercise training modulates heat shock protein response in diabetic rats. *Journal of Applied Physiology*, Vol. 97, pp. 605-611

Baldwin, A.S., Jr. (1996). The NF-κB and IκB proteins: new discoveries and insights. *Annual Review of Immunology*, Vol. 14, pp. 649-683

Beck, K.F.; Eberhardt, W.; Frank, S.; Huwiler, A.; Messmer, U.K.; Muhl, H. & Pfeilschifter, J. (1999). Inducible NO synthase: role in cellular signalling. *Journal of Experimental Biology*, Vol. 202, pp. 645-653

Beere, H.M. (2004). "The stress of dying": the role of heat shock proteins in the regulation of apoptosis. *Journal of Cell Science*, Vol. 117, Pt 13, pp. 2641–2651

Benou, C.; Wang, Y.; Imitola, J.; VanVlerken, L.; Chandras, C.; Karalis, K.P. & Khoury, S,J. (2005). Corticotropin-releasing hormone contributes to the peripheral inflammatory response in experimental autoimmune encephalomyelitis. *Journal of Immunology*, Vol. 174, pp. 5407-5413

Boucher, J.L.; Custot, J.; Vadon, S.; Delaforge, M.; Lepoivre, M.; Tenu, J.P.; Yapo, A. & Mansuy, D. (1994). N$^{\omega}$-hydroxyl-L-arginine, an intermediate in the L-arginine to nitric oxide pathway, is a strong inhibitor of liver and macrophage arginase. *Biochemical and Biophysical Research Communications*, Vol. 203, pp. 1614-1621

Boucher, J.L.; Moali, C. & Tenu, J.P. (1999). Nitric oxide biosynthesis, nitric oxide synthase inhibitors and arginase competition for L-arginine utilization. *Cellular and Molecular Life Sciences*, Vol. 55, pp. 1015-1028

Brennan, L.; Corless, M.; Hewage, C.; Malthouse, J.P.; McClenaghan, N.H.; Flatt, P.R. & Newsholme, P. (2003). ^{13}C-NMR analysis reveals a link between L-glutamine metabolism, D-glucose metabolism and gamma-glutamyl cycle activity in a clonal pancreatic β-cell line. *Diabetologia*, Vol. 46, pp. 1512-1521

Brennan, L.; Shine, A.; Hewage, C.; Malthouse, J.P.; Brindle, K.M.; McClenaghan, N.; Flatt, P.R. & Newsholme, P. (2002). A nuclear magnetic resonance-based demonstration of substantial oxidative L-alanine metabolism and L-alanine-enhanced glucose metabolism in a clonal pancreatic beta-cell line: metabolism of L-alanine is important to the regulation of insulin secretion. *Diabetes*, Vol. 51, pp. 1714-1721

Calderwood, S.K.; Mambula, S.S.; Gray, P.J., Jr. & Theriault, J.R. (2007a). Extracellular heat shock proteins in cell signaling. *Federation of European Biochemical Societies Letters*, Vol. 581, N° 19, pp. 3689–3694

Calderwood, S.K.; Theriault, J.; Gray, P.J. & Gong, J. (2007b). Cell surface receptors for molecular chaperones. *Methods*, Vol. 43, N° 3, pp. 199–206

Campbell, I.L.; Hobbs, M.V.; Dockter, J.; Oldstone, M.B. & Allison, J. (1994). Islet inflammation and hyperplasia induced by the pancreatic islet-specific overexpression of interleukin-6 in transgenic mice. *American Journal of Pathology*, Vol. 145, pp. 157-166

Cardozo, A.K.; Kruhoffer, M.; Leeman, R.; Orntoft, T. & Eizirik, D.L. (2001). Identification of novel cytokine-induced genes in pancreatic β-cells by high-density oligonucleotide arrays. *Diabetes*, Vol. 50, pp. 909-920

Carvalho-Filho, M.A.; Ueno, M.; Hirabara, S.M.; Seabra, A.B.; Carvalheira, J.B.; de Oliveira, M.G.; Velloso, L.A.; Curi, R. & Saad, M.J. (2005). S-Nitrosation of the insulin receptor, insulin receptor substrate 1, and protein kinase B/Akt: a novel mechanism of insulin resistance. *Diabetes*, Vol. 54, pp. 959-967

Castillo, L.; Chapman, T.E.; Sanchez, M.; Yu, Y.M.; Burke, J.F.; Ajami, A.M.; Vogt, J. & Young, V.R. (1993). Plasma arginine and citrulline kinetics in adults given adequate and arginine-free diets. *Proceedings of the National Academy of Sciences of the U.S.A.*, Vol. 90, pp. 7749-7753

Chan, J.Y.; Ou, C.C.; Wang, L.L. & Chan, S.H. (2004). Heat shock protein 70 confers cardiovascular protection during endotoxemia via inhibition of nuclear factor-κB activation and inducible nitric oxide synthase expression in the rostral ventrolateral medulla. *Circulation*, Vol. 110, N° 23, pp. 3560–3566

Chan, O.; Inouye, K.; Akirav, E.; Park, E.; Riddell, M.C.; Vranic, M. & Matthews, S.G. (2005). Insulin alone increases hypothalamus-pituitary-adrenal activity, and diabetes lowers peak stress responses. *Endocrinology*, Vol. 146, pp. 1382-1390

Chang, C.I.; Liao, J.C. & Kuo, L. (1998). Arginase modulates nitric oxide production in activated macrophages. *American Journal of Physiology. Heart and Circulatory Physiology*, Vol. 274, pp. H342-348

Chang, W.K.; Yang, K.D. & Shaio, M.F. (1999). Effect of glutamine on Th1 and Th2 cytokine responses of human peripheral blood mononuclear cells. *Clinical Immunology*, Vol. 93, pp. 294-301

Chen, F.; Castranova, V.; Shi, X. & Demers, L.M. (1999). New insights into the role of nuclear factor-κB, a ubiquitous transcription factor in the initiation of diseases. *Clinical Chemistry*, Vol. 45, pp. 7-17

Chen, H.; Li, X. & Epstein, P.N. (2005). MnSOD and catalase transgenes demonstrate that protection of islets from oxidative stress does not alter cytokine toxicity. *Diabetes*, Vol. 54, pp. 1437-1446

Chen, H.W.; Kuo, H.T.; Wang, S.J.; Lu, T.S. & Yang, R.C. (2005). In vivo heat shock protein assembles with septic liver NF-κB/I-κB complex regulating NF-κB activity. *Shock*, Vol. 24, N° 3, pp. 232-238

Choi, S.E.; Choi, K.M.; Yoon, I.H.; Shin, J.Y.; Kim, J.S.; Park, W.Y.; Han, D.J.; Kim, S.C.; Ahn, C.; Kim, J.Y.; Hwang, E.S.; Cha, C.Y.; Szot, G.L.; Yoon, K.H. & Park, C.G. (2004). IL-6 protects pancreatic islet β cells from pro-inflammatory cytokines-induced cell death and functional impairment in vitro and in vivo. *Transplantation Immunology*, Vol. 13, pp. 43-53

Chung, J.; Nguyen, A.K.; Henstridge, D.C.; Holmes, A.G.; Chan, M.H.; Mesa, J.L.; Lancaster, G.I.; Southgate, R.J.; Bruce, C.R.; Duffy, S.J.; Horvath, I.; Mestril, R.; Watt, M.J.; Hooper, P.L.; Kingwell, B.A.; Vigh, L.; Hevener, A. & Febbraio, M.A. (2008). HSP72 protects against obesity-induced insulin resistance. *Proceedings of the National Academy of Sciences of the U.S.A.*, Vol. 105, N° 5, pp. 1739-1744.

Corraliza, I.M.; Soler, G.; Eichmann, K. & Modolell, M. (1995). Arginase induction by suppressors of nitric oxide synthesis (IL-4, IL-10 and PGE$_2$) in murine bone-marrow-derived macrophages. *Biochemical and Biophysical Research Communications*, Vol. 206, pp. 667-673

Cunningham, G.A.; McClenaghan, N.H.; Flatt, P.R. & Newsholme, P. (2005). L-Alanine induces changes in metabolic and signal transduction gene expression in a clonal rat pancreatic β-cell line and protects from pro-inflammatory cytokine-induced apoptosis. *Clinical Science (London)*, Vol. 109, pp. 447-455

Cunningham, J.M.; Mabley, J.G. & Green, I.C. (1997). Interleukin 1β-mediated inhibition of arginase in RINm5F cells. *Cytokine*, Vol. 9, pp. 570-576

Curi, R.; Newsholme, P.; Pithon-Curi, T.C.; Pires-de-Melo, M.; Garcia, C.; Homem-de-Bittencourt, P.I., Jr.; Guimarães, A.R. (1999). Metabolic fate of glutamine in lymphocytes, macrophages and neutrophils. *Brazilian Journal of Medical and Biological Research*, Vol. 32, pp. 15-21

Currie, G.A. (1978). Activated macrophages kill tumour cells by releasing arginase. *Nature*, Vol. 273, pp. 758-759

Daghigh, F.; Fukuto, J.M. & Ash, D.E. (1994). Inhibition of rat liver arginase by an intermediate in NO biosynthesis, N^G-hydroxy-L-arginine: implications for the regulation of nitric oxide biosynthesis by arginase. *Biochemical and Biophysical Research Communications*, Vol. 202, pp. 174-180

Dahlquist, G. (2006). Can we slow the rising incidence of childhood-onset autoimmune diabetes? The overload hypothesis. *Diabetologia*, Vol. 49, pp. 20-24

Darville, M.I. & Eizirik, D.L. (1998). Regulation by cytokines of the inducible nitric oxide synthase promoter in insulin-producing cells. *Diabetologia*, Vol. 41, pp. 1101-1108

De Maio A. (2011). Extracellular heat shock proteins, cellular export vesicles, and the Stress Observation System: A form of communication during injury, infection, and cell damage : It is never known how far a controversial finding will go! Dedicated to Ferruccio Ritossa. *Cell Stress and Chaperones*, Vol. 16, N° 3, pp. 235-249

DiCosmo, B.F.; Picarella, D. & Flavell, R.A. (1994). Local production of human IL-6 promotes insulitis but retards the onset of insulin-dependent diabetes mellitus in non-obese diabetic mice. *International Immunology*, Vol. 6, pp. 1829-1837

DiGirolamo, M.; Newby,F.D. & Lovejoy, J. (1992). Lactate production in adipose tissue: a regulated function with extra-adipose implications. *Federation of American Societies for Experimental Biology Journal*, Vol. 6, N° 7, pp. 2405-2412

Dillon, E.L.; Knabe, D.A. & Wu, G. (1999). Lactate inhibits citrulline and arginine synthesis from proline in pig enterocytes. *American Journal of Physiology. Gastrointestinal and Liver Physiology*, Vol. 276, N°5 Pt 1, pp. G1079-G1086

Domínguez, C.; Ruiz, E.; Gussinye, M. & Carrascosa A. (1998). Oxidative stress at onset and in early stages of type I diabetes in children and adolescents. *Diabetes Care*, Vol. 21, pp. 1736-1742

Drenth, J.P.; Van Uum, S.H.; Van Deuren, M.; Pesman, G.J.; Van der Ven-Jongekrijg, J. & Van der Meer, J.W. (1995). Endurance run increases circulating IL-6 and IL-1ra but downregulates ex vivo TNF-α and IL-1β production. *Journal of Applied Physiology*, Vol. 79, pp. 1497-1503

Dröge, W. (2002). Free radicals in the physiological control of cell function. *Physiological Reviews*, Vol. 82, pp. 47-95

Eizirik, D.L. & Mandrup-Poulsen, T. (2001). A choice of death - the signal-transduction of immune-mediated β-cell apoptosis. *Diabetologia*, Vol. 44, pp. 2115-2133

Elenkov, I.J. & Chrousos, G.P. (1999). Stress hormones, Th1/Th2 patterns, pro/anti-inflammatory cytokines and susceptibility to disease. *Trends in Endocrinology and Metabolism*, Vol. 10, N° 9, pp. 359-368

Elenkov, I.J.; Webster, E.L.; Torpy, D.J. & Chrousos, G.P. (1999). Stress, corticotropin-releasing hormone, glucocorticoids, and the immune/inflammatory response: acute and chronic effects. *Annals of the New York Academy of Sciences*, Vol. 876, pp. 1-11 (see discussion in pp. 11-13)

Febbraio, M.A.; Mesa, J.L.; Chung, J.; Steensberg, A.; Keller, C.; Nielsen, H.B.; Krustrup, P.; Ott, P.; Secher, N.H. & Pedersen, B.K. (2004). Glucose ingestion attenuates the exercise-induced increase in circulating heat shock protein 72 and heat shock protein 60 in humans. *Cell Stress and Chaperones*, Vol. 9, N° 4, pp. 390-396

Febbraio, M.A.; Ott, P.; Nielsen, H.B.; Steensberg, A.; Keller, C.; Krustrup, P.; Secher, N.H. & Pedersen, B.K. (2002a). Exercise induces hepatosplanchnic release of heat shock protein 72 in humans. *Journal of Physiology*, Vol. 544, Pt 3, pp. 957–962

Febbraio, M.A.; Steensberg, A.; Walsh, R.; Koukoulas, I; Van Hall, G.; Saltin, B. & Pedersen, B.K. (2002b). Reduced glycogen availability is associated with an elevation in HSP72 in contracting human skeletal muscle. *Journal of Physiology*, Vol. 538, Pt 3, pp. 911–917

Fehrenbach, E.; Niess, A.M.; Voelker, K.; Northoff, H. & Mooren, F.C. (2005). Exercise intensity and duration affect blood soluble HSP72. *International Journal of Sports Medicine*, Vol. 26, N° 7, pp. 552–557

Feinstein, D.L; Galea, E.; Aquino, D.A.; Li, G.C.; Xu, H. & Reis DJ. (1996). Heat shock protein 70 suppresses astroglial-inducible nitric-oxide synthase expression by decreasing NF-κB activation. *Journal of Biological Chemistry*, Vol. 271, N° 30, pp. 17724–17732

Fisher-Wellman, K. & Bloomer, R.J. (2009). Acute exercise and oxidative stress: a 30 year history. Dynamic Medicine, Vol. 8, pp. 1

Flodstrom, M.; Niemann, A.; Bedoya, F.J.; Morris, S.M. & Eizirik, D.L. (1995). Expression of the citrulline-nitric oxide cycle in rodent and human pancreatic β-cells: induction of argininosuccinate synthetase by cytokines. *Endocrinology*, Vol. 136, pp. 3200-3206

Flodstrom, M.; Tsai, D.; Fine, C.; Maday, A. & Sarvetnick, N. (2003). Diabetogenic potential of human pathogens uncovered in experimentally permissive β-cells. *Diabetes*, Vol. 52, pp. 2025-2034

Forman, B.M.; Tontonoz, P.; Chen, J.; Brun, R.P.; Spiegelman, B.M. & Evans RM. (1995). 15-deoxy-$\Delta^{12,14}$-prostaglandin J_2 is a ligand for the adipocyte determination factor PPARγ. *Cell*, Vol. 83, pp. 803-812

Gelain, D.P.; de Bittencourt Pasquali, M.A.; Comim, C.; Grunwald, M.S.; Ritter, C.; Tomasi, C.D.; Alves, S.C.; Quevedo, J.; Dal-Pizzol, F.; Fonseca Moreira, J.C. (2011). Serum HSP70 Levels, Oxidant Status and Mortality in Sepsis. *Shock*, Feb 15 [Epub ahead of print], DOI: 10.1097/SHK.0b013e31820fe704

Giannoukakis, N.; Rudert, W.A.; Trucco, M. & Robbins, P.D. (2000). Protection of human islets from the effects of interleukin-1β by adenoviral gene transfer of an IκB repressor. *Journal of Biological Chemistry*, Vol. 275, pp. 36509-36513

Gill, D.J.; Low, B.C. & Grigor, M.R. (1996). Interleukin-1β and tumor necrosis factor-α stimulate the cat-2 gene of the L-arginine transporter in cultured vascular smooth muscle cells. *Journal of Biological Chemistry*, Vol. 271, pp. 11280-11283

Gonzalez, B. & Manso, R. (2004). Induction, modification and accumulation of HSP70s in the rat liver after acute exercise: early and late responses. *Journal of Physiology*, Vol. 556, N° Pt 2, pp. 369–385

Gotoh, T. & Mori, M. (1999). Arginase II downregulates nitric oxide (NO) production and prevents NO-mediated apoptosis in murine macrophage-derived RAW 264.7 cells. *Journal of Cell Biology*, Vol. 144, pp. 427-434

Granger, D.L.; Hibbs, J.B.; Perfect, J.R. & Durack, D.T. (1990). Metabolic fate of L-arginine in relation to microbiostatic capability of murine macrophages. *Journal of Clinical Investigation*, Vol. 85, pp. 264-273

Gutierrez, L.L.P.; Maslinkiewicz, A.; Curi, R. & Homem de Bittencourt, P.I., Jr. (2008). Atherosclerosis: a redox-sensitive lipid imbalance suppressible by cyclopentenone prostaglandins. *Biochemical Pharmacology*, Vol. 75, N° 12, pp. 2245-2262

Hamiel, C.R.; Pinto, S.; Hau, A. & Wischmeyer, P.E. (2009). Glutamine enhances heat shock protein 70 expression via increased hexosamine biosynthetic pathway activity. *American Journal of Physiology. Cell Physiology*, Vol. 297, N° 6, pp. C1509-C1519

Hamilton, K.L.; Staib, J.L.; Phillips, T.; Hess, A.; Lennon, S.L. & Powers, S.K. (2003). Exercise, antioxidants, and HS P72: protection against myocardial ischemia/reperfusion. *Free Radical Biology and Medicine*, Vol. 34, N° 7, pp. 800–809

Harris, M.B. & Starnes, J.W. (2001). Effects of body temperature during exercise training on myocardial adaptations. *American Journal of Physiology. Heart and Circulatory Physiology*, Vol. 280, N° 5, pp. H2271–H2280

Hattori, Y.; Campbell, E.B. & Gross, S.S. (1994). Argininosuccinate synthetase mRNA and activity are induced by immunostimulants in vascular smooth muscle. Role in the regeneration or arginine for nitric oxide synthesis. *Journal of Biological Chemistry*, Vol. 269, pp. 9405-9408

Heck, T.G.; Schöler, C.M. & Homem de Bittencourt, P.I., Jr. (2011). HSP70 expression: does it a novel fatigue signalling factor from immune system to the brain? *Cell Biochemistry and Function*, Vol. 29, N° 3, pp. 215-26

Hecker, M.; Nematollahi, H.; Hey, C.; Busse, R. & Racke, K. (1995). Inhibition of arginase by NG-hydroxy-L-arginine in alveolar macrophages: implications for the utilization of L-arginine for nitric oxide synthesis. *Federation of European Biochemical Societies Letters*. Vol. 359, pp. 251-254

Hecker, M.; Schott, C.; Bucher, B.; Busse, R. & Stoclet, J.C. (1995). Increase in serum NG-hydroxy-L-arginine in rats treated with bacterial lipopolysaccharide. *European Journal of Pharmacology*, Vol. 275, pp. R1-R3.

Heimberg, H.; Heremans, Y.; Jobin, C.; Leemans, R.; Cardozo, A.K; Darville, M. & Eizirik, D.L. (2001). Inhibition of cytokine-induced NF-κB activation by adenovirus-mediated expression of a NF-κB super-repressor prevents β-cell apoptosis. *Diabetes*, Vol. 50, pp. 2219-2224

Henderson, B. (2010). Integrating the cell stress response: a new view of molecular chaperones as immunological and physiological homeostatic regulators. *Cell Biochemistry and Function*, Vol. 28, N° 1, 1–14

Hernando, R. & Manso, R. (1997). Muscle fibre stress in response to exercise: synthesis, accumulation and isoform transitions of 70-kDa heat-shock proteins. *European Journal of Biochemistry*, Vol. 243, N° 1–2, pp. 460–467

Hirabara, S.M.; Silveira, L.R.; Alberici, L.C.; Leandro, C.V.; Lambertucci, R.H.; Polimeno, G.C.; Cury Boaventura, M.F.; Procopio, J.; Vercesi, A.E. & Curi, R. (2006). Acute effect of fatty acids on metabolism and mitochondrial coupling in skeletal muscle. *Biochimica et Biophysica Acta*, Vol. 1757, pp. 57-66

Homem de Bittencourt, P.I., Jr. & Curi, R. (2001). Antiproliferative prostaglandins and the MRP/GS-X pump role in cancer immunosuppression and insight into new strategies in cancer gene therapy. *Biochemical Pharmacology*, Vol. 62, N° 7, pp. 811-819.

Homem de Bittencourt, P.I., Jr.; Lagranha, D.J.; Maslinkiewicz, A.; Senna, S.M.; Tavares, A.M.; Baldissera, L.P.; Janner, D.R.; Peralta, J.S.; Bock, P.M.; Gutierrez, L.L.; Scola, G.; Heck, T.G.; Krause, M.S.; Cruz, L.A.; Abdalla, D.S.; Lagranha, C.J.; Lima, T. & Curi, R. (2007). LipoCardium: endothelium-directed cyclopentenone prostaglandin-based liposome formulation that completely reverses atherosclerotic lesions. *Atherosclerosis*, Vol. 193, pp. 245-258

Hooper, P.L. & Hooper, J.J. (2005). Loss of defense against stress: diabetes and heat shock proteins. *Diabetes Technology and Therapeutics*, Vol. 7, N° 1, pp. 204-208

Hunt, C. & Morimoto, R.I. (1985). Conserved features of eukaryotic hsp70 genes revealed by comparison with the nucleotide sequence of human hsp70. *Proceedings of the National Academy of Sciences of the U.S.A.*, Vol. 82, N° 19, pp. 6455-6459

Ianaro, A.; Ialenti, A.; Maffia, P.; Di Meglio, P.; Di Rosa, M. & Santoro, M.G. (2003). Anti-inflammatory activity of 15-deoxy-$\Delta^{12,14}$-PGJ$_2$ and 2-cyclopenten-1-one: role of the heat shock response. *Molecular Pharmacology*, Vol. 64, pp. 85-93

Jang, H.J.; Kwak, J.H.; Cho, E.Y; We, Y.; Lee, Y.H.; Kim, S.C. & Han, D.J. (2008). Glutamine induces heat-shock protein-70 and glutathione expression and attenuates ischemic damage in rat islets. *Transplantation Proceedings*, Vol. 40, N°8, pp. 2581-2584

Jessop, D.S.; Douthwaite, J.A.; Conde, G.L.; Lightman, S.L.; Dayan, C.M. & Harbuz, M.S. (1997). Effects of Acute Stress or Centrally Injected Interleukin-1β on Neuropeptide Expression in the Immune System. *Stress*, Vol. 2, pp. 133-144

Kampinga, H.H.; Hageman, J.; Vos, M.J.; Kubota, H.; Tanguay,R.M.; Bruford, E.A.; Cheetham, M.E.; Chen, B. & Hightower, L.E. (2009). Guidelines for the nomenclature of the human heat shock proteins. *Cell Stress and Chaperones*, Vol. 14, N° 1, pp. 105-111.

Karlsen, A.E.; Heding, P.E.; Frobose, H.; Ronn, S.G.; Kruhoffer, M.; Orntoft, T.F.; Darville, M.; Eizirik, D.L.; Pociot, F.; Nerup, J.; Mandrup-Poulsen, T. & Billestrup, N. (2004). Suppressor of cytokine signalling (SOCS)-3 protects β cells against IL-1β-mediated toxicity through inhibition of multiple nuclear factor-κB-regulated pro-apoptotic pathways. *Diabetologia*, Vol. 47, pp. 1998-2011

Karlsen, A.E.; Ronn, S.G.; Lindberg, K.; Johannesen, J.; Galsgaard, E.D.; Pociot, F.; Nielsen, J.H.; Mandrup-Poulsen, T.; Nerup, J. & Billestrup, N. (2001). Suppressor of cytokine signaling 3 (SOCS-3) protects β-cells against interleukin-1β- and interferon-γ-mediated toxicity. *Proceedings of the National Academy of Sciences of the U.S.A.* Vol. 98, pp. 12191-12196

Kayani, A.C.; Close, G.L.; Broome, C.S.; Jackson, M.J. & McArdle, A. (2008). Enhanced recovery from contraction-induced damage in skeletal muscles of old mice following treatment with the heat shock protein inducer 17-(allylamino)-17-demethoxygeldanamycin. *Rejuvenation Research*, Vol. 11, N° 6, pp. 1021–1030

Kelly, D.A.; Tiidus, P.M.; Houston, M.E. & Noble, E.G. (1996). Effect of vitamin E deprivation and exercise training on induction of HSP70. *Journal of Applied Physiology*, Vol. 81, N° 6, pp. 2379–2385

Kim, Y.M.; de Vera, M.E.; Watkins, S.C. & Billiar, T.R. (1997). Nitric oxide protects cultured rat hepatocytes from tumor necrosis factor-α-induced apoptosis by inducing heat shock protein 70 expression. *Journal of Biological Chemistry*, Vol. 272, N° 2, pp. 1402–1411

Kliewer, S.A.; Lenhard, J.M.; Willson, T.M.; Patel, I.; Morris, D.C. & Lehmann JM (1995). A prostaglandin J$_2$ metabolite binds peroxisome proliferator-activated receptor γ and promotes adipocyte differentiation. *Cell*, Vol. 83, pp. 813–819

Knowles, R.G. & Moncada, S. (1994). Nitric oxide synthases in mammals. *Biochemical Journal*, Vol. 298, Pt 2, pp. 249–258

Krause, M.S. & Homem de Bittencourt, P.I., Jr. (2008). Type 1 diabetes: can exercise impair the autoimmune event? The L-arginine/glutamine coupling hypothesis. *Cell Biochemistry and Function*, Vol. 26, N° 4, pp. 406-433

Krause, M.S.; Oliveira Junior, L.P.; Silveira, E.M.; Vianna, D.R.; Rossato, J.S.; Almeida, B.S.; Rodrigues, M.F.; Fernandes, A.J.M.; Costa, J.A.B.; Curi, R. & Homem de Bittencourt, P.I., Jr. (2007). MRP1/GS-X pump ATPase expression: is this the explanation for the cytoprotection of the heart against oxidative stress-induced redox imbalance in comparison to skeletal muscle cells? *Cell Biochemistry and Function*, Vol. 25, N° 1, pp. 23-32

Kregel, K.C. & Moseley, P.L. (1996). Differential effects of exercise and heat stress on liver HSP70 accumulation with aging. *Journal of Applied Physiology*, Vol. 80, N° 2, pp. 547-551

Kutlu, B.; Cardozo, A.K.; Darville, M.I.; Kruhoffer, M.; Magnusson, N.; Orntoft, T. & Eizirik, D.L. (2003). Discovery of gene networks regulating cytokine-induced dysfunction and apoptosis in insulin-producing INS-1 cells. *Diabetes*, Vol. 52, pp. 2701-2719

Lagranha, C.J.; Levada-Pires, A.C.; Sellitti, D.F.; Procópio, J.; Curi, R. & Pithon-Curi, T.C. (2008). The effect of glutamine supplementation and physical exercise on neutrophil function. *Amino Acids*, Vol 34, N°3, pp. 337-346

Lancaster, G.I. & Febbraio, M.A. (2005). Exosome-dependent trafficking of HSP70: a novel secretory pathway for cellular stress proteins. *Journal of Biological Chemistry*, Vol. 280, N° 24, pp. 23349-23355

Lancaster, G.I.; Moller, K.; Nielsen, B.; Secher, N.H.; Febbraio, M.A. & Nybo, L. (2004). Exercise induces the release of heat shock protein 72 from the human brain in vivo. Cell Stress and Chaperones, Vol. 9, N° 3, pp. 276-280

Lenzen, S.; Drinkgern, J. & Tiedge, M. (1996). Low antioxidant enzyme gene expression in pancreatic islets compared with various other mouse tissues. *Free Radical Biology and Medicine*, Vol. 20, pp. 463-466

Li, M.; Peterson. S.; Husney, D.; Inaba, M.; Guo, K.; Kappas, A.; Ikehara, S. & Abraham, N.G. (2007). Long-lasting expression of HO-1 delays progression of type I diabetes in NOD mice. *Cell Cycle*, Vol. 6, pp. 567-571

Ligthart-Melis, G.C.; van de Poll, M.C.; Boelens, P.G.; Dejong, C.H.; Deutz, N.E. & van Leeuwen, P.A. (2008). Glutamine is an important precursor for de novo synthesis of arginine in humans. *American Journal of Clinical Nutrition*, Vol. 87, N° 5, pp. 1282-1289

Lindquist, S. & Craig, E.A. (2004). The heat-shock proteins. *Annual Review of Genetics*, Vol. 22, pp. 631-677

Locke, M.; Noble, E.G.; Tanguay, R.M.; Field, M.R.; Ianuzzo, S.E. & Ianuzzo, C.D. (1995). Activation of heat-shock transcription factor in rat heart after heat shock and exercise. *American Journal of Physiology. Cell Physiology*, Vol. 268, N° 6 Pt 1, pp. C1387–C1394

Loï, C.; Zazzo, J.F.; Delpierre, E.; Niddam, C.; Neveux, N.; Curis, E.; Arnaud-Battandier, F. & Cynober, L. (2009). Increasing plasma glutamine in postoperative patients fed an arginine-rich immune-enhancing diet - a pharmacokinetic randomized controlled study. *Critical Care Medicine*, Vol. 37, N° 2, pp. 501-509.

Lovejoy, J.; Newby, F.D.; Gebhart, S.S. & DiGirolamo, M. (1992). Insulin resistance in obesity is associated with elevated basal lactate levels and diminished lactate appearance following intravenous glucose and insulin. *Metabolism*, Vol. 41, N°1, pp. 22-27

MacDonald, M.J. (1995). Feasibility of a mitochondrial pyruvate malate shuttle in pancreatic islets. Further implication of cytosolic NADPH in insulin secretion. *Journal of Biological Chemistry*, Vol. 270, pp. 20051-20058

Malaisse, W.J.; Blachier, F.; Mourtada, A.; Camara, J.; Albor, A.; Valverde, I. & Sener, A. (1989). Stimulus-secretion coupling of arginine-induced insulin release. Metabolism of L-arginine and L-ornithine in pancreatic islets. *Biochimica et Biophysica Acta*, Vol. 1013, pp. 133-143

Malaisse, W.J.; Malaisse-Lagae, F.; Sener, A. & Pipeleers, D.G. (1982). Determinants of the selective toxicity of alloxan to the pancreatic B cell. *Proceedings of the National Academy of Sciences of the U.S.A.*, Vol. 79, pp. 927-930

Mambula, S.S.; Stevenson, M.A.; Ogawa, K. & Calderwood, S.K. (2007). Mechanisms for Hsp70 secretion: crossing membranes without a leader. *Methods*, Vol. 43, N° 3, pp. 168–175

Mandrup-Poulsen, T. (2010). IAPP boosts islet macrophage IL-1 in type 2 diabetes. *Nature Immunology*, Vol. 11, N°10, pp. 881-883

Mandrup-Poulsen, T.; Helqvist, S.; Wogensen, L.D.; Mølvig, J.; Pociot, F.; Johannesen, J. & Nerup, J. (1990). Cytokine and free radicals as effector molecules in the destruction of pancreatic β cells. *Current Topics in Microbiology and Immunology*, Vol. 164, pp. 169-193

Mathews, C.E. & Leiter, E.H. (1999). Constitutive differences in antioxidant defense status distinguish alloxan-resistant and alloxan-susceptible mice. *Free Radical Biology and Medicine*, Vol. 27, pp. 449-455

Matthews, G.D.; Gould, R.M. & Vardimon, L. (2005). A single glutamine synthetase gene produces tissue-specific subcellular localization by alternative splicing. *Federation of European Biochemical Societies Letters*. Vol. 579, pp. 5527-5534

Maxwell, S.R.; Thomason, H.; Sandler, D.; Leguen, C.; Baxter, M.A.; Thorpe, G.H. & Jones, A.F. (1997). Antioxidant status in patients with uncomplicated insulin-dependent and non-insulin-dependent diabetes mellitus. *European Journal of Clinical Investigation*, Vol. 27, N°6, pp. 484-490

McGillis, J.P.; Park, A.; Rubin-Fletter, P.; Turck, C.; Dallman, M.F. & Payan, D.G. (1989). Stimulation of rat B-lymphocyte proliferation by corticotropin-releasing factor. *Journal of Neuroscience Research*, Vol. 23, pp. 346-352

Michalska, M.; Wolf, G.; Walther, R. & Newsholme, P. (2010). Effects of pharmacologic inhibition of NADPH oxidase and iNOS on pro-inflammatory cytokine, palmitic acid or H_2O_2-induced mouse islet or clonal pancreatic beta cell dysfunction. *Bioscience Reports*, Vol. 30, pp. 445-453

Milne, K.J. & Noble, E.G. (2002). Exercise-induced elevation of HSP70 is intensity dependent. *Journal of Applied Physiology*, Vol. 93, N° 2, pp. 561–568

Modolell, M.; Corraliza, I.M.; Link, F.; Soler, G. & Eichmann, K. (1995). Reciprocal regulation of the nitric oxide synthase/arginase balance in mouse bone marrow-derived macrophages by TH1 and TH2 cytokines. *European Journal of Immunology*, Vol. 25, pp. 1101-1104

Mohan, I.K. & Das, U.N. (1998). Effect of L-arginine-nitric oxide system on chemical-induced diabetes mellitus. *Free Radical Biology and Medicine*, Vol. 25, pp. 757-765

Moinard, C.; Belabed, L.; Gupta, S.; Besson, V.; Marchand-Verrecchia, C.; Chaumeil, J.C.; Cynober, L. & Charrueau, C. (2006). Arginine-enriched diet limits plasma and muscle glutamine depletion in head-injured rats. *Nutrition*, Vol. 22, pp. 1039-1044

Moncada, S.; Palmer, R.M. & Higgs, E.A. (1991). Nitric oxide: physiology, pathophysiology, and pharmacology. *Pharmacological Reviews*, Vol. 43, pp. 109-142

Morgan, D.; Oliveira-Emilio, H.R.; Keane, D.; Hirata, A.E.; Santos da Rocha, M.; Bordin, S.; Curi, R.; Newsholme, P. & Carpinelli, A.R. (2007). Glucose, palmitate and pro-inflammatory cytokines modulate production and activity of a phagocyte-like NADPH oxidase in rat pancreatic islets and a clonal β cell line. *Diabetologia*, Vol. 50, pp. 359-369

Mori, M. & Gotoh, T. (2000). Regulation of nitric oxide production by arginine metabolic enzymes. *Biochemical and Biophysical Research Communications*, Vol. 275, pp. 715-719

Mori, M. (2007). Regulation of nitric oxide synthesis and apoptosis by arginase and arginine recycling. *Journal of Nutrition*, Vol. 137, pp. 1616S-1620S

Morris, S.M.; Kepka-Lenhart, D. & Chen, L.C. (1998). Differential regulation of arginases and inducible nitric oxide synthase in murine macrophage cells. *American Journal of Physiology. Endocrinology and Metabolism*, Vol. 275, pp. E740-E747

Morton, J.P.; Maclaren, D.P.; Cable, N.T.; Campbell, I.T.; Evans, L.; Bongers, T.; Griffiths, R.D.; Kayani, A.C.; McArdle, A. & Drust, B. (2007). Elevated core and muscle temperature to levels comparable to exercise do not increase heat shock protein content of skeletal muscle of physically active men. *Acta Physiologica* (Oxford), Vol. 190, N° 4, pp. 319–327

Moynagh, P.N. (2005). The NF-κB pathway. *Journal of Cell Science*, Vol. 118, pp. 4589-4592

Multhoff, G. (2007). Heat shock protein 70 (Hsp70): membrane location, export and immunological relevance. *Methods*, Vol. 43, N° 3, pp. 229–237

Munder, M.; Eichmann, K. & Modolell, M. (1998). Alternative metabolic states in murine macrophages reflected by the nitric oxide synthase/arginase balance: competitive regulation by CD4+ T cells correlates with Th1/Th2 phenotype. *Journal of Immunology*, Vol. 160, pp. 5347-5354

Munder, M.; Eichmann, K.; Moran, J.M.; Centeno, F.; Soler, G. & Modolell, M. (1999). Th1/Th2-regulated expression of arginase isoforms in murine macrophages and dendritic cells. *Journal of Immunology*, Vol. 163, pp. 3771-3777

Murlasits, Z.; Cutlip, R.G.; Geronilla, K.B.; Rao, K.M.; Wonderlin, W.F. & Always, S.E. (2006). Resistance training increases heat shock protein levels in skeletal muscle of young and old rats. *Experimental Gerontology*, Vol. 41, N° 4, pp. 398–406

Murphy, C. & Newsholme, P. (1998). Importance of glutamine metabolism in murine macrophages and human monocytes to L-arginine biosynthesis and rates of nitrite or urea production. *Clinical Science* (London), Vol. 95, pp. 397-407

Murphy, C. & Newsholme, P. (1998). Importance of glutamine metabolism in murine macrophages and human monocytes to L-arginine biosynthesis and rates of nitrite or urea production. *Clinical Science (London)*, Vol. 95, pp. 397-407

Nagasaki, A.; Gotoh, T.; Takeya, M.; Yu, Y.; Takiguchi, M.; Matsuzaki, H.; Takatsuki, K. & Mori, M. (1996). Coinduction of nitric oxide synthase, argininosuccinate synthetase, and argininosuccinate lyase in lipopolysaccharide-treated rats. RNA blot, immunoblot, and immunohistochemical analyses. *Journal of Biological Chemistry*, Vol. 271, pp. 2658-2662

Nakamura, H.; Nakamura, K. & Yodoi, J. (1997). Redox regulation of cellular activation. *Annual Review of Immunology*, Vol. 15, pp. 351-369

Newsholme P.; Homem de Bittencourt, P.I., Jr.; O' Hagan, C.; DeVito, G.; Murphy, C. & Krause, M.S. (2009a). Exercise and possible molecular mechanisms of protection from vascular disease and diabetes: the central role of ROS and nitric oxide. *Clinical Science* (London), Vol. 118, pp. 341–349

Newsholme P., Morgan D., Rebelato, E., Oliveira-Emilio H.C., Procopio J., Curi R. and Carpinelli A. (2009b) Insights into the critical role of NADPH oxidase(s) in the normal and dysregulated pancreatic beta cell. *Diabetologia*, Vol.52, pp. 2489-2498

Newsholme, P.; Gordon, S. & Newsholme, E.A. (1987). Rates of utilization and fates of glucose, glutamine, pyruvate, fatty acids and ketone bodies by mouse macrophages. *Biochemical Journal*, Vol. 242, pp. 631-636

Newsholme, P.; Haber, E.; Hirabara, S.; Rebelato, E.; Propcopio, J.; Morgan, D.; Oliveira-Emilio, H.; Carpinelli, A & Curi, R. (2007). Diabetes associated cell stress and dysfunction - Role of mitochondrial and non-mitochondrial ROS production and activity. *Journal of Physiology*, Vol. 583, pp. 9-24

Newsholme, P.; Lima, M.M.; Procopio, J.; Pithon-Curi, T.C.; Doi, S.Q.; Bazotte, R.B. & Curi, R. (2003). Glutamine and glutamate as vital metabolites. *Brazilian Journal of Medical and Biological Research*, Vol. 36, pp. 153-163

Newsholme, P.; Procópio, J.; Lima, M.M.; Pithon-Curi, T.C. & Curi R. (2003). Glutamine and glutamate - their central role in cell metabolism and function. *Cell Biochemisry and Function*, Vol. 21, pp. 1-9

Nieman, D.C. & Pedersen, B.K. (1999). Exercise and immune function. Recent developments. *Sports Medicine*, Vol. 27, pp. 73-80

Noble, E.G.; Milne, K.J. & Melling, C.W. (2008). Heat shock proteins and exercise: a primer. *Applied Physiology, Nutrition and Metabolism*, Vol. 33, N° 5, pp. 1050–1065

Nomikos, I.N.; Prowse, S.J.; Carotenuto, P. & Lafferty, K.J. (1986). Combined treatment with nicotinamide and desferrioxamine prevents islet allograft destruction in NOD mice. *Diabetes*, Vol. 35, pp. 1302-1304

Nussler, A.K.; Billiar, T.R.; Liu, Z.Z. & Morris, S.M., Jr. (1994). Coinduction of nitric oxide synthase and argininosuccinate synthetase in a murine macrophage cell line. Implications for regulation of nitric oxide production. *Journal of Biological Chemistry*, Vol. 269, pp. 1257-1261

Ogawa, F.; Shimizu, K.; Hara, T. ; Muroi, E.; Hasegawa, M.; Takehara, K. & Sato, S. (2008). Serum levels of heat shock protein 70, a biomarker of cellular stress, are elevated in patients with systemic sclerosis: association with fibrosis and vascular damage. *Clinical and Experimental Rheumatology*, Vol. 26, N° 4, pp. 659–662

Oliveira, H.R.; Verlengia, R.; Carvalho, C.R.; Britto, L.R.; Curi, R. & Carpinelli, A.R. (2003). Pancreatic β-cells express phagocyte-like NAD(P)H oxidase. *Diabetes*, Vol. 52, pp. 1457-1463

Palmer, J.P.; Benson, J.W.; Walter, R.M. & Ensinck, J.W. (1976). Arginine-stimulated acute phase of insulin and glucagon secretion in diabetic subjects. *Journal of Clinical Investigation*, Vol. 58, pp. 565-570

Paroo, Z. & Noble, E.G. (1999). Isoproterenol potentiates exercise-induction of Hsp70 in cardiac and skeletal muscle. *Cell Stress and Chaperones*, Vol. 4, N° 3, pp. 199-204

Paroo, Z.; Dipchand, E.S. & Noble, E.G. (2002b). Estrogen attenuates postexercise HSP70 expression in skeletal muscle. *American Journal of Physiology. Cell Physiology*, Vol. 282, N° 2, pp. C245-C251

Paroo, Z.; Haist, J.V.; Karmazyn, M. & Noble, E.G. (2002a). Exercise improves postischemic cardiac function in males but not females: consequences of a novel sex-specific heat shock protein 70 response. *Circulation Research*, Vol. 90, N° 8, pp. 911-917

Paroo, Z.; Tiidus, P.M. & Noble, E.G. (1999). Estrogen attenuates HSP 72 expression in acutely exercised male rodents. *European Journal of Applied Physiology and Occupational Physiology*, Vol. 80, N° 3, pp. 180-184

Parry-Billings, M.; Leighton, B.; Dimitriadis, G.D.; Bond, J. & Newsholme, E.A. (1990). Effects of physiological and pathological levels of glucocorticoids on skeletal muscle glutamine metabolism in the rat. *Biochemical Pharmacology*, Vol. 40, pp. 1145-1148

Pedersen, B.K. & Hoffman-Goetz, L. (2000). Exercise and the immune system: regulation, integration, and adaptation. *Physiological Reviews*, Vol. 80, pp. 1055-1081

Pedersen, B.K. & Steensberg, A. (2002). Exercise and hypoxia: effects on leukocytes and interleukin-6-shared mechanisms? *Medicine Science in Sports and Exercise*, Vol. 34, pp. 2004-2013

Pedersen, B.K.; Ostrowski. K.; Rohde, T. & Bruunsgaard, H. (1998). The cytokine response to strenuous exercise. *Canadian Journal of Physiology and Pharmacology*, Vol. 76, N° 5, pp. 505-511

Pedersen, B.K.; Steensberg, A. & Schjerling, P. (2001). Muscle-derived interleukin-6: possible biological effects. *Journal of Physiology*, Vol. 536, pp. 329-337

Piatti, P.M.; Monti, L.D.; Valsecchi, G.; Magni, F.; Setola, E.; Marchesi, F.; Galli-Kienle, M.; Pozza, G. & Alberti, K.G. (2001). Long-term oral L-arginine administration improves peripheral and hepatic insulin sensitivity in type 2 diabetic patients. *Diabetes Care*, Vol. 24, pp. 875-880

Pieper, G.M. & Dondlinger, L.A. (1997). Plasma and vascular tissue arginine are decreased in diabetes: acute arginine supplementation restores endothelium-dependent relaxation by augmenting cGMP production. *Journal of Pharmacology and Experimental Therapeutics*, Vol. 283, pp. 684-691

Pithon-Curi, T.C.; De Melo, M.P. & Curi, R. (2004). Glucose and glutamine utilization by rat lymphocytes, monocytes and neutrophils in culture: a comparative study. *Cell Biochemistry and Function*, Vol. 22, pp. 321-326

Piva, R.; Gianferretti, P.; Ciucci, A.; Taulli, R.; Belardo, G. & Santoro, M.G. (2005). 15-Deoxy-$\Delta^{12,14}$-prostaglandin J_2 induces apoptosis in human malignant B cells: an effect associated with inhibition of NF-κB activity and down-regulation of antiapoptotic proteins. *Blood*, Vol. 105, pp. 1750-1758

Rabinovitch, A. & Suarez-Pinzon, W.L. (1998). Cytokines and their roles in pancreatic islet β-cell destruction and insulin-dependent diabetes mellitus. *Biochemical Pharmacology*, Vol. 55, pp. 1139-1149

Rabinovitch, A.; Suarez, W.L.; Thomas, P.D.; Strynadka, K. & Simpson, I. (1992). Cytotoxic effects of cytokines on rat islets: evidence for involvement of free radicals and lipid peroxidation. *Diabetologia*, Vol. 35, pp. 409-413

Rabinovitch, A.; Suarez-Pinzon, W.L; Strynadka, K.; Lakey, J.R. & Rajotte, R.V. (1996). Human pancreatic islet β-cell destruction by cytokines involves oxygen free radicals and aldehyde production. *Journal of Clinical Endocrinology and Metabolism*, Vol. 81, pp. 3197-3202

Ran, R.; Lu, A.; Zhang, L.; Tang, Y.; Zhu, H.; Xu, H.; Feng, Y.; Han, C.; Zhou, G.; Rigby, A.C. & Sharp, F.R. (2004). Hsp70 promotes TNF-mediated apoptosis by binding IKK gamma and impairing NF-kappa B survival signaling. *Genes and Development*, Vol. 18, $N°$ 12, pp. 1466-1481

Rieneck, K.; Bovin, L.F.; Josefsen, K.; Buschard, K.; Svenson, M. & Bendtzen, K. (2000). Massive parallel gene expression profiling of RINm5F pancreatic islet β-cells stimulated with interleukin-1β. *Acta Pathological, Microbiologica, et Immunologica Scandinavica*, Vol. 108, pp. 855-872

Rocič, B.; Vucič, M.; Knezevič-Cuča, J.; Radica, A.; Pavlič-Renar, I.; Profozič, V. & Metelko, Z. (1997). Total plasma antioxidants in first-degree relatives of patients with insulin-dependent diabetes. *Experimental and Clinical Endocrinology and Diabetes*, Vol. 105, $N°$ 4, pp. 213-217

Rohde, T.; MacLean, D.A.; Richter, E.A.; Kiens, B. & Pedersen, B.K. (1997). Prolonged submaximal eccentric exercise is associated with increased levels of plasma IL-6. *American Journal of Physiology. Endocrinology and Metabolism*, Vol. 273, pp. E85-E91

Rossi, A.; Kapahi, P.; Natoli, G.; Takahashi, T.; Chen, Y.; Karin, M. & Santoro, M.G. (2000). Anti-inflammatory cyclopentenone prostaglandins are direct inhibitors of IκB kinase. *Nature*, Vol. 403, $N°$ 6765, pp. 103-108

Rothe, H.; Hausmann, A. & Kolb, H. (2002). Immunoregulation during disease progression in prediabetic NOD mice: inverse expression of arginase and prostaglandin H synthase 2 *vs.* interleukin-15. *Hormone and Metabolic Research*, Vol. 34, pp. 7-12

Rutschman, R.; Lang, R.; Hesse, M.; Ihle, J.N.; Wynn, T.A. & Murray, P.J. (2001). Cutting edge: Stat6-dependent substrate depletion regulates nitric oxide production. *Journal of Immunology*, Vol. 166, pp. 2173-2177

Salo, D.C.; Donovan, C.M. & Davies, K.J. (1991). HSP70 and other possible heat shock or oxidative stress proteins are induced in skeletal muscle, heart, and liver during exercise. *Free Radical Biology and Medicine*, Vol. 11, $N°$ 3, pp. 239-246

Santini, S.A.; Marra, G.; Giardina, B.; Cotroneo, P.; Mordente, A.; Martorana, G.E.; Manto, A. & Ghirlanda, G. (1997). Defective plasma antioxidant defenses and enhanced susceptibility to lipid peroxidation in uncomplicated IDDM. *Diabetes*, Vol. 46, pp. 1853-1858

Scarim, A.L.; Heitmeier, M.R. & Corbett, J.A. (1998). Heat shock inhibits cytokine-induced nitric oxide synthase expression by rat and human islets. *Endocrinology*, Vol. 139, $N°$ 12, pp. 5050-5057

Silveira, E.M.; Rodrigues, M.F.; Krause, M.S.; Vianna, D.R.; Almeida, B.S.; Rossato, J.S.; Oliveira Junior, L.P.; Curi, R. & Homem de Bittencourt, P.I., Jr. (2007) Acute exercise stimulates macrophage function: possible role of NF-κB pathways. *Cell Biochemistry and Function*, Vol. 25, N° 1, pp. 63–73

Simar, D.; Malatesta, D.; Badiou, S.; Dupuy, A.M. & Caillaud, C. (2007). Physical activity modulates heat shock protein-72 expression and limits oxidative damage accumulation in a healthy elderly population aged 60-90 years. *Journals of Gerontology. Series A, Biological Sciences and Medical Sciences*, Vol. 62, N° 12, pp. 1413–1419

Simmons, W.W.; Closs, E.I.; Cunningham, J.M.; Smith, T.W. & Kelly, R.A. (1996). Cytokines and insulin induce cationic amino acid transporter (CAT) expression in cardiac myocytes. Regulation of L-arginine transport and no production by CAT-1, CAT-2A, and CAT-2B. *Journal of Biological Chemistry*, Vol. 271, pp. 11694-11702

Simopoulos, A.P. (2006). Evolutionary aspects of diet, the ω-6/ω-3 ratio and genetic variation: nutritional implications for chronic diseases. *Biomedicine and Pharmacotherapy*, Vol. 60, pp. 502-507

Singh, V.K. & Leu, S.J. (1990). Enhancing effect of corticotropin-releasing neurohormone on the production of interleukin-1 and interleukin-2. *Neuroscience Letters*, Vol. 120, pp. 151-154

Singleton, K.D. & Wischmeyer, P.E. (2008). Glutamine induces heat shock protein expression via O-glycosylation and phosphorylation of HSF-1 and Sp1. Journal of Parenteral and Enteral Nutrition, Vol. 32, N° 4, pp. 371-376

Sipetic, S.; Vlajinac, H.; Marinkovi, J.; Kocev, N.; Milan, B.; Ratkov, I. & Sajic, S. (2007). Stressful life events and psychological dysfunctions before the onset of type 1 diabetes mellitus. *Journal of Pediatric Endocrinology and Metabolism*, Vol. 20, pp. 527-534

Skidmore, R.; Gutierrez, J.A.; Guerriero, V., Jr. & Kregel, K.C. (1995). HSP70 induction during exercise and heat stress in rats: role of internal temperature. *American Journal of Physiology. Regulatory, Integrative and Comparative Physiology*, Vol. 268, N° 1 Pt 2, pp. R92–R97

Smolka, M.B.; Zoppi, C.C.; Alves, A.A.; Silveira, L.R.; Marangoni, S.; Pereira-Da-Silva, L.;Novello, J.C. & Macedo, D.V. (2000). HSP72 as a complementary protection against oxidative stress induced by exercise in the soleus muscle of rats. *American Journal of Physiology. Regulatory, Integrative and Comparative Physiology*, Vol. 279, N° 5, pp. R1539–R1545

Smukler, S.R.; Tang, L.; Wheeler, M.B. & Salapatek, A.M. (2002). Exogenous nitric oxide and endogenous glucose-stimulated β-cell nitric oxide augment insulin release. *Diabetes*, Vol. 51, pp. 3450-3460

Soltesz, G. (2003). Diabetes in the young: a paediatric and epidemiological perspective. *Diabetologia*, Vol. 46, pp. 447-454

Spinas, G.A. (1999). The Dual Role of Nitric Oxide in Islet β-Cells. *News in Physiological Sciences*, Vol. 14, pp. 49-54

Staib, J.L.; Quindry, J.C.; French, J.P.; Criswell, D.S. & Powers, S.K. (2007). Increased temperature, not cardiac load, activates heat shock transcription factor 1 and heat shock protein 72 expression in the heart. *American Journal of Physiology. Regulatory, Integrative and Comparative Physiology*, Vol. 292, N° 1, pp. R432–R439

Stickings, P.; Mistry, S.K.; Boucher, J.L.; Morris, S.M. & Cunningham, J.M. (2002). Arginase expression and modulation of IL-1β-induced nitric oxide generation in rat and human islets of Langerhans. *Nitric Oxide*, Vol. 7, pp. 289-296

Suarez-Pinzon, W.L.; Strynadka, K. & Rabinovitch, A. (1996). Destruction of rat pancreatic islet β-cells by cytokines involves the production of cytotoxic aldehydes. *Endocrinology*, Vol. 137, pp. 5290-5296

Sumoski, W.; Baquerizo, H. & Rabinovitch, A. (1989). Oxygen free radical scavengers protect rat islet cells from damage by cytokines. *Diabetologia*, Vol. 32, pp. 792-796

Sun, Y. & MacRae, T.H. (2005). The small heat shock proteins and their role in human disease. *Federation of European Biochemical Societies Letters*, Vol. 272, N° 11, pp. 2613-2627.

Suzuki, K.; Yamada, M.; Kurakake, S.; Okamura, N.; Yamaya, K.; Liu, Q.; Kudoh, S.; Kowatari, K.; Nakaji, S. & Sugawara, K. (2000). Circulating cytokines and hormones with immunosuppressive but neutrophil-priming potentials rise after endurance exercise in humans. *European Journal of Applied Physiology*, Vol. 81, pp. 281-287

Tavaria, M.; Gabriele, T.; Anderson, R.L.; Mirault, M.E.; Baker, E.; Sutherland, G. & Kola, I. (1995). Localization of the gene encoding the human heat shock cognate protein, HSP73, to chromosome 11. *Genomics*, Vol. 29, N° 1, pp. 266–268

Tavaria, M.; Gabriele, T.; Kola. I & Anderson, R.L. (1996). A hitchhiker's guide to the human Hsp70 family. *Cell Stress and Chaperones*, Vol. 1, N° 1, pp. 23–28

Tenu, J.P.; Lepoivre, M.; Moali, C.; Brollo, M.; Mansuy, D. & Boucher, J.L. (1999). Effects of the new arginase inhibitor N$^{\omega}$-hydroxy-nor-L-arginine on NO synthase activity in murine macrophages. *Nitric Oxide*, Vol. 3, pp. 427-438

Tupling, A.R.; Bombardier, E.; Stewart, R.D.; Vigna, C. & Aqui, A.E. (2007). Muscle fiber type-specific response of Hsp70 expression in human quadriceps following acute isometric exercise. *Journal of Applied Physiology*, Vol. 103, N° 6, pp. 2105-2111

Vabulas, R.M.; Ahmad-Nejad, P.; Ghose, S.; Kirschning, C.J.; Issels, R.D & Wagner. H. (2002). HSP70 as endogenous stimulus of the Toll/interleukin-1 receptor signal pathway. *Journal of Biological Chemistry*, Vol. 277, N° 17, pp. 15107–15112

Van de Poll, M.C.; Ligthart-Melis, G.C.; Boelens, P.G.; Deutz, N.E.; van Leeuwen, P.A. & Dejong, C.H. (2007). Intestinal and hepatic metabolism of glutamine and citrulline in humans. *Journal of Physiology*, Vol. 581(Pt 2), pp. 819-827

Vasilijević, A.; Buzadzič, B.; Korač, A.; Petrovič, V.; Jankovič, A.; Micunovič, K. & Korač, B. (2007). The effects of cold acclimation and nitric oxide on antioxidative enzymes in rat pancreas. *Comparative Biochemistry and Physiology. C: Toxicology and Pharmacology*, Vol. 145, pp. 641-647

Velmurugan, K.; Alam, J.; McCord, J.M. & Pugazhenthi, S. (2009). Synergistic induction of heme oxygenase-1 by the components of the antioxidant supplement Protandim. *Free Radical Biology and Medicine*, Vol. 46, pp. 430-440

Vermeulen, M.A.; van de Poll, M.C.; Ligthart-Melis, G.C.; Dejong, C.H.; van den Tol, M.P.; Boelens, P.G. & van Leeuwen, P.A. (2007). Specific amino acids in the critically ill patient--exogenous glutamine/arginine: a common denominator? *Critical Care Medicine*, Vol. 35, pp. S568-S576

Wachlin, G.; Heine, L.; Klöting, I.; Dunger, A.; Hahn, H.J. & Schmidt, S. (2002). Stress response of pancreatic islets from diabetes prone BB rats of different age. *Autoimmunity*, Vol. 35, N° 6, pp. 389-395

Waddington, S.N.; Mosley, K.; Cook, H.T.; Tam, F.W. & Cattell, V. (1998). Arginase AI is upregulated in acute immune complex-induced inflammation. *Biochemical and Biophyssical Research Communications*, Vol. 247, pp. 84-87

Wadt, K.A.; Larsen, C.M.; Andersen, H.U.; Nielsen, K.; Karlsen, A.E. & Mandrup-Poulsen, T. (1998). Ciliary neurotrophic factor potentiates the β-cell inhibitory effect of IL-1β in rat pancreatic islets associated with increased nitric oxide synthesis and increased expression of inducible nitric oxide synthase. *Diabetes*, Vol. 47, pp. 1602-1608

Walsh, R.C.; Koukoulas, I.; Garnham, A.; Moseley, P.L.; Hargreaves, M. & Febbraio, M.A. (2001). Exercise increases serum Hsp72 in humans. *Cell Stress and Chaperones*, Vol. 6, pp. 386-393

Wei, L.H.; Jacobs, A.T.; Morris, S.M., Jr. & Ignarro, L.J. (2000). IL-4 and IL-13 upregulate arginase I expression by cAMP and JAK/STAT6 pathways in vascular smooth muscle cells. *American Journal of Physiology. Cell Physiology*. Vol. 279, pp. C248-C256

Wierusz-Wysocka, B.; Wysocki, H.; Byks, H.; Zozulińska, D.; Wykretowicz, A. & Kaźmierczak, M. (1997). Metabolic control quality and free radical activity in diabetic patients. *Diabetes Research and Clinical Practice*, Vol. 27, pp. 193-197

Wilmore, D. (2004). Enteral and parenteral arginine supplementation to improve medical outcomes in hospitalized patients. *Journal of Nutrition*, Vol. 134, pp. 2863S-2867S (see discussion in 2895S)

Winyard, P.G. & Blake, D.R. (1997). Antioxidants, redox-regulated transcription factors, and inflammation. *Advances in Pharmacology*, Vol. 38, pp. 403-421

Wischmeyer, P.E.; Kahana, M.; Wolfson, R.; Ren, H.; Musch, M.M. & Chang, E.B. (2001). Glutamine reduces cytokine release, organ damage, and mortality in a rat model of endotoxemia. *Shock*, Vol. 16, pp. 398-402

Wischmeyer, P.E.; Riehm, J.; Singleton, K.D.; Ren, H.; Musch, M.W.; Kahana, M. & Chang, E.B. (2003). Glutamine attenuates tumor necrosis factor-alpha release and enhances heat shock protein 72 in human peripheral blood mononuclear cells. *Nutrition*, Vol. 19, N° 1, pp. 1-6

Wisloff, U.; Najjar, S.M.; Ellingsen, O.; Haram, P.M.; Swoap, S.; Al-Share, Q.; Fernstrom, M.; Rezaei, K.; Lee, S.J.; Koch, L.G. & Britton, S.L. (2005). Cardiovascular risk factors emerge after artificial selection for low aerobic capacity. *Science*, Vol. 307, pp. 418-420

Wu, G. & Morris, S.M. (1998). Arginine metabolism: nitric oxide and beyond. *Biochemical Journal*, Vol. 336, Pt 1, pp. 1-17

Wu, G.; Bazer, F.W.; Davis, T.A.; Kim, S.W.; Li, P.; Marc Rhoads, J.; Carey Satterfield, M.; Smith, S.B.; Spencer, T.E. & Yin, Y. (2009). Arginine metabolism and nutrition in growth, health and disease. *Amino Acids*, vol 37, pp. 153-168

Wu, G.; Knabe, D.A. & Kim, S.W. (2004). Arginine nutrition in neonatal pigs. *Journal of Nutrition*, Vol. 134, pp. 2783S-2790S (see discussion in 2796S-2797S)

Yabunaka, N.; Ohtsuka, Y.; Watanabe, I.; Noro, H.; Fujisawa, H. & Agishi, Y. (1995). Elevated levels of heat-shock protein 70 (HSP70) in the mononuclear cells of patients with non-insulin-dependent diabetes mellitus. *Diabetes Research and Clinical Practice*, Vol. 30, N° 2, pp. 143-147

Zhang, Y.; Zou, Z.; Li, Y.K.; Yuan, H.B. & Shi, X.Y. (2009). Glutamine-induced heat shock protein protects against renal ischaemia-reperfusion injury in rats. *Nephrology* (Carlton), Vol. 14, N° 6, pp. 573-580

Ziegler, T.R.; Ogden, L.G.; Singleton, K.D.; Luo, M.; Fernandez-Estivariz, C.; Griffith, D.P.; Galloway, J.R. & Wischmeyer, P.E. (2005). Parenteral glutamine increases serum heat shock protein 70 in critically ill patients. *Intensive Care Medicine*, Vol. 31, N° 8, pp. 1079–1086

Zingarelli, B.& Cook, J.A. (2005). Peroxisome proliferator-activated receptor-gamma is a new therapeutic target in sepsis and inflammation. *Shock*, Vol. 23, N° 5, pp. 393-399

2

Altering Trends in the Epidemiology of Type 1 Diabetes Mellitus in Children and Adolescents

Elisavet Efstathiou and Nicos Skordis
Paediatric Endocrine Unit, Department of Paediatrics,
Makarios Hospital, Nicosia
Cyprus

1. Introduction

Diabetes mellitus is a group of metabolic diseases characterised by chronic hyperglycemia resulting from defects in insulin secretion and/or insulin action, or both [1]. The history of diabetes dates back to 1550 BC as the polyuric states were described in an Egyptian papyrus, where treatment was given with a four day decoction of bones, wheat, grain, grit and earth. The term diabetes was coined by Aretaeus of Cappadocia in the 2nd century AD for conditions causing increased urine output. The sweet taste of diabetic urine was noted in the 5th century AD by Indian physicians and in 1776, Matthew Dobson confirmed that diabetic serum and urine contained sugar. The revolution in the history of Diabetes was the discovery of insulin by Banting, Best and colleagues in 1922 (http://wwunix.oit.umass.edu/~abhu000/diabetes/index.html).

Type 1 diabetes mellitus (T1DM) is one of the most common endocrine metabolic disorders in children and adolescence worldwide with serious acute and chronic complications. It has been proven that T1DM represents the ending result of an autoimmune destruction of the pancreatic islet beta cells in genetically susceptible individuals exposed to certain but still unclear environmental factors. The precise cause of T1DM is not known. However, multiple genetic and environmental risk factors seem to play an important role in the genesis of the disease. The genetic background is complex and difficult to be explained by the involvement of HLA gene region alone. On the other hand viral and nutritional factors changing continuously from country to country, may contribute to the etiology of T1DM. There is no doubt that monitoring temporal trends and incidence of T1DM contribute to the international effort to determine the exact pathogenesis of the disease and it is of critical public health importance. All these temporal trends in the incidence of T1DM have provided significant clues for understanding the disease, most likely reflecting environmental changes more than genetic changes and detecting the factors that implicated in this increase.

In this chapter we review the changing trends in the epidemiology of T1DM and we present data on the rising incidence of T1DM in Greek Cypriot population.

2. Incidence-changing trends

The prevalence of T1DM greatly varies between different countries, within countries, and between different ethnic populations. The global variation of the incidence of T1DM is evaluated by grouping the populations with very low (<1/100.000 per yr), low (1-4/100.000 per yr), intermediate (5-9.99/100.000 per yr), high (10-19.99/100.000 per yr) and very high (>20/100.000 per yr) incidence [2]. The different annual incidence rates of T1DM comparing different countries of the world (0.1 to 57.6 per 100000) are displayed in figure 1 [1]. The highest incidence is observed in the Scandinavian countries, where Finland has the highest one reported while there is a gradual decrease in countries located closer to equator [3]. However in some areas such as Puerto Rico, Kuwait and Sardinia there is an unexplained highly increased incidence [4]. The lowest incidence in the world is observed in China, where an enormous geographic variation in the development risk is observed [5]. A long time ago, during the 5th century BC, Hippocrates described diabetes as a 'rare condition' while later on Arataeus the Cappadocian described it as 'not being frequent among men' (http://wwunix.oit.umass.edu/~abhu000/diabetes/index.html). Nowadays the incidence of T1DM increases dramatically throughout the world and it is estimated that it may reach the status of an epidemic in the 21st century [6].

A number of 37 studies from 27 countries confirmed the increased incidence for the period 1960-96 in T1DM with an upward tendency in another 12 countries. The global average annual increase was 3.0% per year with a more pronounced relative increase in the populations with lower incidence [7]. If these trends continue, the number of new cases T1DM in children younger than five years of age may double in some regions between 2005 and 2020 and prevalent cases in children under 15 years will rise by 70 % [8].

The need for rigorous epidemiological studies to monitor the trends of T1DM in children less than 15 year of age led to the creation of the World Health Organization (WHO) - sponsored Diabetes Mondiale (DIAMOND) [2] Project and the EURODIAB study [9].

The data from the WHO project for the incidence of T1DM worldwide DIAMOND showed a large geographic variability. This study group was based on 43,013 cases of T1DM from a study population of 84 million children aged 14 year old or less during the period 1990-1999 in 114 populations from 57 countries. During this time the average annual increase in incidence was 2.8% (95% CI 2.4%–3.2%) with a slightly higher rate during 1995 to 1999, 3.4% (95% CI 2.7%–4.3%) than during 1990 to 1994, 2.4% (95% CI 1.3%–3.4%). An increase in the incidence of T1DM was observed in the populations studied (4.0% in Asia, 3.2% in Europe, and 5.3% in North America) with the exception of Central America and the West Indies, where T1D is less prevalent, and where the trend was a decrease of 3.6% [10].

It is of interest that several reports have shown an increase in the incidence of T1DM worldwide. This tendency implicates an increasing influence of environmental trigger factors against a background of genetic susceptibility. The geographic and ethnic variations mirror the prevalence of susceptibility genes or that of contributing environmental factors, or both. Nevertheless this increasing incidence rate in such a short period cannot be solely attributed to genetic shifts.

The EURODIAB ACE study group examined the trends in the incidence of T1DM from 1989 to 1994. The study was based on 16,362 cases of T1D in 44 European centres and Israel covering a population of 28 million children [9]. There were enormous variations in the annual incidence rate with 3.2/100,000 person-years in the Former Yugoslav Republic of Macedonia to 40.2/100,000 person-years in two regions of Finland. During this time the annual increase in the incidence rate of T1D was 3.4% (95% CI 2.5%–4.4%) although the rate of increase was noted to be higher in some central European countries. The rates of increase were found to be the highest in the youngest age group: ages 0 to 4 years (6.3%, 95% CI 1.5%–8.5%), 5 to 9 years (3.1%, 95% CI 1.5%–4.8%), and 10 to 14 years (2.4%, 95% CI 1.0%–3.8%).

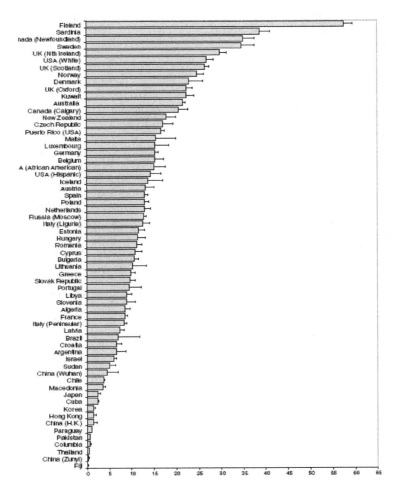

Fig. 1. Mean Annual Incidence rates for T1DM comparing different countries in the world as seen in reference 1.

Furthermore one of the most notable and recent, in the United States, includes a population-based study of incidence rates of T1DM from 10 study locations by The SEARCH for Diabetes in Youth Study. The Search Group found an overall incidence of T1DM in children 0–19 of 24.3 per 100,000 person years with the highest rates observed among the 5–9 and 10–14 age groups with rates of 22.9 and 33.9 per 100,000 respectively [11].

A recent study from Saudi Arabia over an 18 year period, has shown an average incidence of 27.52/100000/year increasing from 18.05/100000/year in the first 9 years of the study period to 36.99/100000/year in the next 9 years [12]. Significant increase in incidence of T1DM was also observed in Lower Silesia during the period 2000-2005 with an increase from 10.43/100000 in 2000 to 13.49/100000 in 2005 [13].

Additionally in Scotland two studies by Patterson and co-workers [14-15] have shown an increasing incidence from 13, 8/100000/year between 1968 and 1976 and up to

21,0/100000/year from 1977 to 1983 for children aged less than 19 year old. Another study for the same population found that the incidence of T1DM had increased from 22,7/100000 in 1984 to 26,0/100000 in 1993 and this increase of about 2% a year, though small, is statistically significant and the effect over 10 years is a large increase [16]. An important increase in incidence of T1DM was also observed in Saxony between the five year periods 1999-2003 and 2004-2008 with estimated rates 15.7/100000 and 19.2/100000 respectively [17].

In our study we have ascertained the mean annual incidence on T1DM in the Greek Cypriot population during the period 1990 - 1999 in children younger than 15 years of age. During this period the incidence of T1DM was 10.76 /100000[18]. In order to identify an increase in the incidence of T1DM in our country, as occurred in the majority of the populations worldwide, we had performed an analysis of the newly diagnosed cases until the end of the year 2004. There was a statistically significant increase in the incidence during the period 2000-2004 with an estimated mean overall incidence 11.9/100000[19]. We had subsequently extended this work by adding the new cases of the five year period 2005 – 2009 in order to document this rising trend by comparing the incidence between the two decades (1990-1999 vs 2000-2009). We have observed a rising trend of the mean incidence from 10.76/100.000 at the first decade (1990-1999) of the study up to 14.4/100.000 at the second decade (2000-2009). According to Wilcoxon two-sample test this increasing trend of incidence during the 20 years analysed is statistically significant (p-value=0.0091). The mean incidence rate for each 5 year- period in accordance with the population data (population below the age of 15yr) is presented in figure 2.   The overall mean incidence of T1DM, in the Greek Cypriot population was 12.46/100000 during the twenty-year period 1990-2009.   This raised incidence classifies Cyprus among the countries with high incidence of T1DM.

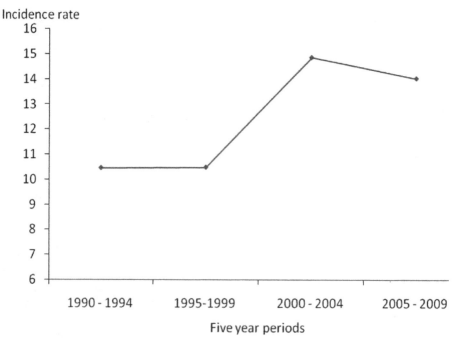

Fig. 2. Different annual incidence rates during five year periods.

Additionally this rising incidence was more pronounced among children who manifested the disease before the age of 5yr. Table 1 shows the percentage of newly diagnosed T1DM cases expressed as age group in accordance with the international standards.

Period at Diagnosis	Age Group (years)					
	0-4		5-9		10-14	
	n	%	n	%	n	%
1990-1999	31	19.0 (13.0-25.0)	66	40.5 (33.0-48.0)**	66	40.5 (33.0-48.0)**
2000-2009	55	26.4 (20.4-32.4)	77	37.0 (30.4-43.6)*	76	36.5 (30.0-43.0)*
1990-2009	86	23.2 (18.9-27.5)	143	38.5 (33.5-43.5)**	142	38.3 (33.4-43.2)**

Table 1. Age of diagnosis in total and in the three age groups. Binomial test performed to compare proportions compared to "0-4 year" age group: * $p<0.01$, **$p<0.001$

3. Age of onset

T1DM formerly called as juvenile diabetes it is one of the most common chronic disease of youth as 80% of individuals with T1DM are younger than 20 year of age [20-21]. The age of manifestation of childhood onset T1DM has a bimodal allotment with one peak at 4 to 6 years of age and a second in early puberty (10 to 14 years of age) [22-23]. Recent studies report a higher rate of increase among children younger than 5 years than in children between 5 and 15 years of age [24-25]. This may be related to an earlier onset of clinical manifestation or to a true increase in the causative factors of the disease.

Although the clinical appearance occurs at all ages [21] one fourth of individuals with T1DM are diagnosed as adults [26]. Up to 10% of adults primarily supposed to have type 2 diabetes are found to have antibodies associated with T1D [27] and beta cell destruction in adults seems to take place at a much slower rate than in young T1D cases, often delaying the need for insulin therapy after diagnosis.

4. Gender differences

Although most autoimmune diseases are more common in females, there appears to be no gender difference in the overall incidence of childhood T1DM [11].

However, a gender influence on the age of onset has been reported, in select populations. Some data reported from Europe suggest a female predominance in lower risk populations, and slight male excess in the high risk groups [3]. Furthermore many reports showed that older male adults of European origin (≥15 to 40 years of age) are more likely to develop T1DM than females of similar age and geographic location with an approximate 3:2 male to female ratio [28-30]. The same 3:2 male to female ratio also was reported in children younger than 6 years of age in an observational study from Boston [31]. Based on our data it seems that more males develop T1DM at younger age, whereas female predominate during the peripubertal period as shown in figure 3.

5. Seasonal variation at onset and birth

The first report of seasonal variation in the manifestation of T1DM was presented by Franklin Adams in 1926[32] although a consistent picture on the real seasonality of the disease has not been established. The increased incidence of T1DM diagnosis during

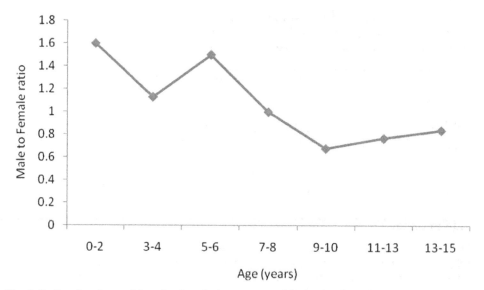

Fig. 3. Ratio of males and females in relation to year of diagnosis (at 2-yr intervals).

Autumn and Winter months could support the hypothesis that infections may act as participating factors in the clinical onset of the disease, possibly accelerating an autoimmune process that may have been initiated months or years before [33]. Based on the average temperature record in our island, the newly diagnosed cased were grouped according to the month of diagnosis as follow: November, December, January, and February were defined as cold months, October, March, April and May as neutral months and, June, July , August and September, as warm months. More children were significantly diagnosed with T1DM during the cold months compared to those who manifested the disease during the warm months (p<0.001), whereas no difference was observed in the incidence between neutral and cold months ((p>0.05) throughout the study period (1990-2009) as depicted in Table 2. A recent study on seasonal variation in DM in 53 countries has suggested that seasonality in the diagnosis of T1DM occurs and that the pattern of seasonality appears to be related to the geographical position, at least as far as the northern/southern hemisphere dichotomy is concerned [34].

Period at Diagnosis	Month at Diagnosis					
	Cold Months		Neutral Months		Warm Months	
	n	%	n	%	n	%
1990-1999	64	38.6 (31.2-46.0)	61	36.7 (29.4-44.0)*	41	24.7 (18.1-31.3)****
2000-2009	82	39.4 (32.8-46.0)	67	32.2 (25.9-38.5)**	59	28.4 (22.3-34.5)***
1990-2009	146	39.0 (34.1-43.9)	128	34.2 (29.4-39.0)*	100	26.7 (22.2-31.2)****

Table 2. Percentage of children diagnosed with T1DM at cold months, neutral months and warm months. Binomial test performed to compare proportions compared to "Cold Months" group: * NS (p>0.05), ** p<0.05, *** p<0.01, ****p<0.001

A seasonal variation of birth has been also observed in children who developed T1DM later in life in many countries, which suggests that environmental factors during pregnancy, in the neonatal period or very early in life play a role in its development. Several studies from Europe [35-37] and Israel [38] showed higher rates of T1DM among youth born in spring and lower rates among youth born in winter. Although McKinney maintained that there is no relationship between T1DM diagnosis and date of birth[39]. It has been suggested that seasonability pattern may be explained by reduced vitamin D production [40] during the critical intrauterine and neonatal periods of life.

6. Genotype

The genetics of T1DM cannot be classified according to a specific model of inheritance. Susceptibility to autoimmune T1DM is determined by multiple genes with HLA genes having the strongest known association.   HLA antigens are present on the surface of the leucocytes and participate in some immune reactions. The genes coding for these antigens are located on chromosome 6. The class II sub region of HLA consists of the DR, DQ, and DP loci. These class II molecules are involved to the immune destruction of the pancreatic beta cells because they participate in the presentation of the antigen to the helper T cell, which initiates the immune reaction.

Inheritance of HLA-DR3 and HLA-DR4 appears to confer a 2 to 3 fold increased risk for the development of T1DM. When both HLA-DR3 and HLA-DR4 are inherited the relative risk for the development of T1DM is increased by 7-10 folds. It is estimated that 48 percent of the familial aggregation can now be ascribed to known loci, and the Major Histocompatibility Complex (MHC) contributes 41 percent [41]. As an example, siblings with the highest risk HLA DR and DQ alleles, who inherit both HLA regions identical by descent to their diabetic sibling, may have a risk of developing anti-islet autoimmunity as high as 80 percent and a similar long-term risk of diabetes[42].   Moreover HLA DR2 and HLA DR5 are both protective in most studies. Furthermore, stronger associations of DM1 have been reported with other MHC loci: HLA-DQA1 and DQB1 antigens[43].

In our effort to detect the genetic susceptibility of Greek Cypriot population to DM1, we studied 101 DM1 patients with age of onset less than 15 years through HLA serological typing for the DR and DQ1 alleles and compared them to 209 healthy controls. Our findings support the strong association of HLA-DR4 and DR3 with DM1. The most frequent allelic combination was that of HLA-DR3/DR4 (27%) followed by that of DR2/DR4 (21.6%). The percentage of HLA antigens in patients with DM1 and controls are shown in figure 4. The protective role of HLA-DR5 was shown, whereas the presence of HLA-DR2 is neutral, in contrast with most findings among Caucasian population where DR2 is protective.   In addition, high resolution testing of the DR4 and DR3 alleles revealed the predominant presence of the DRB1*0403 (0% vs 36%), similar frequency of the DRB1*0402 in both groups (19% vs 14%) and that the DRB1*301 was the only DR3 allele detected. The DQB1 alleles present in our T1DM patients as shown in figure 5 were nearly exclusively DQB1*0201 and DQB1*0302 [44]. The relative risk of developing T1DM in children carrying the DQB1*0201 and the DQB1*0302 alleles is 5.05 and 2.56 respectively whereas the protective role of DQB1*0301 is documented.

Furthermore, although most T1D cases occur in individuals without a family history of the disease, T1D is strongly influenced by genetic factors. The lifelong risk of T1DM is markedly

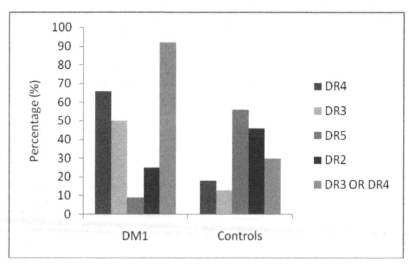

Fig. 4. HLA antigens in DM1 patients and controls.

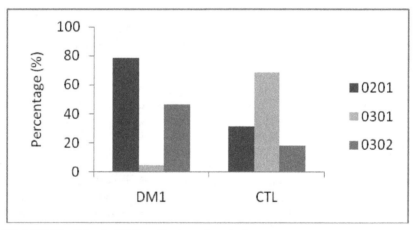

Fig. 5. HLA DQ B1 alleles in DM1 patients and controls.

increased in close relatives of a patient with T1DM, averaging about 6 percent in offspring, 5 percent in siblings and 50 percent in identical twins (versus 0.4 percent in subjects with no family history) [45-46]. T1DM is 2-3 times more common in the offspring of diabetic men (3.6-8.5%) compared with diabetic woman (1.3-3.6%) [1]. A monozygotic twin of a patient with type 1 diabetes has a higher risk of diabetes than a dizygotic twin, and the risk in a dizygotic twin sibling is similar to that in non-twin siblings [46].

Additionally age at onset is inversely related to the proportion of HLA haplotypes, and young children with T1DM show the greatest HLA-associated genetic risk. Siblings of children with onset of T1D before the age of 5 years have a 3- to 5-fold greater cumulative risk of diabetes by age 20 years compared with siblings of children diagnosed between 5 and 15 years of age [47]. Several reports suggest a higher proportion of lower risk haplotypes and in association with the decreased age at onset of T1DM are consisted with a major environmental effect on the development of the disease [48-51].

T1DM is associated with other autoimmune diseases such as thyroiditis, celiac disease, autoimmune gastritis and Addison disease [52]. The coexistence of these autoimmune diseases is associated to genes within the MHC complex [52].

7. Other risk factors

The variations in the incidence of T1DM in different countries its rising in rich and developed countries have raised questions about changes in environmental risk factors that may either initiate or accelerate the autoimmune process leading to pancreatic β-pancreatic cell destruction.

Reports have linked several environmental factors to an increased risk of T1DM; however, none of these have associations have verified and many have been contradicted by other studies. They include: viral infections in infancy and early childhood, maternal viral infection during pregnancy [53], early exposure to cow's milk and other nutritional factors [54], chemical contamination of food and water [55], high birth weight and an increase in body mass index [56].

Viruses that have been associated with T1DM as environmental triggers include enteroviruses, mumps, rubella, cytomegalovirus, rotavirus and Epstein-Barr virus. The one proven environmental virus trigger T1DM is congenital rubella [57]. Many epidemiological studies have been supported the involvement of enteroviruses, especially the Coxsackie B viruses in the aetiology which appears to trigger β cell autoimmunity [58-59]. Furthermore it has been hypothesized that excessive weight gain and increase in insulin resistance in early childhood is trigger event which initiates the autoimmunity leading to β cell destruction and this Accelerator Hypothesis has been supported by several epidemiological studies [56, 60-61].

A number of dietary factors may influence the development of T1DM in infants at high risk for T1DM. Early introduction to the infant diet of cattle proteins, lack or short lasting breast feeding might be reasons for development of immunological reaction leading to the destruction of pancreatic beta cells [62]. In two large prospective cohort studies of newborns at high risk for T1DM diabetes (either a first degree relative [63-64] or a high risk HLA genotype) [63], first exposure to cereal before age three months [63-64] or after seven months [63] was associated with an increased risk of developing autoantibodies (IA) compared to infants whose first exposure was between ages four to six months. The increased risk was associated with gluten-containing cereals in one study [64], but with either gluten or rice-containing cereals in the other [63].

On the other hand Vitamin D and omega-3 fatty acids may have a protective role. A case control study in seven European countries suggested that supplementation with vitamin D in early infancy can protect against development of T1DM [65]. A similar protective effect was found in a birth-cohort study of over 10,000 children [66]. Moreover preliminary studies in animals sustain a protective role of omega-3 fatty acids in the inflammatory reaction associated with autoimmune islet cell damage [67-68].

In conclusion there is no doubt that the incidence of T1DM is increasing dramatically. Data from large epidemiological studies worldwide indicate that the incidence of T1DM has been increasing by 2% to 5% worldwide [69] and this is of concern because of its health and resource implications. This rising incidence of T1DM in young children has been confirmed to a genetically susceptible subgroup of the population (48). The heightened proportion of lower risk hapltotypes and decreased median age at onset of T1DM within the subgroup are consistent with a major environmental effect on Diabetes development (50).

8. Epilogue

It is a an actuality that significant advances have been made in the clinical care of T1DM, which ultimately improved the clinical outcomes. However much more need to be done to find a cure for T1DM. In the absence of an ideal therapy Diabetes will always be a hurdle in the quality of life of these children. Moreover the increasing incidence is of concern because of its health and resource implications. There is a great research potential and more studies are required to identify the environmental factors that trigger the autoimmune destruction of the pancreatic beta cell particularly in some populations and individuals, who are not genetically predisposed to develop T1DM. These environmental triggers if ever identified could potentially be targeted for new preventive strategies and optimal intervention.

9. References

[1] Craig, M.E., A. Hattersley, and K.C. Donaghue, *Definition, epidemiology and classification of diabetes in children and adolescents*. Pediatr Diabetes, 2009. 10 Suppl 12: p. 3-12.

[2] Karvonen, M., et al., *Incidence of childhood type 1 diabetes worldwide. Diabetes Mondiale (DiaMond) Project Group*. Diabetes Care, 2000. 23(10): p. 1516-26.

[3] Green, A., E.A. Gale, and C.C. Patterson, *Incidence of childhood-onset insulin-dependent diabetes mellitus: the EURODIAB ACE Study*. Lancet, 1992. 339(8798): p. 905-9.

[4] Eisenbarth, G.S., *Immunology of type 1 diabetes*. 2nd ed. 2004: Plenum Publishers.

[5] Yang, Z., et al., *Childhood diabetes in China. Enormous variation by place and ethnic group*. Diabetes Care, 1998. 21(4): p. 525-9.

[6] Silink, M., *Childhood diabetes: a global perspective*. Horm Res, 2002. 57 Suppl 1: p. 1-5.

[7] Onkamo, P., et al., *Worldwide increase in incidence of Type I diabetes--the analysis of the data on published incidence trends*. Diabetologia, 1999. 42(12): p. 1395-403.

[8] Patterson, C.C., et al., *Incidence trends for childhood type 1 diabetes in Europe during 1989-2003 and predicted new cases 2005-20: a multicentre prospective registration study*. Lancet, 2009. 373(9680): p. 2027-33.

[9] *Variation and trends in incidence of childhood diabetes in Europe. EURODIAB ACE Study Group*. Lancet, 2000. 355(9207): p. 873-6.

[10] *Incidence and trends of childhood Type 1 diabetes worldwide 1990-1999*. Diabet Med, 2006. 23(8): p. 857-66.

[11] Dabelea, D., et al., *Incidence of diabetes in youth in the United States*. JAMA, 2007. 297(24): p. 2716-24.

[12] Al-Mendalawi, M.D., et al., *Incidence trends of childhood type 1 diabetes in eastern Saudi Arabia*. Saudi Med J, 2010. 31(9): p. 1074-5; author reply 1074-5.

[13] Zubkiewicz-Kucharska, A. and A. Noczynska, *[Epidemiology of type 1 diabetes in Lower Silesia in the years 2000-2005]*. Pediatr Endocrinol Diabetes Metab, 2010. 16(1): p. 45-9.

[14]   Patterson, C.C., et al., *Increasing prevalence of diabetes mellitus in children.* Br Med J (Clin Res Ed), 1983. 287(6386): p. 213-4.

[15]   Patterson, C.C., et al., *Geographical variation in the incidence of diabetes mellitus in Scottish children during the period 1977-1983.* Diabet Med, 1988. 5(2): p. 160-5.

[16]   Rangasami, J.J., et al., *Rising incidence of type 1 diabetes in Scottish children, 1984-93. The Scottish Study Group for the Care of Young Diabetics.* Arch Dis Child, 1997. 77(3): p. 210-3.

[17]   Galler, A., et al., *Incidence of childhood diabetes in children aged less than 15 years and its clinical and metabolic characteristics at the time of diagnosis: data from the Childhood Diabetes Registry of Saxony, Germany.* Horm Res Paediatr, 2010. 74(4): p. 285-91.

[18]   Skordis, N., et al., *The incidence of type 1 diabetes mellitus in Greek-Cypriot children and adolescents in 1990-2000.* Pediatr Diabetes, 2002. 3(4): p. 200-4.

[19]   Toumba, M., et al., *Rising incidence of type 1 diabetes mellitus in children and adolescents in Cyprus in 2000-2004.* Pediatr Diabetes, 2007. 8(6): p. 374-6.

[20]   Liese, A.D., et al., *The burden of diabetes mellitus among US youth: prevalence estimates from the SEARCH for Diabetes in Youth Study.* Pediatrics, 2006. 118(4): p. 1510-8.

[21]   Thunander, M., et al., *Incidence of type 1 and type 2 diabetes in adults and children in Kronoberg, Sweden.* Diabetes Res Clin Pract, 2008. 82(2): p. 247-55.

[22]   Felner, E.I., et al., *Genetic interaction among three genomic regions creates distinct contributions to early- and late-onset type 1 diabetes mellitus.* Pediatr Diabetes, 2005. 6(4): p. 213-20.

[23]   Elamin, A., et al., *Epidemiology of childhood type I diabetes in Sudan, 1987-1990.* Diabetes Care, 1992. 15(11): p. 1556-9.

[24]   Karvonen, M., J. Pitkaniemi, and J. Tuomilehto, *The onset age of type 1 diabetes in Finnish children has become younger. The Finnish Childhood Diabetes Registry Group.* Diabetes Care, 1999. 22(7): p. 1066-70.

[25]   Schoenle, E.J., et al., *Epidemiology of type I diabetes mellitus in Switzerland: steep rise in incidence in under 5 year old children in the past decade.* Diabetologia, 2001. 44(3): p. 286-9.

[26]   Haller, M.J., M.A. Atkinson, and D. Schatz, *Type 1 diabetes mellitus: etiology, presentation, and management.* Pediatr Clin North Am, 2005. 52(6): p. 1553-78.

[27]   Turner, R., et al., *UKPDS 25: autoantibodies to islet-cell cytoplasm and glutamic acid decarboxylase for prediction of insulin requirement in type 2 diabetes. UK Prospective Diabetes Study Group.* Lancet, 1997. 350(9087): p. 1288-93.

[28]   Gale, E.A. and K.M. Gillespie, *Diabetes and gender.* Diabetologia, 2001. 44(1): p. 3-15.

[29]   Weets, I., et al., *The incidence of type 1 diabetes in the age group 0-39 years has not increased in Antwerp (Belgium) between 1989 and 2000: evidence for earlier disease manifestation.* Diabetes Care, 2002. 25(5): p. 840-6.

[30]   Pundziute-Lycka, A., et al., *The incidence of Type I diabetes has not increased but shifted to a younger age at diagnosis in the 0-34 years group in Sweden 1983-1998.* Diabetologia, 2002. 45(6): p. 783-91.

[31]   Quinn, M., et al., *Characteristics at diagnosis of type 1 diabetes in children younger than 6 years.* J Pediatr, 2006. 148(3): p. 366-71.

[32] Adams, F., *The seasonal variation in the onset of acute diabetes. The age and sex factors in 1000 diabetic patients.* Arch Intern Med, 1926. 37: p.:861-864.

[33] Jun, H.S. and J.W. Yoon, *A new look at viruses in type 1 diabetes.* Diabetes Metab Res Rev, 2003. 19(1): p. 8-31.

[34] Moltchanova, E.V., et al., *Seasonal variation of diagnosis of Type 1 diabetes mellitus in children worldwide.* Diabet Med, 2009. 26(7): p. 673-8.

[35] Vaiserman, A.M., et al., *Seasonality of birth in children and young adults (0-29 years) with type 1 diabetes in Ukraine.* Diabetologia, 2007. 50(1): p. 32-5.

[36] Jongbloet, P.H., et al., *Seasonality of birth in patients with childhood diabetes in The Netherlands.* Diabetes Care, 1998. 21(1): p. 190-1.

[37] Samuelsson, U., C. Johansson, and J. Ludvigsson, *Month of birth and risk of developing insulin dependent diabetes in south east Sweden.* Arch Dis Child, 1999. 81(2): p. 143-6.

[38] Laron, Z., et al., *Month of birth and subsequent development of type I diabetes (IDDM).* J Pediatr Endocrinol Metab, 1999. 12(3): p. 397-402.

[39] McKinney, P.A., *Seasonality of birth in patients with childhood Type I diabetes in 19 European regions.* Diabetologia, 2001. 44 Suppl 3: p. B67-74.

[40] Mohr, S.B., et al., *The association between ultraviolet B irradiance, vitamin D status and incidence rates of type 1 diabetes in 51 regions worldwide.* Diabetologia, 2008. 51(8): p. 1391-8.

[41] Todd, J.A., et al., *Robust associations of four new chromosome regions from genome-wide analyses of type 1 diabetes.* Nat Genet, 2007. 39(7): p. 857-64.

[42] Aly, T.A., et al., *Extreme genetic risk for type 1A diabetes.* Proc Natl Acad Sci U S A, 2006. 103(38): p. 14074-9.

[43] Thorsby, E. and K.S. Ronningen, *Particular HLA-DQ molecules play a dominant role in determining susceptibility or resistance to type 1 (insulin-dependent) diabetes mellitus.* Diabetologia, 1993. 36(5): p. 371-7.

[44] Stylianou, C.H., Apsiotou, N., Stavrou, S., Demetriades, M., Kyriakou, A., Costeas, P., Skordis, N., *Detection of HLA-DR and DQB1 alleles, which predispose to diabetes mellitus type 1 in the Greek Cypriot population.* Hormone Research, 2003. 60((Suppl I)): p. 136.

[45] Atkinson, M.A. and N.K. Maclaren, *The pathogenesis of insulin-dependent diabetes mellitus.* N Engl J Med, 1994. 331(21): p. 1428-36.

[46] Redondo, M.J., et al., *Genetic determination of islet cell autoimmunity in monozygotic twin, dizygotic twin, and non-twin siblings of patients with type 1 diabetes: prospective twin study.* BMJ, 1999. 318(7185): p. 698-702.

[47] Gillespie, K.M., E.A. Gale, and P.J. Bingley, *High familial risk and genetic susceptibility in early onset childhood diabetes.* Diabetes, 2002. 51(1): p. 210-4.

[48] Gillespie, K.M., et al., *The rising incidence of childhood type 1 diabetes and reduced contribution of high-risk HLA haplotypes.* Lancet, 2004. 364(9446): p. 1699-700.

[49] Hermann, R., et al., *Temporal changes in the frequencies of HLA genotypes in patients with Type 1 diabetes--indication of an increased environmental pressure?* Diabetologia, 2003. 46(3): p. 420-5.

[50] Gale, E.A., *The rise of childhood type 1 diabetes in the 20th century.* Diabetes, 2002. 51(12): p. 3353-61.

[51] Vehik, K., et al., *Trends in high-risk HLA susceptibility genes among Colorado youth with type 1 diabetes.* Diabetes Care, 2008. 31(7): p. 1392-6.

[52] Tsirogianni, A., E. Pipi, and K. Soufleros, *Specificity of islet cell autoantibodies and coexistence with other organ specific autoantibodies in type 1 diabetes mellitus.* Autoimmun Rev, 2009. 8(8): p. 687-91.

[53] Dahlquist, G.G., et al., *Maternal enteroviral infection during pregnancy as a risk factor for childhood IDDM. A population-based case-control study.* Diabetes, 1995. 44(4): p. 408-13.

[54] Akerblom, H.K., et al., *Dietary manipulation of beta cell autoimmunity in infants at increased risk of type 1 diabetes: a pilot study.* Diabetologia, 2005. 48(5): p. 829-37.

[55] Longnecker, M.P. and J.L. Daniels, *Environmental contaminants as etiologic factors for diabetes.* Environ Health Perspect, 2001. 109 Suppl 6: p. 871-6.

[56] Hypponen, E., et al., *Obesity, increased linear growth, and risk of type 1 diabetes in children.* Diabetes Care, 2000. 23(12): p. 1755-60.

[57] McIntosh, E.D. and M.A. Menser, *A fifty-year follow-up of congenital rubella.* Lancet, 1992. 340(8816): p. 414-5.

[58] Rewers, M. and P. Zimmet, *The rising tide of childhood type 1 diabetes--what is the elusive environmental trigger?* Lancet, 2004. 364(9446): p. 1645-7.

[59] Salminen, K., et al., *Enterovirus infections are associated with the induction of beta-cell autoimmunity in a prospective birth cohort study.* J Med Virol, 2003. 69(1): p. 91-8.

[60] Betts, P., et al., *Increasing body weight predicts the earlier onset of insulin-dependant diabetes in childhood: testing the 'accelerator hypothesis' (2).* Diabet Med, 2005. 22(2): p. 144-51.

[61] Evertsen, J., R. Alemzadeh, and X. Wang, *Increasing incidence of pediatric type 1 diabetes mellitus in Southeastern Wisconsin: relationship with body weight at diagnosis.* PLoS One, 2009. 4(9): p. e6873.

[62] Virtanen, S.M. and M. Knip, *Nutritional risk predictors of beta cell autoimmunity and type 1 diabetes at a young age.* Am J Clin Nutr, 2003. 78(6): p. 1053-67.

[63] Norris, J.M., et al., *Timing of initial cereal exposure in infancy and risk of islet autoimmunity.* JAMA, 2003. 290(13): p. 1713-20.

[64] Ziegler, A.G., et al., *Early infant feeding and risk of developing type 1 diabetes-associated autoantibodies.* JAMA, 2003. 290(13): p. 1721-8.

[65] *Vitamin D supplement in early childhood and risk for Type I (insulin-dependent) diabetes mellitus. The EURODIAB Substudy 2 Study Group.* Diabetologia, 1999. 42(1): p. 51-4.

[66] Hypponen, E., et al., *Intake of vitamin D and risk of type 1 diabetes: a birth-cohort study.* Lancet, 2001. 358(9292): p. 1500-3.

[67] Kleemann, R., et al., *Impact of dietary fat on Th1/Th2 cytokine gene expression in the pancreas and gut of diabetes-prone BB rats.* J Autoimmun, 1998. 11(1): p. 97-103.

[68] Krishna Mohan, I. and U.N. Das, *Prevention of chemically induced diabetes mellitus in experimental animals by polyunsaturated fatty acids.* Nutrition, 2001. 17(2): p. 126-51.

[69] Maahs, D.M., et al., *Epidemiology of type 1 diabetes.* Endocrinol Metab Clin North Am, 2010. 39(3): p. 481-97.

3

The Enlarging List of Phenotypic Characteristics That Might Allow the Clinical Identification of Families at Risk for Type 1 Diabetes

Elena Matteucci and Ottavio Giampietro
Department of Internal Medicine, University of Pisa
Italy

1. Introduction

Type 1 diabetes is a chronic metabolic disease whose aetiology and pathogenesis remain not completely understood. Current criteria for the diagnosis of diabetes are: 1) haemoglobin A1c $\geq$ 6.5% (assayed using a method that is certified by the National Glycohemoglobin Standardization Program, NGSP, and standardised or traceable to the Diabetes Control and Complications Trial, DCCT, reference assay), 2) fasting plasma glucose (FPG) $\geq$ 126 mg/dl, 3) 2-hour plasma glucose $\geq$ 200 mg/dl during an oral glucose tolerance test (OGTT, 75 g), 4) a random plasma glucose $\geq$ 200 mg/dl (American Diabetes Association, 2011). The classification of diabetes includes: type 1 diabetes, type 2 diabetes, other specific types of diabetes due to other causes, and gestational diabetes mellitus. Type 2 diabetes, which is usually associated with obesity and older age, results from insulin resistance and progressive failure of pancreatic beta-cell function. Type 1 diabetes, which has usually an abrupt onset in younger people, is an organ-specific autoimmune disease characterised by absolute insulin deficiency resulting from beta-cell destruction. However, autoimmunity may not be the primary cause: environmental triggers are believed to precipitate type 1 diabetes in genetically susceptible individuals (van Belle et al., 2011). The overall incidence of type 1 diabetes is increasing; the majority of the increase is observed in the youngest age group, which also appeared to be the heaviest (Evertsen et al., 2009). Indeed, the accelerator hypothesis (Wilkin, 2009) suggests that type 1 and type 2 diabetes are the same disorder of insulin resistance set against different genetic backgrounds. Three processes could variably accelerate the loss of beta cells through apoptosis: constitution, insulin resistance, and autoimmunity. None of these accelerators leads to diabetes without excess weight, which causes an increase in insulin resistance and, thus, the weakening of glucose control. In turn, the glucotoxicity accelerates beta-cell apoptosis directly and by inducing beta-cell immunogens and autoimmunity in genetically predisposed subjects. Insulitis is commonly observed in recent-onset type 1 diabetes, but it does not uniformly affect all insulin-containing islets (differences in islet function?). It has been suggested that under increased insulin demand (puberty, adolescence, high sugar intake, etc.) a population of islets may be more prone to dysfunction or death, thereby attracting antigen presenting cells and promoting insulitis in susceptible individuals (Rowe et al., 2011). In a genome-wide association study, 41 distinct genomic locations provided evidence for association with type 1 diabetes in the meta-analysis (Barrett et al., 2009). The Type 1 Diabetes Genetics Consortium (T1DGC) has recruited families with at least two siblings who have type 1 diabetes in order to identify genes that determine an individual's risk of type 1 diabetes. T1DBase is the web-based resource focused on the genetics and genomics of type 1 diabetes susceptibility (https://www.t1dgc.org) that provides the updated table of human loci associated with type 1 diabetes (Table 1).

Chromosome	Gene of interest	Abbreviation
1p13.2	Protein tyrosine phosphatase, non-receptor type 22	PTPN22
1q31.2	Regulator of G-protein signalling 1	RGS1
2q12	Interleukin 18 receptor accessory protein	IL18RAP
2q24.2	Interferon induced with helicase C domain 1	IFIH1
2q33.2	Cytotoxic T-lymphocyte-associated protein 4	CTLA4
3p21.31	Chemokine (C-C motif) receptor 5	CCR5
4q27	Interleukin 2	IL2
5p13		
6p21.31 6p21.33	Major histocompatibility complexes	HLA-B, -A, -DRB1, -DQB1, -DPB1
6q15	similar to BTB and CNC homology 1, basic leucine zipper transcription factor 2	BACH2
6q23.3	similar to Tumor necrosis factor, α-induced protein 3	TNFAIP3
6q25.3	T-cell activation Rho GTPase-activating protein	TAGAP
10p15.1	Interleukin 2 receptor, α	IL2RA
10p15.1	Protein kinase C, θ	PRKCQ
11p15.5	Insulin II	INS
12q13.2		
12q13.3	Kinesin family member 5A	KIF5A
12q24.12		
15q25.1		
16p13.3		
18p11.21	Protein tyrosine phosphatase, non-receptor type 2	PTPN2
18q22.2	CD226 antigen	CD226
21q22.3		
22q13.1		

(from: http://t1dbase.org/page/PosterView/display/poster_id/386)

Table 1. Human loci associated with type 1 diabetes.

With regards to the causative environmental triggers that have been implicated in the pathogenesis of type 1 diabetes, they have been recently reviewed (van Belle et al., 2011; Vehik & Dabelea, 2011) and include particularly viral infections, gut microbic flora and other bacteria, early life feeding patterns, wheat proteins, and vitamin D.

The Enlarging List of Phenotypic Characteristics That Might Allow the Clinical Identification of
Families at Risk for Type 1 Diabetes

63

2. Identifying individuals at risk for type 1 diabetes

In Europe, the number of adults with diabetes was expected to reach 55.2 million (8.5% of the adult population) in 2010; about 112,000 children and adolescents were estimated to have type 1 diabetes mellitus (http://www.diabetesatlas.org/content/europe).

Most diabetic cases are complex diseases resulting from interactions between genetic and environmental determinants in genetically predisposed individuals. Empirical evidence suggests a architecture of many genetic loci with many variants of small effect (Wray & Goddard, 2010). Genome-wide association studies have suggested that the majority of susceptible loci have small contributions to phenotypic variation and therefore there should be a large number of susceptibility loci involved in the genetic basis of complex diseases (consistent with the polygenic model). Moreover, the differentiation of sporadic and familial cases has implied that most complex diseases are genetically heterogeneous. Family history has a high positive predictive value, but a low negative predictive value. Yang et al. (2010) have shown that 1) the proportion of sporadic cases depends on disease prevalence and heritability of the underlying liability scale, and 2) a large proportion of sporadic cases is expected under the polygenic model due to the low prevalence rates of common complex genetic diseases. Thus, the causal mechanisms cannot be inferred from the observed proportion of sporadic cases alone. The prediction of disease risk to relatives from many risk loci or markers requires a model that combines the effects of these loci. The constrained multiplicative, Odds and Probit models fitted data on risk to relatives, but it is difficult to distinguish between them until genetic variants that explain the majority of the known genetic variance are identified (Wray & Goddard, 2010). Hence, genetic risk modelling to derive prediction of individual risk and risk to relatives are still difficult to reconcile.

In most individuals with autoimmune type 1 diabetes, beta cell destruction is a chronically progressive and very slow process that starts long before overt disease. During this "silent" phase, autoantibodies are produced and self-reactive activated lymphocytes infiltrate the islets of Langerhans (Rowe et al., 2011). Autoantibodies that target self-antigens in the insulin-secreting beta cells of the pancreas include: islet cell autoantibodies (ICA), insulinoma-associated antigen-2 antibodies (IA-2A), antibodies against the related antigen IA-2 beta (IA-2β), insulin autoantibodies (IAA), autoantibodies to the 65kDa isoform of glutamic acid decarboxylase 65 (GADA), and the recently identified autoantibodies to the zinc transporter 8 (ZnT8A) (Table 2).

Islet autoantibodies are potent tools for the prediction of type 1 diabetes and are the basis for recruitment in prevention trials and immunointervention trials. In the general childhood population in Finland, one-time screening for GADA and IA-2A was capable of identifying about 60% of those individuals who will develop type 1 diabetes over the subsequent 27 years; both positive and negative seroconversions occurred over time reflecting a dynamic process of beta cell autoimmunity, but positivity for at least two diabetes-associated autoantibodies represented in most cases a point of no return (Knip et al., 2010). So far, however, the place of autoantibody-based risk assessment in routine clinical practice is limited because no proven therapeutic interventions is available for people at high risk of progression to type 1 diabetes. Until therapies modulating the disease process become available, the benefit to individual patients is questionable - awareness of risk is rather useless or even stressful - and diabetes antibody testing does not yet have a role in clinical care (Bingley, 2010). It is considered likely that islet-related autoantibodies are not directly pathogenetic, whereas autoreactive CD4 and CD8 T cells mediate beta cell damage.

Therefore, standardised autoantibody screenings should be combined with the detection of autoreactive T cells. Unfortunately, none of the currently available T cell assays satisfies all the features of a good assay: small blood sample required, simplicity, specificity, low intra- and inter-assay variability (Fierabracci, 2011). Notwithstanding recent developments based on immunosorbent spot and immunoblotting techniques, the International Workshops of the Immunology Diabetes Society concluded that T cell results are still inconclusive and novel approaches are currently being investigated.

In conclusion, it may be that in the future combination screening predicts type 1 diabetes clinical onset, but actually genetic risk, serum autoantibody profiling and T cell assays are uneconomical when applied in the general population.

Autoantibodies against	Abbreviation	Method
38-kDa glycated islet cell membrane-associated protein	GLIMA	Immunoprecipitation
51-kDa aromatic-L-amino-acid decarboxylase	AADC	Immunoprecipitation
52-kDa rat insulinoma	52-kDa RIN	Immunoblot
Aminoacyl-tRNA synthetase	ARS	ELISA*
Carbonic anydrase II	CA II	ELISA*
Carboxypeptidase H	CPHA	Radiobinding assay
Chymotrypsinogen-related 30-kDa pancreatic		Immunoblot analysis
DNA topoisomerase II	TopIIA	ELISA* and Western blot
Ganglioside GM2-1	GM2-1	Indirect immunoperoxidase technique
Gangliosides GM1, 2, 3, etc.		*ELISA
Glucose type-2 transporter	GLUT2	Western blot
Glutamic acid decarboxylase	GADA	Radiobinding assay, ELISA*
Heat shock proteins	HSP	*ELISA
Insulin	IAA	Radiobinding assay
Insulinoma-associated antigen-2	IA-2A	Radiobinding assay, ELISA*
Insulinoma-associated antigen 2β	IA-2β	Radiobinding assay
Islet cell	ICA	Indirect immunofluorescence
Islet cell surface	ICSA	Radiobinding assay
Proinsulin	PIAA	Radiobinding assay
Zinc transporter 8	ZnT8	Radiobinding assay

* Enzyme linked immunosorbent assay

Table 2. List of islet autoantibodies detected in type 1 diabetes (modified from Winter & Schatz, 2011).

3. Phenotyping type 1 diabetes families

Translational research aims to integrate basic life science (genomics, transcriptomics, proteomics, and metabolomics) with insights gained from clinical experience to comprehensively study complex biological system and complex human diseases. Translation requires, among others, methods that relate molecular and cellular phenotypes to clinical characteristics (Bebek et al., 2011). Indeed, the correlation between quantitative phenotypes and traits allows for a more efficient use of the genetic information; hence the importance of accurate family phenotyping studies. Unaffected family members can contribute as much to the analysis as individuals with the disease diagnosis. For example, the finding of cognitive deficits in individuals with schizophrenia and in the clinically unaffected relatives of these individuals suggested that these deficits are part of the innate underlying distinct differences that make some individuals vulnerable to schizophrenia. Examining these complementary biological phenotypes in genetic studies has been found to provide valuable information about the pathway that connects genotype to clinical disease (Almasy et al., 2008). Similarly, large-scale genetic fine mapping and genotype-phenotype associations implicated polymorphisms in the IL2RA region in type 1 diabetes: IL2RA type 1 diabetes susceptibility genotypes were associated with lower circulating levels of the biomarker, soluble IL-2RA (Lowe et al., 2007). However, despite the theoretical advantages of quantitative trait analysis and testing of multiple plausible domains, some matters have emerged since quantitative traits may not be the most relevant phenotypes to investigate in search for the genetic etiology of disease. Identifying the "best" phenotype for genetic studies needs to survey family members and examine coexisting features and familial segregation patterns. A focus on careful assessment of the most genetically relevant phenotypes has been recommended (Brzustowicz & Bassett, 2008).

Over the years, our research efforts have sought primarily to gain a comprehensive understanding of the common phenotypic elements that characterise families with a sporadic case of type 1 diabetes. Here we provide a research-based overview of these familial peculiarities that include multifaceted, easily detectable, clinical perturbations: physical (BMI), cardiovascular (blood pressure response to exercise and circadian blood pressure pattern), biochemical (fasting plasma glucose, HbA1c, lipids, homeostasis model assessment of insulin sensitivity, plasma markers of oxidative damage), cellular (cellular markers of oxidative damage, transplasma membrane electron transport systems, mitochondrial membrane potential), and immunological (lymphocyte subsets).

4. Body weight in type 1 diabetes families

According to epidemiological findings and the accelerator hypothesis, the prevalence of overweight in preadolescent children is increasing, it tracks into adulthood and may increase diabetes and cardiovascular disease risk in adulthood. The risk of childhood obesity seems to increase with exposure to diabetes or cigarette smoke in utero, high birth weight, rapid weight gain in infancy, and shorter breastfeeding duration. The Diabetes Autoimmunity Study in the Young (DAISY) examined longitudinally 1,718 children from birth that were at increased risk for type 1 diabetes (Lamb et al., 2010). Gender, diabetes exposure in utero, size for gestational age, weight gain in the first year of life, and total breastfeeding duration (inverse) showed significant association with higher childhood BMI. Mediation analysis suggested that 1) the protective effect of breastfeeding duration on childhood BMI was largely mediated by slower infant weight gain, and 2) the increased risk of higher childhood BMI associated with exposure to diabetes in utero was partially explained by greater birth size. Maternal obesity before pregnancy and weight gain during pregnancy significantly predicted increased risk of persistent multiple positivity for islet autoantibodies in offspring with high genetic susceptibility for type 1 diabetes (Rasmussen et al., 2009). A systematic review and meta-analysis (12 studies) indicated that high birth weight and increased weight gain during the first year of life were associated with an increased risk of type 1 diabetes in later life (Harder et al., 2009).

Metabolic demand and insulin resistance have been suggested to be involved in the development of type 1 diabetes (Evertsen et al., 2009; Wilkin, 2009), but the evidence is not consistent across the studies. In 1650 prospectively followed children of mothers or fathers with type 1 diabetes (BABYDIAB cohort), islet autoantibodies-positive children were not insulin resistant (based on homeostasis model assessment of insulin resistance, HOMA-IR) and did not have increased BMI around and early after seroconversion (Winkler at al., 2009). In this study, of 777 children with HOMA-IR measurements, 84 developed islet antibodies during the study: analysis of HOMA-IR by age showed no significant difference between islet autoantibody-positive and islet autoantibody-negative children, with a tendency towards a lower HOMA-IR in the antibody-positive children compared with the antibody-negative children.

In a primary school health program in Pisa we screened 869 primary school children (448 M, 421 F, mean age 118±5 months): height, weight, four skinfolds, and four circumferences were measured; a family-reported questionnaire was used to determine family composition, history, and lifestyle (Giampietro et al., 2002). The percentages of children who could be considered overweight (BMI ≥ 95th percentile of age- and sex-specific National Health and Nutrition Examination Survey I, NHANES I, reference data) were boys, 10.0%, and girls, 9.3%. It emerged that offspring BMI was correlated with birth weight, parental BMI and scholarship level, children blood pressure, and hours per day spent in television viewing. Family history for diabetes was associated with higher BMI, skinfold thickness at the subscapular area (SSF), waist circumference, and upper thigh. Family history for hypertension was associated with higher SSF/skinfold thickness at the triceps area (TCF) ratio. We concluded that anthropometric and anamnestic data on child and family yield more accurate estimates of risk profile: fat distribution seems relevant for metabolic and cardiovascular disorders.

Since our initial investigations on type 1 diabetes families, we found that first degree relatives' BMI tended to be higher when compared with healthy control subjects who had no first-degree relative with type 1 diabetes, although the difference did not always reach statistical significance (Matteucci & Giampietro, 2000a; Matteucci et al. 2004a, 2004b; Matteucci et al. 2006). In recent years, on the contrary, the difference in BMI between unaffected siblings of type 1 diabetic probands and healthy control subjects has reached the statistical significance (Figure 1, Matteucci et al., 2010).

This finding probably reflects the trend toward increasing body weight and obesity in the general population, declining physical activity and unhealthy dietary habits that we have documented (Matteucci et al., 2004b, 2007, 2008). However, the emerging difference in BMI between unaffected relatives and control subjects suggests that additional factors are operative in type 1 diabetes families, which remain unknown. The single nucleotide polymorphism rs9939609 in the fat mass and obesity associated gene (FTO) region on chromosome 16q12, which increases the risk of childhood obesity and type 2 diabetes, did not alter susceptibility to type 1 diabetes (Field et al., 2007). Although increased early growth was associated with disease risk in various European populations, any role of infant feeding in this association remained unclear (EURODIAB Substudy 2 Study Group, 2002). Scientific evidences suggested associations of allelic variations in the Vitamin D receptor gene and phenotypes related to body weight, glucose homeostasis, diabetes and

The Enlarging List of Phenotypic Characteristics That Might Allow the Clinical Identification of
Families at Risk for Type 1 Diabetes

67

its vascular complications (Reis et al., 2005). Whatever the case, our data in adult members of type 1 diabetes families highlight that the 'familial' predisposition to overweight remains throughout life.

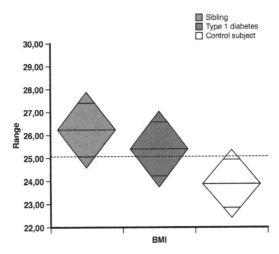

Fig. 1. Body mass index (BMI) in control subjects, type 1 diabetic patients and their siblings (Matteucci et al., 2010).

5. Familial cardiovascular abnormalities

Diabetes and hypertension are strongly associated although the role of glycaemia in promoting hypertension is a matter of debate (Invitti, 2003). HbA1c variability predicts not only incident microalbuminuria and progression of established renal disease but also cardiovascular disease events in patients with type 1 diabetes (Wadén et al., 2009). Moreover, HbA1c concentration predicts cardiovascular disease and all-cause mortality in adults without diabetes (Khaw et al., 2004). In healthy non-diabetic and non-hypertensive men, fasting plasma glucose is independently associated with blood pressure at rest and during exercise and development of elevated blood pressure after 7-years follow-up (Biornholt et al., 2003). Usually, in type 1 diabetes families, parental hypertension has been associated with diabetic nephropathy in adult and young offspring (Viberti et al., 1987; Marcovecchio et al., 2010), but the familial/hereditary factors that have an impact on diabetic nephropathy have not been so far identified. In a large homogeneous population from the Finnish Diabetic Nephropathy study, a cluster of parental hypertension, cardiovascular disease, cardiovascular mortality, and type 1 diabetes was associated with diabetic nephropathy in offspring with type 1 diabetes. It seemed that the more the traits clustered in family, the higher the risk for diabetes nephropathy (Thorn et al., 2007).

In this regard it is noteworthy that enhanced sodium/lithium countertransport and sodium/hydrogen exchange had been suggested to predict diabetic nephropathy (Walker et al., 1990; Ng et al, 1990). However, we found evidence contradicting this favourite hypothesis. Indeed, our data demonstrated convincingly that sodium/hydrogen exchange activity was significantly higher in type 1 diabetes with no difference among the two groups of diabetic patients with and without nephropathy. Moreover, enhanced sodium/hydrogen exchange activity was also a common feature of nondiabetic first-degree relatives of type 1 diabetic patients with no difference among the corresponding groups of relatives. The association between antiport activities of diabetic probands and their relatives suggested that the altered activity of the transporter was primarily determined by familial factors whose nature remained to be clarified (Matteucci & Giampietro, 2000b).

Generally, the observation of raised arterial blood pressure in relatives of type 1 diabetes patients was based on history, a single measurement of arterial blood pressure, or a 24-h ambulatory record; we were first to evaluate the response to ergometer exercise (Matteucci et al., 2006). Blood pressure response to exercise had been evaluated as a predictor of future hypertension and cardiovascular disease (Sharabi et al., 2001). Moreover, the heritability for resting blood pressure and blood pressure response to exercise was under investigation (An et al., 2000). We identified an abnormal blood pressure response to exercise testing not only in type 1 diabetic probands but also in asymptomatic normotensive non-diabetic relatives of type 1 diabetics, in which it was associated with indices of metabolic syndrome and oxidative damage. Furthermore, in healthy normotensive non-diabetic control subjects without family history of type 1 diabetes, strong associations were found 1) between resting systolic blood pressure and fasting plasma glucose as well as fasting plasma insulin levels, and 2) between systolic blood pressure response to exercise and HbA1c levels (Matteucci et al., 2006).

In a recent study, we performed 24-hour ambulatory blood pressure monitoring in type 1 diabetes families with the primary aim of investigating the circadian variability of blood pressure and the ambulatory arterial stiffness index in healthy siblings of type 1 diabetes patients vs healthy control subjects who had no first-degree relative with type 1 diabetes (Matteucci et al., 2010). Secondary aims of the study were to explore the influence of both cardiovascular autonomic function and erythrocyte electron transfer activity as oxidative marker on the ambulatory blood pressure profile. Indeed, human erythrocytes possess a transplasma ferricyanide reductase activity (measured as the erythrocyte velocity of ferricyanide reduction) that transfers reducing equivalents from intracellular reductants to extracellular oxidants (Matteucci & Giampietro, 2000c) and belongs to the ubiquitous transplasma membrane electron transport systems. Transplasma membrane electron transport activities have been related to the regulation of vital cellular processes and to the pathogenesis of various human disorders (Lane & Lawen, 2009) and exist also in endothelial cells where they have been suggested to regulate redox status and possibly atherogenesis through regulation of haeme oxygenase-1 expression (Lee et al., 2009).

We found that systolic blood pressure midline-estimating statistic of rhythm and pulse pressure were higher in type 1 diabetes patients and correlated positively with diabetes duration and the rate of oxidant-induced erythrocyte electron transfer to extracellular ferricyanide. Autonomic dysfunction was associated with diastolic blood pressure ecphasia and increased ambulatory arterial stiffness index. Siblings had higher BMI (Figure 1), lower insulin sensitivity (Figure 2), larger systolic blood pressure amplitude (Figure 3), and higher ambulatory arterial stiffness index than controls. Daytime systolic blood pressure was positively, independently associated with BMI and erythrocyte electron transfer to extracellular ferricyanide. Among non-diabetic people, there was a significant correlation between ambulatory arterial stiffness index and fasting plasma glucose. We concluded that siblings of type 1 diabetes patients exhibited a cluster of sub-clinical metabolic abnormalities associated with consensual perturbations in blood pressure variability. Moreover, our

The Enlarging List of Phenotypic Characteristics That Might Allow the Clinical Identification of
Families at Risk for Type 1 Diabetes

69

findings supported, in a clinical setting, the proposed role of transplasma membrane
electron transport systems in vascular pathobiology.

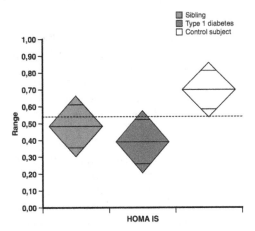

Fig. 2. Homeostasis model assessment of insulin sensitivity (HOMA-IS) in the same study
groups (Matteucci et al., 2010).

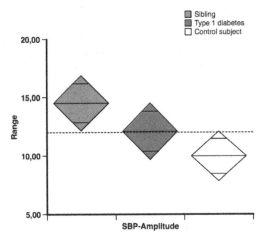

Fig. 3. Systolic blood pressure amplitude (SBP-Amplitude) in the same study groups
(Matteucci et al., 2010).

6. Biochemical phenotype and redox balance in type 1 diabetes relatives

Our studies over the years have linked family history of type 1 diabetes (first-degree
kinship) with multiple biochemical abnormalities. Since 2000 we documented metabolic
perturbations in nondiabetic relatives: parents differed from age-matched control subjects in
the higher plasma concentrations of glucose and Lipoprotein (a); their fibrinogen was
borderline but did not reach any statistical significance; in turn, siblings of type 1 diabetes

patients differed from age-matched control subjects in the higher levels of Lipoprotein (a) (Matteucci et al., 2000a). In the same study, we investigated the redox status and antioxidant defences in these families.

The premises were the following:

- enhanced levels of free radicals found in diabetes mellitus and impaired glucose tolerance has long been assumed to be related to chronically elevated glucose levels (Baynes and Thorpe, 1999; Vijayalingam et al., 1996),

- oxidative stress was suggested to play a primary role in the pathogenesis of diabetes and its complications but Authors still discussed whether oxidation preceded the appearance of complications or it merely reflected their presence (Baynes and Thorpe, 1999).

We suggested an alternative hypothesis, i.e. that oxidative stress preceded diabetes mellitus. In the case, indirect evidence for increased oxidative stress could be also detectable in non-diabetic relatives of type 1 diabetic patients. In order to provide evidence of a familial imbalance between radical production and antioxidant defences, we investigated indices of glucose and lipid metabolism, markers of plasma and cell lipid peroxidation, a novel marker of oxidant-induced protein damage, and the effects of oxygen radicals on erythrocytes of patients with type 1 diabetes and their relatives. We measured blood creatinine, glucose, HbA1c, cholesterol, triglycerides, Lipoprotein (a), fibrinogen, malondialdehyde, and advanced oxidation protein products. Erythrocyte response to oxidative stress (3-h-incubation at 37°C with or without a radical generating system) was evaluated by measuring erythrocyte glutathione, erythrocyte malodialdehyde, and haemolysis. Plasma and erythrocyte malodialdehyde were found to be significantly elevated in diabetics and relatives than in controls. Basal erythrocyte glutathione was lower in diabetics and incubations of cells caused in diabetics a decrease in erythrocyte glutathione of lesser degree than in control subjects, while a significant increase in haemolysis. Among relatives, haemolysis was increased both at baseline and after incubation. Plasma malodialdehyde was associated with blood glucose, creatinine, and fibrinogen; basal erythrocyte malodialdehyde with plasma Lipoprotein (a), fibrinogen, and plasma malodialdehyde. Basal erythrocyte glutathione content correlated with serum glucose and erythrocyte malodialdehyde production.

In that occasion, we were pioneers of the research on redox balance in type 1 diabetes families. We presented first evidence that markers of lipoprotein metabolism (Lipoprotein (a)), oxidative stress (plasma and erythrocyte malodialdehyde), and cellular fragility (haemolysis) are abnormal in non diabetic relatives of type 1 diabetics supporting the view that familial elements even precede diabetes. It seemed reasonable that the same biologic markers considered major predictors of cardiovascular disease could also trace familial susceptibility to type 1 diabetes, just as they have been associated with the development of type 2 diabetes (Matteucci et al., 2000a).

Based on the finding of elevated circulating markers of lipid peroxidation and increased cellular fragility, we decided to complete and integrate our investigation with further biochemical measurements of possible first-chain initiating or stimulating factors in order to evaluate, in the same families, the contribution of extracellular antioxidants to the increased oxidative stress. We also aimed to understand the eventual relationship between oxidative stress and the abnormal sodium/hydrogen exchange activity previously observed

The Enlarging List of Phenotypic Characteristics That Might Allow the Clinical Identification of
Families at Risk for Type 1 Diabetes

71

(Matteucci et al., 2001). We were unable to find out any abnormalities in circulating metal ions (such as iron, transferrin, ferritin, copper, and ceruloplasmin) or extracellular antioxidant defences (such as serum uric acid, albumin, bilirubin,) that could favour oxidative stress in non-diabetic relatives of type 1 patients. On the contrary, we confirmed our previous finding of a generalised increase in sodium/hydrogen exchange activity. The rate of amiloride-sensitive hydrogen efflux from erythrocytes was significantly associated with both erythrocyte glutathione content and some markers of radical-induced damage such as plasma advanced oxidation protein products and malondialdehyde, erythrocyte osmotic fragility, and erythrocyte malondialdehyde accumulation under oxidative stress. Hence, this additional study provided the first *in vivo* demonstration of a significant association between oxidative stress and sodium/hydrogen exchange upregulation. The familiarly overactive sodium/hydrogen exchange itself could be viewed as further evidence pointing to the presence in these families of a redox disequilibrium where oxidation seems to be prevailing.

Taken into account that:

- mitochondria are the cellular site of oxidation-reduction reactions and energy transfer processes; mitochondrial dysfunction is believed to play a role in the development of diabetes and its complications because of the active generation of free radicals (Maiese et al., 2007),
- a reactive oxygen species-mediated long-term 'memory' of hyperglycaemic stress has been reported in the mitochondria of endothelial cells (Ihnat et al., 2007), but impairment of mitochondrial function has been also observed in subjects with family history of type 2 diabetes before the onset of impaired glucose tolerance (Petersen et al., 2004),

in the last step of our research we measured the mitochondrial membrane potential in peripheral blood granulocytes from type 1 diabetic patients and their unaffected siblings using the mitochondrial indicator 5,5',6,6'-tetra chloro-1,1',3,3'-tetraethylbenzimidazolyl-carbocyanine iodide (JC-1) in conjunction with flow cytometry (Matteucci et al., 2011). This was the first study to examine mitochondrial membrane potential of circulating leukocytes in type 1 diabetes families and to document consistent evidence for mitochondrial hyperpolarisation that was highest in type 1 diabetic patients and intermediate in their siblings. Fasting plasma glucose was the only correlate of leukocyte mitochondrial membrane potential. Confirming previous observations in type 1 diabetes families, siblings had fasting plasma glucose slightly higher than control subjects yet lower HbA1c levels. The combination of higher mean fasting plasma glucose, lower homeostasis model assessment of insulin sensitivity (HOMA-IS) and lower HbA1c levels suggested that siblings had both impaired basal glucose clearance rate and enhanced insulin-stimulated muscle glucose disposal.

We hypothesised that in type 1 diabetes families, radical-induced mitochondrial membrane potential oscillations may be synchronized toward polarized states. The positive association between mitochondrial membrane potential oscillations and fasting plasma glucose within the range from normal to dysglycemic conditions suggested that hyperglycaemic challenge implied increased glucose metabolisation, enhanced oxidant formation and hyperpolarisation of the mitochondrial membrane.

It is noteworthy that succination of proteins, which is an irreversible chemical modification of cysteine by the Krebs cycle intermediate fumarate, is increased by hyperpolarisation of the inner mitochondrial membrane and develops in concert with mitochondrial and oxidative stress in diabetes (Frizzell et al., 2011).

7. Immunological functions in type 1 diabetes families

Although type 1 diabetes is a T-cell–mediated autoimmune disease, until a few years ago relatively few studies have attempted to associate T-cell autoreactivity with disease progression, in comparison with efforts directed on monitoring autoantibodies, and those that have been performed were largely limited to CD4 T-cells (Roep, 2008). Currently, islet epitope-specific CD8 T cells are believed to have a pivotal role in the destruction process. Unfortunately, monitoring multiple epitope-specific CD8 T cell populations poses many technical problems. Recently, monitoring of CD8 T cells reactive to beta-cell-derived antigens has been performed using the combinatorial quantum dot technique, which has been validated using peripheral blood cells from recent-onset type 1 diabetic patients, their siblings, and control subjects (Velthuis et al., 2010). Moreover, during the progression of autoimmune diabetes, memory autoreactive regulatory CD8 T cells can be expanded that could effectively suppress the expansion of dominant and subdominant effectors (Khadra et al., 2010). Increasing evidence shows the significance of CD4 and CD8 regulatory T cells, expressing the marker CD25 or IL-2 receptor, in autoimmune disease models. On the contrary, very few study have dealt with the role of CD23 or low affinity IgE receptor. In 2004, given that abnormalities in redox balance clustered in type 1 diabetes families and the intracellular redox status seemed to modulate immune function, we aimed to investigate the relationship between oxidative stress and immunologic features. We measured oxidative markers, serum pro-inflammatory cytokines, soluble cytokine receptors, and subsets of peripheral blood lymphocytes (by varying combinations of CD4, CD8, CD23, and CD25) from type 1 patients, low-risk (i.e. without underlying islet autoimmunity) non-diabetic first-degree relatives of diabetic patients, and healthy subjects (Matteucci et al., 2004a). In these families, protein and lipid oxidation was confirmed from reduced sulfhydryl groups, increased advanced oxidation protein products, increased plasma and erythrocyte malondialdehyde. Relatives had decreased counts of monocytes, of cells coexpressing CD23 and CD25, and of CD25$^+$ cells in peripheral blood. Patients with type 1 diabetes had similar defects and, in addition, showed decreased counts of peripheral CD4$^+$CD8$^+$ lymphocytes and increased serum levels of soluble receptors for IL-6 and IL-2. This was the first demonstration of leukocyte abnormalities in low-risk T1DM relatives, also presenting signs of oxidative stress. Moreover, our study reported first evidence that the oxidative stress observed in type 1 diabetes families was correlated to immunological hallmarks suggestive of different immunoregulatory mechanisms. A crucial question remained open: did the alteration in immune functions follow the altered intracellular redox status or vice versa?

More recently, we have characterised CD26 expression of T cell subsets in patients with type 1 diabetes because 1) high expression of CD26 among CD8$^+$ T cells has been suggested to be a marker of effective long-term memory T cell formation typical of acute resolved viral infections (Ibegbu et al., 2009), and 2) an increased risk of persistent viral infections, such as hepatitis C (HCV), was reported among diabetic patients (Lonardo et al., 2009).

No significant difference was seen in percentages or absolute numbers of CD4$^+$CD26$^+$, CD4$^+$CD26$^-$, CD8$^+$CD26$^+$, and CD8$^+$CD26$^-$ between type 1 diabetes and control people.

The Enlarging List of Phenotypic Characteristics That Might Allow the Clinical Identification of
Families at Risk for Type 1 Diabetes

73

However, the fluorescence intensity of CD26 expression on CD8+ lymphocytes revealed a significant decrease in type 1 diabetic patients compared with control subjects. Mean fluorescence of CD8+CD26+ cells was inversely correlated with the absolute number of CD4+CD26- cells (Matteucci et al., 2010). We interpreted the finding (low expression of CD26 among CD8+ T cells in type 1 diabetes) as indicating a defect in successfully developed long-term memory CD8+ T cells or in CD8+ T cells activation, even though the negative association with the number of CD4+CD26- T cell does not support a recent activation of peripheral T cells. We intend to continue research in this field in consideration of the immunomodulating role of the multifunctional CD26 (Ohnuma et al., 2011).

8. Concluding remarks

Today, there is a great need to integrate molecular biology with whole organ physiology. Findings from molecular and cellular studies must be brought back to intact organ systems without loosing the physiological context (Königshoff et al., 2011). This is especially true in the field of metabolic diseases where the study of individual proteins and signalling pathways in detail may not be easily translated to the intact organism. Taken into account the enlarging list of phenotypic characteristics that might allow the early clinical identification of families possibly at risk for sporadic cases of type 1 diabetes, many questions await an answer. We suggest the two main (in our opinion) issues.

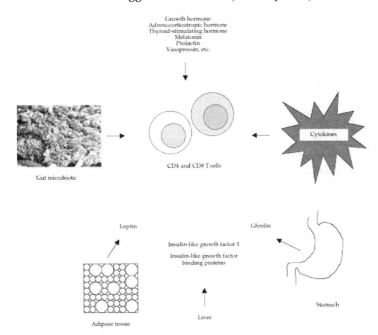

Fig. 4. Some of the potential mechanisms linking metabolic syndrome and T cell maintenance.

First question: may insulin-resistance be the common denominator of the observed familial peculiarities? And therefore, second question: could an early correction of one/some of these common clinical abnormalities modify the natural history of the disease and thence its epidemiology? The data above summarised suggest to consider also alternative ways beyond the traditional immuno-based interventions so far extensively investigated in the field of type 1 diabetes. There is increasing attention to the role of metabolic syndrome and immune responses as well as to the relation between the immune and neuroendocrine systems (Figure 4). The adipocyte-derived proinflammatory hormone leptin can affect the survival and proliferation of autoreactive CD4 T cells (Matarese et al., 2008; Galgani et al., 2010). Immune and neuroendocrine systems have bidirectional communications (Kelley et al., 2007; Berczi et al., 2009). Growth hormone and ghrelin are expressed in immune cells, which in turn bear receptors for these hormones (Hattori, 2009). Leptin, ghrelin, insulin-like growth factor 1, insulin-like growth factor binding protein 3, and cytokines regulate both thymopoiesis and maintenance of T cells. Therefore, elucidation of metabolic syndrome, T cell metabolism, hormones, and microbiota may lead to new insights into the maintenance of proper immune responses (Hsu & Mountz, 2010).

At the present state of knowledge and given the current diabetes epidemic, it would seem reasonable that proper, more realistic, public health interventions (by general and family practitioners) are designed that address general issues such as feeding, lifestyle, overweight, 'borderline' blood pressure, impaired fasting glucose, etc. These health interventions, beyond the conventional boundaries that have for so long limited the visual field, might have a favourable cost-benefit ratio.

9. References

Almasy, L., Gur, R.C., Haack, K., Cole, S.A., Calkins, M.E., Peralta, J.M., Hare, E., Prasad, K., Pogue-Geile, M.F., Nimgaonkar, V., Gur, RE. (2008). A genome screen for quantitative trait loci influencing schizophrenia and neurocognitive phenotypes. *The American Journal of Psychiatry*, Vol. 165, N. 9: 1185–1192.

American Diabetes Association. (2011). Standards of medical care in diabetes-2011. *Diabetes Care*, Vol. 34, N. Supplement 1: S11-S61.

An, P., Rice, T., Pérusse, L., Borecki, I.B., Gagnon, J., Leon, A.S., et al. (2000). Complex segregation analysis of blood pressure and heart rate measured before and after a 20-week endurance exercise training program: the HERITAGE Family Study. *American Journal of Hypertension*, Vol. 13, N. 5 Pt1: 488-497.

Barrett, J.C., Clayton, D.G., Concannon, P., Akolkar, B., Cooper, J.D., Erlich, H.A., Julier, C., Morahan, G., Nerup, J., Nierras, C., Plagnol, V., Pociot, F., Schuilenburg, H., Smyth, D.J., Stevens, H., Todd, J.A., Walker, N.M., Rich, S.S.; Type 1 Diabetes Genetics Consortium. (2009). Genome-wide association study and meta-analysis find that over 40 loci affect risk of type 1 diabetes. *Nature Genetics*, Vol. 4, N. 6: 703-707.

Baynes, J.W., Thorpe, S.R. (1999). Role of oxidative stress in diabetic complications. A new perspective on an old paradigm. *Diabetes*, Vol. 48, N. 1: 1-9.

Bebek, G., Koyutürk, M., Chance, M.R., Price, N.D. (2011). Integrative –omics for translational sciente. In: *Biocomputing 2011. Proceedings of Pacific Symposium*, date of access 2011-03-17, available from: <http://eproceedings.worldscinet.com/ 9789814335058/9789814335058_0001.html>. Berczi, I., Quintanar-Stephano, A., Kovacs, K. (2009). Neuroimmune regulation in immunocompetence, acute illness, and healing. *Annals of the New York Academy of Sciences*, Vol. 1153: 220-239.

The Enlarging List of Phenotypic Characteristics That Might Allow the Clinical Identification of
Families at Risk for Type 1 Diabetes

75

Bingley, P. J. (2010). Clinical application of diabetes antibody testing. *The Journal of Clinical Endocrinology and Metabolism*, Vol. 95, N. 1: 25-33.

Biornholt, J., Erikssen, G., Kjeldsen, S.E., Bodegård, J., Thaulow, E., Erikssen, J. (2003) Fasting blood glucose is independently associated with resting and exercise blood pressure and development of elevated blood pressure. *Journal of Hypertension*, Vol. 21, N. 7: 1383-1389.

Brzustowicz, L.M., Bassett, A.S. (2008). Phenotype matters: the case for careful characterization of relevant traits. *The American Journal of Psychiatry*, Vol. 165, N. 9: 1196–1198.

EURODIAB Substudy 2 Study Group. (2002). Rapid early growth is associated with increased risk of childhood type 1 diabetes in various European populations. *Diabetes Care*, Vol. 25, N. 10: 1755-1760.

Evertsen, J., Alemzadeh, R., Wang, X. (2009). Increasing incidence of pediatric type 1 diabetes mellitus in Southeastern Wisconsin: relationship with body weight at diagnosis. *PLoS ONE*, Vol. 4, N. 9: e6873.

Field, S.F., Howson, J.M., Walker, N.M., Dunger, D.B., Todd, J.A. (2007). Analysis of the obesity gene FTO in 14,803 type 1 diabetes cases and controls. *Diabetologia*, Vol. 50, N. 10: 2218-2220.

Fierabracci, A. (2011). The potential of multimer technologies in type 1 diabetes prediction strategies. *Diabetes/Metabolism Research and Reviews*, Vol. 27, N. 3: 216-229.

Frizzell, N., Lima, M., Baynes, J.W. (2011). *Free Radical Research*, Vol. 45, N. 1: 101-109.

Galgani, M., Procaccini, C., De Rosa V., Carbone, F., Chieffi, P., La Cava, A., Matarese, G. (2010). Leptin modulates the survival of autoreactive CD4+ T cells through the nutrient/energy-sensing mammalian target of rapamycin signaling pathway. *Journal of Immunology*, Vol. 185, N. 12: 7474-7479.

Giampietro, O., Virgone, E., Carneglia, L., Griesi, E., Calvi, D., Matteucci, E. (2002). Anthropometric indices of school children and familiar risk factors. *Preventive Medicine*, Vol. 32, N. 5: 492-498.

Harder, T., Roepke, K., Diller, N., Stechling, Y., Dudenhausen, J.W., Plagemann, A. (2009). Birth weight, early weight gain, and subsequent risk of type 1 diabetes: systematic review and meta-analysis. *American Journal of Epidemiology*, Vol. 169, N. 12: 1428-1436.

Hattori, N. (2009). Expression, regulation and biological actions of growth hormone (GH) and ghrelin in the immune system. *Growth hormone and IGF Research*, Vol. 19, N. 3: 187-197.

Hsu, H.C., Mountz, J.D. (2010). Metabolic syndrome, hormones, and maintenance of T cells during aging. *Current Opinion in Immunology*, Vol. 22, N. 4: 541-548.

Ibegbu, C.C., Xu, Y.X., Fillos, D., Radziewicz, H., Grakoui, A., Kourtis, A.P. (2009). Differential expression of CD26 on virus-specific CD8(+) T cells during active, latent and resolved infection. *Immunology*, Vol. 126, N. 3:346-353.

Ihnat, M.A., Thorpe, J.E., Kamat, C.D., Szabó, C., Green, D.E., Warnke, L.A., et al. (2007). Reactive oxygen species mediate a cellular 'memory' of high glucose stress signalling. *Diabetologia*, Vol. 50, N. 7: 1523-1531.

Invitti, C. (2003). Can glycaemia affect blood pressure? *Journal of Hypertension*, Vol. 21, N. 7: 1265-1267.

Kelley, K.W., Weigent, D.A., Kooijman, R. (2007). Protein hormones and immunity. *Brain, Behavior, and Immunity*, Vol. 21, N. 4: 384-392.

Khadra, A., Tsai, S., Santamaria, P., Edelstein-Keshet, L. (2010). On how monospecific memory-like autoregulatory CD8+ T cells can blunt diabetogenic autoimmunity: a computational approach. *Journal of Immunology*, Vol. 185, N. 10: 5962-5972.

Khaw, K.-T., Wareham, N., Bingham, S., Luben, R., Welch, A., Day, N. (2004). Association of hemoglobin A1c with cardiovascular disease and mortality in adults: the European Prospective Investigation into cancer in Norfolk. *Annals of Internal Medicine*, Vol. 141, N. 6: 413-420.

Knip, M., Korhonen, S., Kulmala, P., Veijola, R., Reunanen, A., Raitakari, O.T., Viikari, J., Akerblom, H.K. (2010). Prediction of type 1 diabetes in the general population. *Diabetes Care*, Vol. 33, N. 6: 1206-1212.

Königshoff, M., Uhl, F., Gosens, R. (2011). From molecule to man: integrating molecular biology with whole organ physiology in studying respiratory disease. *Pulmonary Pharmacology & Therapeutics*, doi:10.1016/j.pupt.2011.02.002.

Lamb, M.M., Dabelea, D., Yin, X., Ogden, L.G., Klingensmith, G.J., Rewers, M., Norris, J.M. (2010). Early-life predictors of higher body mass index in healthy children. *Annals of Nutrition & Metabolism*, Vol. 56, N. 1: 16-22.

Lane, D.J., Lawen, A. (2009). Ascorbate and plasma membrane electron transport-Enzymes vs efflux. *Free Radical Biology & Medicine*, Vol. 47, N. 5:485-495.

Lee, S., Li, R., Kim, B., Palvolgyi, R., Ho, T., Yang, Q.Z., Xu, J., Szeto, W.L., Honda, H., Berliner, J.A. (2009). Ox-PAPC activation of plasma membrane electron transport (PMET) system increases expression of heme oxygenase 1 (HO-1) in human aortic endothelial cell (HAEC). *Journal of Lipid Research*, Vol. 50, N. 2:265-274.

Lonardo, A., Adinolfi, L.E., Petta, S., Craxì, A., Loria, P. (2009). Hepatitis C and diabetes: the inevitable coincidence? *Expert Review of Anti-Infective Therapy*, Vol. 7, N. 3:293-308.

Lowe, C.E., Cooper, J.D., Brusko, T., Walker, N.M., Smyth, D.J., Bailey, R., Bourget, K., Plagnol, V., Field, S., Atkinson, M., Clayton, D.G., Wicker, L.S., Todd, J.A. (2007). Large-scale genetic fine mapping and genotype-phenotype associations implicate polymorphism in the IL2RA region in type 1 diabetes. *Nature Genetics*, Vol. 39, N. 9: 1074-1082.

Maiese, K., Morhan, S.D., Chong, Z.Z. (2007). Oxidative stress biology and cell injury during type 1 and type 2 diabetes mellitus. *Current Neurovascular Research*, Vol. 4, N. 1: 63-71.

Marcovecchio, M.L., Tossavainen, P.H., Acerini, C.L., Barrett, T.G., Edge, J., Neil, A., Shield, J., Widmer, B., Dalton, R.N., Dunger, D.B. (2010). Maternal but not paternal association of ambulatory blood pressure with albumin excretion in young offspring with type 1 diabetes. *Diabetes Care*, Vol. 33, N. 2: 366-371.

Matarese, G., Procaccini, C., De Rosa V. (2008). The intricate interface between immune and metabolic regulation: a role for leptin in the pathogenesis of multiple sclerosis? *Journal of Leukocyte Biology*, Vol. 84, N. 4: 893-899.

Matteucci, E., Consani, C., Masoni, M.C., Giampietro, O. (2010). Circadian blood pressure variability in type 1 diabetic subjects and their nondiabetic siblings – influence of erythrocyte electron transfer. *Cardiovascular Diabetology*, 9: 61 (http://www.cardiab.com/content/9/1/61).

The Enlarging List of Phenotypic Characteristics That Might Allow the Clinical Identification of
Families at Risk for Type 1 Diabetes

77

Matteucci, E., Ghimenti, M., Consani, C., Di Beo, S., Giampietro, O. (2010). About CD26 CD8 lymphocytes in type 1 diabetes. *Scandinavian Journal of Immunology*, Vol. 71, N. 2: 123-124.

Matteucci, E., Ghimenti, M., Consani, C., Masoni, M.C., Giampietro, O. (2011). Exploring mitochondrial membrane potential in type 1 diabetes families. *Cell Biochemistry and Biophysics*, Vol. 59, N. 2: 121-126.

Matteucci, E., Giampietro, O. (2000a). Oxidative stress in families of type 1 diabetic patients. *Diabetes Care*, Vol. 23, N. 8, 1182-1186.

Matteucci, E., Giampietro, O. (2000b). Erythrocyte sodium/hydrogen exchange activity and albuminuria in families of type 1 diabetic patients. *Diabetes Care*, Vol. 23, N. 3, 418-420.

Matteucci, E., Giampietro, O. (2000c). Transmembrane electron transfer in diabetic nephropathy. *Diabetes Care*, Vol. 23, N. 7, 994-999.

Matteucci, E., Giampietro, O. (2001). Oxidative stress in families of type 1 diabetic patients: further evidence. *Diabetes Care*, Vol. 24, N. 1, 167-168.

Matteucci, E., Giampietro, O. (2007). Central Italy: unexpected macro- and micro-nutrient deficiencies in regular diet of residents from Pisa province. The potential role of medical education in young people; In: *Malnutrition in the 21th century*, Editor Vesler L.W., pp. 127-145, Nova Science Publishers, Hauppauge NY, U.S.A.

Matteucci, E., Giampietro, O. (2008). Central Italy: physical activity of female residents from Pisa province, In: *Progress in exercise and women's health research*, Editor Coulter J. P., pp. 241-253, Nova Science Publishers, Hauppauge NY, U.S.A.

Matteucci, E., Malvaldi, G., Fagnani, F., Evangelista, I., Giampietro, O. (2004a). Redox status and immune function in type I diabetes families. *Clinical and Experimental Immunology*, Vol. 136, N. 3: 549-554.

Matteucci, E., Passerai, S., Mariotti, M., Fagnani, F., Evangelista, I., Rossi, L., Giampietro, O. (2004b). Dietary habits and nutritional biomarkers in Italian type 1 diabetes families: evidence of unhealthy diet and combined-vitamin-deficient intakes. *European Journal of Clinical Nutrition*, Vol. 59, N. 1: 114-122.

Matteucci, E., Rosada, J., Pinelli, M., Giusti, C., Giampietro, O. (2006). Systolic blood pressure response to exercise in type 1 diabetes families compared with healthy control individuals. *Journal of Hypertension*, Vol. 24, N. 9: 1745-1751.

Ng, L.L., Simmons, D., Frighi, V., Garrido, M.C., Bomford, J., Hockaday, T.D. (1990). Leukocyte Na+/H+ antiport activity in type 1 (insulin-dependent) diabetic patients with nephropathy. *Diabetologia*, Vol. 33, N. 6: 371-377.

Ohnuma, K., Hosono, O., Dang, N.H., Morimoto, C. (2011). Dipeptidyl peptidase in autoimmune pathophysiology. *Advances in Clinical Chemistry*, Vol. 53: 51-84.

Petersen, K.F., Dufour, S., Befroy, D., Garcia, R., Shulman, G.I. (2004). Impaired mitochondrial activity in the insulin-resistant offspring of patients with type 2 diabetes. *The New England Journal of Medicine*, Vol. 350, N. 7: 664-671.

Rasmussen, T., Stene, L.C., Samuelsen, S.O., Cinek, O., Wetlesen, T., Torjesen, P.A., Rønningen, K.S. (2009). Maternal BMI before pregnancy, maternal weight gain during pregnancy, and risk of persistent positivity for multiple diabetes-associated autoantibodies in children with the high-risk HLA genotype: the MIDIA study. *Diabetes Care*, Vol. 32, N. 10: 1904-1906.

Reis, A.F., Hauache, O. M., Velho, G. (2005). Vitamin D endocrine system and the genetic susceptibility to diabetes, obesity and vascular disease. A review of evidence. *Diabetes & Metabolism*, Vol. 31, N. 4: 318-325.

Roep, B.O. (2008). Islet autoreactive CD8 T-cells in type 1 diabetes: licensed to kill? *Diabetes*, Vol. 57, N. 5: 1156.

Rowe, P.A., Campbell-Thompson, M.L., Schatz, D.A., Atkinson, M.A. (2011) The pancreas in human type 1 diabetes. *Seminars in Immunopathology*, Vol. 33, N. 1: 29-43.

Sharabi, Y., Ben-Cnaan, R., Hanin, A., Martonovitch, G., Grossman, E. (2001). The significance of hypertensive response to exercise as a predictor of hypertension and cardiovascular disease. *Journal of Human Hypertension*, Vol. 15, N. 5: 353-356.

Thorn, L.M., Forsblom, C., Fagerudd, J., Pettersson-Fernholm, K., Kilpikari, R., Groop, P.H.; FinnDiane Study Group. (2007). Clustering of risk factors in parents of patients with type 1 diabetes and nephropathy. *Diabetes Care*, Vol. 30, N. 5 :1162-1167.

van Belle, T.L., Coppieters, K.T., von Herrath, M.G. (2011). Type 1 diabetes: etiology, immunology, and therapeutic strategies. *Physiological Reviews*, Vol. 91, N. 1: 79-118.

Vehik, K., Dabelea, D. (2011). The changing epidemiology of type 1 diabetes: why is it going through the roof? *Diabetes/Metabolism Research and Reviews*, Vol. 27, N. 1: 3-13.

Velthuis, J.H., Unger, W.W., Abreu, J.R., Duinkerken, G., Franken, K., Peakman, M., Bakker, A.H., Reker-Hadrup, S., Keymeulen, B., Drijfhout, J.W., Schumacher, T.N., Roep, B.O. (2010). Simultaneous detection of circulating autoreactive CD8+ T-cells specific for different islet cell-associated epitopes using combinatorial MHC multimers. *Diabetes*, Vol. 59, N. 7: 1721-1730.

Viberti, G.C., Keen, H., Wiseman, M.J. (1987). Raised arterial pressure in parents of proteinuric insulin dependent diabetics. *British Medical Journal*, Vol. 295, N. 6597: 515-51.

Vijayalingam, S., Parthiban, A., Shanmugasundaram, K.R., Mohan, V. (1996). Abnormal antioxidant status in impaired glucose tolerance and non-insulin-dependent diabetes mellitus. *Diabetic Medicine*, Vol. 13, N. 8: 715-719.

Wadén, J., Forsblom, C., Thorn, L.M., Gordin, D., Saraheimo, M., Groop, P.H.; Finnish Diabetic Nephropathy Study Group. (2009). A1C variability predicts incident cardiovascular events, microalbuminuria, and overt diabetic nephropathy in patients with type 1 diabetes. *Diabetes*, Vol. 58, N. 11: 2649-2655.

Walker, J.D., Tariq, T., Viberti, G. (1990). Sodium-lithium countertransport activity in red cells of patients with insulin-dependent diabetes and nephropathy and their parents. *British Medical Journal*, Vol. 301, N. 6753: 635-638.

Wilkin, T.J. (2009) The accelerator hypothesis: a review of the evidence for insulin resistance as the basis for type I as well as type II diabetes. *International Journal of Obesity*, Vol. 34, N:1: 210-211.

Winkler, C., Marienfeld, S., Zwilling, M., Bonifacio, E., Ziegler, A.G. (2009). Is islet autoimmunity related to insulin sensitivity or body weight in children of parents with type 1 diabetes? *Diabetologia*, Vol. 51, N. 10: 2072-2078.

Wray, N.M., Goddard, M.E. (2010). Multi-locus models of genetic risk of disease. *Genome Medicine*, Vol. 2 (N. 2): 10.

Yang, J., Visscher, P.M., Wray, N.M. (2010). Sporadic cases are the norm for complex disease. *European Journal of Human Genetics*, Vol. 18, N. 9: 1039-1044.

4

Diabetes Type 1 and 2:
What is Behind a Classification?

Adriana Mimbacas[1] and Gerardo Javiel[2,3]
[1]Instituto de Investigaciones Biológicas Clemente Estable,
Department of Genetics, Human Genetic Group
[2]ASSE-Ministry of Health, Hospital Pasteur
[3]IAMPP-Centro de Asistencia del Sindicato Médico
del Uruguay,(CASMU), Diabetologic Service
Uruguay

1. Introduction

At present, we wonder if the current classification of diabetes agrees with the new advances At the molecular genetic level. Every day we can see an exponential increase of type 1 and 2 diabetes anywhere in the world. On the other hand, although several clinical and biochemical characteristics have been described in order to differentiate between both types of diabetes, this does not seem satisfactory for all cases when facing the patient. These characteristics are: (a) The presence of a strong familiar history of diabetes, obesity, *acanthosis nigricans*, and lack of ketoacidosis and auto-antibodies against antigens of pancreatic b-cells islets supports the diagnosis of type 2 diabetes; (b) In contrast, patients with type 1 diabetes are usually thin and with ketoacidosis; almost 90% of them have auto-antibodies at the onset of the disease.

Nevertheless, in the last decades numerous reports described adults and adolescents (usually from minority groups) presenting ketoacidosis with lack of antibodies and characteristics of type 2 diabetes such as obesity, *acanthosis nigricans* and/or one significant familiar history of diabetes (Pinhas-Hamiel et al., 1997; Pinhas-Hamiel & Zeitler, 1999;).

Until very recently, most children and adolescents diagnosed with the disease were diagnosed as type 1 diabetes; however, there have recently been numerous reports describing an increase in the number of cases of type 2 diabetes in youngsters (Dabelea et al., 1998; Hathout et al., 2001; Neufeld et al., 1998; Pinhas Hamiel et al., 1996; Scott et al., 1997). Epidemiological data suggests that type 1 and 2 diabetes can coexist in the same family (Kolb & Mandrup-Poulsen, 2005; Libman & Becker, 2003).

The potential importance of formulating a specific diagnosis has been emphasized, as this could determine the type of treatment, associated complications, and outcomes (Fagot et al., 2001; Pinhas-Hamiel & Zeitler, 1999). The current criteria for defining diabetes (Asociación Latinoamericana de Diabetes [ALAD], 2010; American Diabetes Association [ADA], 2010) do not always explain neither the evolution of the disease in different patients or the different responses of individuals to treatments. These facts are suggesting the importance of considering the genetic background of individuals for their categorization and subsequent treatment. A highly controversial topic has recently aroused worldwide: is there a new type of diabetes with mixed characteristics of both types? Different authors have identified this variety as "Double Diabetes" or "Hybrid Diabetes" (Libman & Becker, 2003; Mimbacas et al., 2011; Pozzilli & Buzzetti; 2007; Pozzilli & Guglielmi., 2007); but, are we really facing a new type of diabetes unknown before?, or is it a phenomenon not demonstrated until present due to the use of former inappropriate methodologies or instrumentations? If it is a new expression, why does it appear now? Is there an evolutionary process involved? How?

We will try to discuss these subjects in this chapter.

2. Brief history of diabetes mellitus and the evolution of the classification

In order to understand our point of view we must begin with a brief description of diabetes history and classification. The term diabetes (Greek: διαβητη) was coined by Aretaues of Cappadocia. It is derived from the Greek word διβαινειν, diabaínein that literally means "passing through" or "siphon", a reference to one of diabetes' major symptoms—excessive urine production. In 1675, Thomas Willis added the word mellitus, from the Latin meaning "honey", as a reference to the sweet taste of the urine. Matthew Dobson (1776) confirmed that the sweet taste was due to an excess of a kind of sugar in the urine and blood of people with diabetes. The ancient Indians tested for diabetes by observing whether ants were attracted to a person's urine, and called the ailment "sweet urine disease". The Korean, Chinese, and Japanese words for diabetes are based on the same ideographs (糖尿病), which mean "sugar urine disease".

As stated above, although diabetes has been recognized since antiquity, and treatments of different efficiencies have been known in several regions since the Middle Ages and for much longer in legends, the pathogenesis of diabetes has only been understood experimentally since about 1900 (Patlak, 2002a; 2002b). The endocrine role of the pancreas in metabolism, and indeed the existence of insulin, was not further clarified until 1922, when Banting and Best demonstrated that they could reverse induced diabetes in dogs by giving them a pancreatic islets of Langerhans extract of healthy dogs (Banting et al., 1922). However the precise molecular mechanism of the disease is just beginning to be unraveled. Fortunately, the increasing inventory of human genetic variation is easing our understanding of why susceptibility to the common disease varies between individuals and populations (Rotimi & Jorde, 2010), as we shall see.

In terms of classification, the first distinction between different presentations of the disease, as it is currently known, was clearly established by Sir H P Himsworth, and published in January 1936 (Himsworth, 1936). From its very beginning, the different classifications have undergone changes in the attempt to obtain a better adjustment of the organization of diabetes' nosology (Alberti & Zimmet, 1998): (1) Age, which was the main criterion of the first classification, was quickly abandoned because the different forms can appear at any age, although one is more frequently observed in childhood and youth and the other one in adults (at present, type 1 and 2 respectively); (2) Insulin dependence was the new clinical criterion taken into consideration, because it was easy to use in clinical practice and allowed to consider sub-groups with different pathogenic mechanisms; for several years insulin dependence was an indicator of the auto-immune process.

Currently, the classification of Diabetes mellitus (ADA, 2010; ALAD, 2010) contemplates four well-known major groups: (a) Type 1 Diabetes (T1DM), (b) Type 2 (T2DM), (c) Other specific types of diabetes, and (d) Gestational diabetes.

However, on the basis of clinical observations, genetics and molecular research studies carried out in some mixed populations such as those in Latin America (as we shall see below) would point out that this classification is not always adequate; phenotype does not always reflect genotype (Mimbacas et al., 2009).

3. Miscegenated population

In order to support our hypothesis that phenotype is not always a proper indicator of genotype, mainly in miscegenated populations (particularly in multifactorial diseases such as diabetes), we will focus our analysis on the research carried out in our population. We believe that the current classification does not always allow an accurate diagnosis, and therefore the treatment plan is not always the correct one.

Previous research has shown that the Uruguayan population has a particular genetic behavior; in addition to its small size (three millions inhabitants), it presents such a high level of miscegenation that there are individuals that cannot currently identify their ancestors' origin. It has a tri-hybrid origin (Caucasoid, African and Amerindian) but, unlike other Latin-American countries, we do not isolate Amerindian groups (Cardoso et al., 2004; Gascue et al., 2005; Mimbacas et al., 2003, 2004, 2007, 2009; Sans et al., 2011). Thus, this would permit us to think a priori that ethnological factors would (at least in part) cancel each other, therefore eliminating their possible blurring effect on the analysis. When we consider these factors, we can look at our population as an interesting source of information for the study of different issues on diabetes.

Several years ago, we focused our investigation on HLA genes associated with type 1 diabetes; our studies (Mimbacas et al., 2003, 2004) were done both by case-control and parent-cases design. We found a very high frequency of specific alleles (DQB1*0201, DQB1*0302, DR3, DR4) in our population; although the associated alleles were the same as those of the Caucasian population, their frequencies were different; additionally, we also found that almost all of the patients had associated DR3 and DR4 alleles. Continuing with our investigations, we observed that different polymorphisms of other analyzed genes also showed variations when compared with Caucasian populations or with populations from other origin (Fernández et al., 2009; Mimbacas et al., 2007; Soto et al., 2004; Zorrilla et al., 2006).

Conversely, there have been numerous reports describing an increasing number of type 2 diabetes cases in youngsters (Dabelea et al., 1998; Neufeld et al., 1998; Pinhas-Hamiel et al., 1996; Scott et al., 1997). Recently, Lidman and Becker (2003) described the coexistence of types 1 and 2 diabetes in a non-Caucasian individual; afterwards, Pozzili and Buzzetti (2007) described more cases and defined the possibility of a new type of diabetes, proposing more characterization studies in different ethnic groups. In a recent paper (Mimbacas et al., 2011) we described a case report that, according to our criteria, showed this type of presentation of the disease.

In what it has to do with this possibility of a new expression of diabetes, it is important to determine the influence of the genetic and auto-immune factors underlying the consequent destruction of the beta islets, which would pass unnoticed in a classic phenotype.

In the light of an emerging expression of diabetes, and in an attempt to link genetics to the clinic, we continued with our research. On the basis of previous findings and in the clinical evolution of patients, we began to see that in many cases it was very difficult to classify patients into one of the 2 main groups of the current diabetes classification (type 1 or type 2). Another associated observation was that, despite following the international protocols, patients did not always show a good response to treatment.

Therefore, we were interested in testing the hypothesis that genotype does not necessarily result in the disease phenotype. For this purpose, we proposed to determine whether a genetic profile is useful for providing the clinician and the patient with more accurate information, not only for knowing the specific type of diabetes, but also to understand the hyperglycemia pathogenesis and thus treat it more effectively.

For five years we examined a dynamic cohort of clinical histories of diabetes' patients, with a follow up of 86.6% (Mimbacas et al., 2009). At first, patients were classified into two groups: type 1 diabetes and type 2 diabetes according to the American Diabetes Association criteria (ADA, 2004). We analyzed HLADQB1*/DR in all samples and studied the presence of autoantibodies glutamic acid decarboxylase (GADA) and islet cell (ICA). We found surprising results, specifically in patients diagnosed as type 2 diabetes. When we applied the classification grouping the patients as type 1 and type 2 to our data, we found that the phenotype was not correlated with the expected data in all cases. In order to improve our knowledge of the pathogenesis of hyperglycemia and thus implement a more accurate treatment for the patients, we reclassified our sample according to the presence or absence of the genetic and immunological markers (Figure 1).

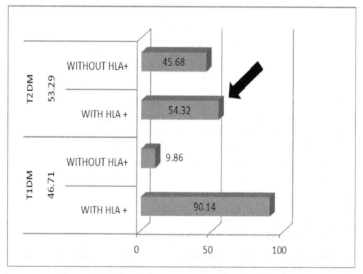

Fig. 1. A high percent of type 2 diabetes have HLA susceptibility gene for type 1 diabetes.

The data obtained shows statistical significant differences, implying that the clinical classification is probably not discriminatory enough for an accurate classification of different types of diabetes (Mimbacas et al., 2009). The methodology implemented in this investigation permitted us to establish that the phenotypic classification did reflect neither the genetic profile nor the immunological disease. The genetic data can help us to provide an accurate definition of the disease, and would therefore give the physician a better possibility of providing an adequate treatment.

Today, a proper differentiation between the different types of diabetes is becoming an increasingly challenging task. The effect of genetic variables on diabetes has been studied for several decades, but there are only a few consistent risk factors identified up to date.

Most of the large scale studies on candidate genes for diabetes published so far have not performed a combined analysis of both types of diabetes; moreover, there are a high number of published papers dealing with this subject but whose populations are not admixed like the Uruguayan one. Thus, we consider that the Uruguayan population is an interesting one to accomplish epidemiological studies, and that it will therefore contribute to the discussion. Unfortunately, currently there are a very few researchers using new advanced methodology, such as genome wide association, in non-Caucasian population; nearly 90% of genome scan studies have been carried out in populations of European ancestry (Rotimi & Jorde, 2010).

4. Overweight and obesity mask a genetic profile associated to type 1 diabetes

As stated above, once diabetes diagnosed, proper classification is the first difficulty of this disease in clinical practice, as future treatment will depend on this. This is partly due to a lack of correlation between phenotype and genotype, and to the possible existence of a new form of diabetes, or a different expression, called "hybrid or double". This may pass inadvertently if the corresponding genetic and immunological analyses are not carried out.

Overweight or obesity is one phenotypic trait that is part of the definition of type 2 diabetes. In our study (Mimbacas et al., 2009) we observed that many patients clinically diagnosed as type 2 with positive HLA show overweight or obesity; we therefore suggested looking for a genetic explanation for this apparent contradiction. Overweight or obesity is indicative of insulin-resistance. The primary disorder type 2 diabetes is considered as an insulin-resistant one with an increase in insulin secretion and a decrease in beta cell secretion after several years (Ruiz, 2011).

On the other hand, the importance of a study on insulin resistance lies in the fact that the underlying process would be a cardiovascular risk factor per se (Howard et al., 1996; Yip et al., 1998).

Despite evidence of a genetic influence, bibliography suggests that the genetic contribution to insulin resistance is the result of several gene variants that are relatively common in the population, each one with only a moderate influence, but with much more stronger effects when they interact. The heterogeneous and polygenic nature of insulin resistance has made the identification of these gene variants a challenging task. However, once these insulin-resistance susceptibility gene variants are identified, they will have far-reaching implications for our comprehension of the molecular and pathophysiologic basis of insulin resistance, type 2 diabetes and related clustered traits, and thus for the treatment and prevention of these endemic disorders (Mercado et al., 2002).

From the molecular point of view, Insulin-Resistance is caused by different metabolic pathways with gene-gene and gene-environment interactions. In order to begin our study, we selected some of the genes found within these pathways; the first selected gene was the Peroxisome Proliferator-Activated Receptor (PPARγ2) gene, which is in turn one of the strongest candidate genes contributing to the susceptibility of type 2 diabetes, especially the

Pro12Ala polymorphism (de Dios & Frechtel, 2011). The PPARγ gene is a key regulator of lipid metabolism and energy balance, and it is implicated in the development of insulin resistance and obesity. It is a member of the nuclear hormone receptor family involved in adipocyte differentiation and gene expression regulation, and it is a transcriptional factor involved in adipogenesis and regulation of adipocyte gene expression. PPARγ plays a role in insulin signaling, insulin resistance and the development of type 2 diabetes mellitus (Chawla et al., 1994; Auwerx, 1999; Zhang et al., 2007)

A splice variant of this gene contains a common amino acid polymorphism, Pro12Ala (carrier frequencies 8–20%, depending on the population) that, depending on the cell lines, reduces the ligand-induced activity of the PPARγ protein by 30–50% (Altshuler et al., 2000; Deeb et al., 1998; Hansen et al., 2006). This missense mutation (involving a C to G substitution at nucleotide 34) results in the exchange of a proline for an alanine in position 12 of the PPARγ2 protein (Yen et al., 1997). This polymorphism has been associated with a reduced risk of development of a type 2 diabetes mellitus (Altshuler et al., 2000; Stumvoll et al., 2001). Many studies have suggested that the mechanism of reduction of the risk of type 2 diabetes mellitus by this polymorphism involves enabling greater insulin sensitivity. The Pro12Ala polymorphism produces a PPARγ2 protein with lower transcriptional activity (Deeb et al., 1998; Kang et al., 2005). The Diabetes Prevention Program (DPP) found that the Ala12 allele influences central obesity and that it is associated with the differences seen in the different treatment groups regarding polyunsaturated fatty acid intake (DPP, 2008).

In recent years, research has identified PPARs as pivotal actors in the transcriptional control of the Uncoupling Protein genes (UCP) (Villarroya et al., 2007). Thus we selected this one as a possible second gene responsible for IR. UCP-2 are mitochondrial transporters present in the inner membrane of the mitochondria of several cells (Das & Elbein, 2006; Villaroya et al., 2007). Their main function is the uncoupling of oxidative phosphorylation in the respiratory chain, preventing the formation of ATP from the energy released by substrate oxidation, and promoting its dissipation as heat.

The UCP would be in charge of the so-called adaptive thermogenesis, i.e. the generation or dissipation of heat to certain stimuli, such as overeating, cold and exercise, thus regulating temperature and body weight. Other functions have been described, in the case of UCP-2, that takes part in the regulation of insulin secretion (inhibiting its secretion by lowering the ATP synthesis through uncoupling), in immunity, and decreased oxidative stress. Their presence in different tissues, together with their energy dissipating role, could be crucial in explaining not only the genesis of obesity, but certain co morbidities (diabetes mellitus type 2) and their treatment.

A common polymorphism (-866G/A) has been associated with obesity, insulin secretion, and type 2 diabetes (Bell et al., 2005; Freeman and Cox, 2006). In what it has to do with the genetic-environmental interaction, several evidences indicate a fatty acid-dependent activation of UCP-2. Direct analysis of regulation of the promoter of the UCP-2 gene in muscle cells indicated that PPARγ and their ligands induce promoter activity (Aubert et al., 1997), while PPAR activators induce UCP-2 mRNA expression in brown adipocytes. Adipose tissue contains large amounts of endogenous triglycerides, which are capable of causing the local generation of free fatty acids after lipolysis. PPAR receptors can provide a mechanism for responsiveness of UCP-2 expression to intracellularly-derived fatty acid.

Thus cross-talk between adrenergic regulation of adipose tissue lipolysis and PPAR induction mechanisms of UCP-2 gene expression may occur, especially in response to noradrenergic stimulus in brown adipocytes (Carmona et al., 1998; Villaroya et al., 2007).

With regard to diabetes, the overexpression of PPARγ causes up regulation of UCP-2 expression and suppresses glucose-stimulated insulin secretion (Ito et al., 2004). However, there are situations where patients can, due to these genes, present the wild type variant and yet remain with their obesity and IR unchanged. Because of this, we selected another gene that may cause IR on the other metabolic pathway: IRS-1.

IRS-1: Genetic variance in the insulin receptor substrate-1 is thought to play a key role in the insulin resistance that characterizes type 2 diabetes. Transfection studies have demonstrated that the most common IRS-1 variant, Arg972, which involves a Gly 224 Arg substitution at codon 972, impairs insulin signaling via the phosphatidylinositol-3 (PI3)-kinase pathway, and in some (but not all) studies this variant has been found with an increased frequency among type 2 diabetic patients (Almind et al., 1993, 1996; Imai et al., 1994; Sesti et al., 2001; Sigal et al., 1996; Zhang et al., 1996). Interestingly, carriers of the Arg972 substitution have been found to have lower fasting insulin and C-peptide levels than noncarriers (Clausen et al., 1995; Stumvoll et al., 2001), suggesting that this IRS-1 variant might also play a role in the secretory capacity of the beta-cells. Indeed, impaired insulin secretion has also been observed in rat insulinoma (RIN) cells overexpressing the Arg972 IRS-1 polymorphism (Porzio et al., 1999), in human islets naturally carrying the variant (Marchetti et al., 2002), and even in normal glucose-tolerant subjects with the Arg972 variant. These observations raise the intriguing hypothesis that genetic defects in the IRS-1/PI3 kinase pathway might also be involved in the inadequate insulin secretion that characterizes type 2 diabetes. More recent studies suggest that the Arg972 IRS-1 variant also plays a role in beta cell survival.

The human Arg972 islets contain a significantly higher number of apoptotic cells than their wild-type counterparts, and they are also resistant to the antiapoptotic effects of insulin (Federici et al., 2003). It has been speculated that apoptosis plays a crucial role in the autoimmune destruction of beta cells characterizing type 1 diabetes (Mathis et al., 2001). An increase in apoptosis might have pathological consequences in diabetes prone individuals, who have an auto-reactive T-cell repertoire that may be activated by the exposed beta-cell antigens. The Arg972 variant of the IRS-1 seems to play a complex role in the pathogenesis of diabetes, affecting both peripheral insulin sensitivity and the functional capacities of the pancreatic beta-cells themselves. In the light of our findings, it is possible to speculate that the same mechanisms —in the presence of a genetically determined predisposition— might also result in, or contribute to, different clinical manifestations of diabetes.

Once we have identified the genes to be analyzed, we decided to test our hypothesis: there are patients with a complex clinical autoimmune disease masked by insulin-resistance which in turn is genetically determined.

The results of our research, although not published yet, were presented in recent meetings in our country and international events as the "1st Latin American Congress: Controversies to Consensus in Diabetes, Obesity and Hypertension [CODHy]" and the "XIV Latin-American Congress of Asociación Latinoamericana de Diabetes [ALAD]" (Fabregat et al., 2010; Farias et al., 2010; Fernández et al., 2010; Mimbacas et al., 2010; Reyes et al., 2010; Souto et al., 2010).

Indeed, all patients tested (presence of HLA and positive susceptibility to type 1 diabetes antibody) with a body mass index >25kg/m^2 and clinical diagnosis of type 2 diabetes were overweight or obese with mutations in one or more of the analyzed genes. Our results indicated that insulin resistance in patients with complex diagnosis may be explained by the occurrence of a mutation in one or more of the analyzed single nucleotide polymorphisms (SNPs).

5. Importance of genetics for the clinician

In the last 15 to 20 years, clinicians have been concerned with grasping the increasing complexity of this disease, with a gradual worldwide increase of its prevalence that has turned it into a pandemic disease. The latest evidence shows that, despite correcting their lifestyle, we cannot always achieve good metabolic control in patients in complex clinical situations.

There is a population, which is probably formed by most of our patients, with clinical features where their phenotype is a good reflection of their genotype; but we are finding with increasingly frequency clinical cases that are difficulty to classify with the current criteria.

In these cases, a high percentage of patients had severe difficulties with their metabolic control. It is precisely here where we need to carry out a proper genetic diagnosis, and eventually an immunologic one, to allow us a broader view of their pathology. Several clinical observations and systematic studies have shown that classical type 1 diabetes, whether in children, late onset in adults, or individuals over 65, can coexist in the same individual with "classic" type 2 diabetes where insulin secretion deficiency and insulin resistance are detected simultaneously (Serrano Rios, 2009). This group of patients is usually referred to a diabetes specialist because the primary care physician cannot decide about or control them. Once reached this stage and after correcting the variables that affect proper metabolic control, such as nutritional plan and regular physical activity, we can see that many of these patients keep having a poor metabolic control. These patients are usually overweight and / or obese with a very erratic response to anti-diabetic drugs alone or in combination, both between them and with insulin.

Complying with the algorithms, we almost always end up giving insulin to our patients, but in many cases this is probably done too late. This was analyzed by many authors that described as final: "therapeutic inertia". They are usually described as patients with a poor adherence to the treatment plan. Also, on average they start insulin treatment before the classical diabetes type 2 patients.

Thus, we are planning to deepen into genetic typing, in order to see if it may help us to understand the etiopathogenesis of these patients, and why they do not have the expected response to the drug treatment.

As stated above, these patients surprisingly had a genotype that does not agree with their phenotype. This was what allowed us as clinicians to begin to understand these facts and to find an explanation (albeit partial) of the poor outcome of each patient.

What are the issues that the clinician should consider for further study of certain patients?

a. Obese patients showing good response to insulin during intercurrence: many of these patients had an intercurrent disease, and with the temporary insulin treatment they achieved a good control (especially in early stages of diagnosis) that may be explained by an improvement in glucotoxicity and / or moderate insulinopenia. In these patients the insulin will be removed based on these myths: (1) Insulin is "ineffective"; (2) Insulin injection increases cardiovascular diseases and hyperinsulinemia; and (3) Insulin causes weight gain. The reluctance we see in these patients insulin is based on misguided or questionable in view of the genetic results we are finding and the matching clinical trials.

b. Poor response to insulin sensitizers: in particular thiazolidinedione but also biguanides.

c. Poor response to secretagogues: it is usually attributed to glucotoxicity, but how much influence does drug response have?

d. Obese patients without dyslipidemia or other elements of metabolic syndrome.
e. Overweight or obese type 2 diabetes patients with hypoglycemia episodes, especially at night.
f. Type 2 Diabetic patients with microangiopathic complications preceding or concomitant to the macrovascular complications.

Already, Nolan and Murphy (2001) posed an approach to the phenotypic and metabolic characterization of insulin-resistant patients, impaired glucose tolerance, or type 2 diabetes, and the use of glutamic acid decarboxylase antibodies (GADA), genetic markers, and models to estimate the insulin-resistance should be considered. These authors discuss the utility of using genetic markers based on population studies for type 2 diabetes mellitus. In what it has to do with the poor response to treatment, we must remember that both therapeutic inefficiency and drug toxicity, which have been seen in some individuals, have been frequently observed. Due to the presence of some drug metabolizing enzymes, drugs can participate as inhibitors or inducers of these enzymes, thereby their variation in activity between individuals. This variability in enzyme activity may reflect the existence of mutations in their genes.

6. Conclusion: What is happening?

The above mentioned points will lead us to review the different mechanisms that may have taken place in the evolutionary processes leading to the current status of this disease. We will consider some possible situations.

a. Researchers are considering the way natural selection is currently operating in humans. The concept of "the survival of the strongest individual" perhaps is no longer valid in the 21st century. Quintana Murci et al. (2007), at the Pasteur Institute (Paris), have looked for answers regarding the mechanisms of human evolution by comparing whole genomes of different populations. They analyzed more than 2.8 million genetic markers in different populations from different ethnic groups collected in the HAPMAP project. They found that 582 genes were subject to "strong selective pressures" during the last 60,000 to 10,000 years. Some of these genes are strongly associated to external features (e.g.: hair, skin color); others are to the response to pathogenic agents or drugs; and others to diseases with different incidences between populations, like diabetes, obesity, or hypertension. Barreiro pointed out that "it is the first time that it can be demonstrated, concerning the whole genome that natural selection participates in the differentiation of the populations" This work is not only useful to satisfy our curiosity, but also to aid in the identification of genes implied in different diseases (Barreiro et al., 2005; 2008).

Well defined since the XV century, clinical knowledge on diabetes gradually increased, and in the end two major distinct types of this pathology were described (1 and 2). In order to understand the current increase of chronic diseases, it is necessary to consider the important relationship between human feeding and human evolution. The regular offer of food that seemed to help human evolution so greatly in the past is also generating a great amount of diseases and their corresponding incapacities (like hemiplegics, aphasia, amputations, etc.). This fact is a true evolutionary paradox (Insua & Fuks, 2003).

Initially, we must consider the importance of the neutralization of positive selective pressure introduced by the availability of nutrients as consequence of human civilization. A good example of the relationship between nutritional factors, diabetes, and population genetics is Szathmary's hypothesis (Marrodán, 2000) for explaining the high incidence of diabetes in several Amerindian populations (USA and Canada), either in reservations or in those adapted to western life.

Diabetes is a genetic-based disease whose manifestation is partly favored by excessive carbohydrate consumption. Possibly, several individuals with a specific genotype would produce insulin faster when faced with higher glucose levels than others; and they would also store this glucose as glycogen or fat more efficiently. This genotype would have been positively selected in a nutritional environment where periods of abundant or shortage of foods oscillate in a critical form. But this capacity for a faster answer to carbohydrate stimulus has a biological cost when food intake is constant. Under this situation, genes increasing insulin production are no longer beneficial to the individual because their carriers become obese, exhausting the physiological capacity of the pancreas, and leading to the subsequent development of diabetes (Marrodán, 2000; Harris, 2002). Variations in diabetes or obesity genes imply that adaptation to fasting was also an important selective agent. Quintana-Murci et al. (2007) pointed out that insulin-regulating genes have been positively selected. Thus, for instance, the ENPP1 gene has a mutation protecting against obesity and type II diabetes. This variant is present in 90% of non-African individuals and it is almost absent in African ones.

The susceptible genotype may have been selected in these populations because unusually frequent fasting periods may have taken place during the initial colonization of 'new worlds'. The abovementioned non-insulin dependent diabetes mellitus has shown a strong genetic component that may include a 'thrifty' genotype(s) (Neel 1962; Zimmet et al., 1990).

The 'thrifty' genotype(s) may have once allowed founding populations to survive both 'feast' and 'famine' conditions for several generations. Individuals carrying these genes would have had an increased efficiency for energy extraction (nutrition) from environmental scarce resources. During times of abundance those individuals with this predisposition would store more energy than those lacking it. When the progress of human civilization assured continuous fat-rich and fiber-poor diets, and a sedentary lifestyle, the 'thrifty' genotype(s) became disadvantageous, leading to obesity, increased insulin resistance, beta cell misbalance, and finally diabetes (Wendorf, 1991; 1992).

What was a selective advantage in past environments is currently, for most people in industrialized countries, an undesired condition. The result is obesity, diabetes, and the metabolic syndrome. For many years, diabetes was considered as a lethal or near-fatal disease by death simply by complications or by difficulties in the reproductive stages, both for men and women. More recently —the use of insulin is a landmark in this subject— reproductive problems and some of their related complications have been solved.

In conclusion, evolutionary or Darwinian medicine considers that many contemporary diseases are associated to incompatibility between current human lifestyles and environments, and those under which human biology was shaped. As the observed difference between the incremental rates of both civilization and evolution is so great, most human evolutionary changes took place when our ancestors were gatherer-hunters. Thus, many characteristics and conducts that had adaptive value in the past may currently have non-adaptive value. Medicine has always tried to improve and look for the patient's cure. It really improved people's health, but in this process populational issues that are beyond the epidemiologic point of view were overlooked. This medical conduct may be explained by the lack of information, or misinterpretation, of the importance of the genetic components of the disease. But this disregarding could be considered also as having iatrogenic elements: we improve the current patient's quality of life, but on the other hand we hamper that of future persons. This process implies the emergence of currently unknown entities. New discoveries have allowed life extension for affected people, with the subsequent appearance of new pathological complications that were not seen before simply because affected individuals passed away before their onset.

b.   Are we witnessing a new type of diabetes, called "double o hybrid" by some authors? We believe that the phenomenon we are watching is simply another expression of the multifactorial nature of this disease. When we analyze populations with an ethnic mixture or of different ethnic origins, we begin to get a glimpse of the products of genetic admixture. This leads us to find a higher proportion of problematic patients that are difficult to classify because, when examining their phenotype, they are affected by certain genes that are masked by others. Hence, we can see families where, according to traditional classification, both entities (type 1 and type 2) coexist. This fusion would be associated with a new and intermediate phenotype (Tuomi, 2005). There are a few studies identifying patients where both type of diabetes overlap (Libman &. Becker, 2003; Pozzilli & Gugliemi, 2009); moreover, Pozzilli and Gugliemi (2007) place this entity in the middle of the double "rainbow" (made up of type 1 and type 2 diabetes).

The "accelerator hypothesis" is a theory that shares this vision. It is a singular, unifying concept, which states that type 1 and type 2 diabetes are the same insulin-resistance disorder set against different genetic backgrounds. This hypothesis does not deny the role of autoimmunity, only its primacy in the process. It distinguishes type 1 and 2 diabetes only by tempo, the faster tempo reflecting the (inevitably) earlier presentation in the more susceptible genotype (Wilkin, 2009).

Recognition that susceptibility arises through the combination of multiple genetic pathways influencing hazardous factors in a nonlinear manner suggests that a 'decanalization' process contributes to the epidemic nature of common genetic diseases. The evolution of the human genome, combined with a marked environmental and cultural perturbation in the past two generations, might lead to the uncovering of cryptic genetic variations that are a major source of disease susceptibility (Gibson, 2009).

This would be also favored by others processes such as an increase of life expectancy and fertility of affected individuals, the globalization phenomena, and increased admixture of different ethnic groups when compared with the past. The last phenomenon is clearly seen in Latin America and mainly in the Uruguayan population as it was stated above.

Regardless of all the arguments presented in this chapter, we think that it is extremely important to introduce the genetic risk profile into the present diabetes classification criteria. This will clearly improve our capability of distinguishing between different types of diabetes or specific presentations.

The effects of genetic traits in diabetes had been studied for decades, but few consistent risk factors have been well established. Currently, most of large scale studies on candidate genes do not combine the analysis of both types of diabetes. Establishing the association between genotype and phenotype would allow a deeper insight into the pathogenesis of the disease. Screening of associated anomalies and the possibility of anticipating future outcomes would be consequently improved.

While for many countries, especially in Latin-America, individual genetic diagnosis can be very expensive to implement, we must realize that we are facing a multifactorial disease.

Thus, although classifications may be useful, they only have relative value. We must keep an open mind to the fact that there are patients that do not fall in any of them, and we must remember that genetics is at the base of diabetes, as there are multiple genes that interact both with the environment and between them. These interactions can result in a somewhat "liar" phenotype. In the preceding sections we saw how mutations in a few genes associated to insulin resistance may mask the presence and/or action of genes causing autoimmune disorders. Moreover, if we take into account the modifications observed with genome scanning, where there are millions of Single Nucleotide Polymorphisms, it is virtually impossible to make a phenotype-based classification.

Although we are aware that understanding the pathogenesis of hyperglycemia or the basis for an effective treatment may be deemed as more important than knowing the type of diabetes we are dealing with, we are currently persuaded that the distinguishing between different types or presentation forms of diabetes based on genetic information is an important task that has turned into our great challenge.

7. Acknowledgment

This chapter could not have been written without the valuable collaboration of graduate and postgraduate students that are part of our research group (in alphabetic list): Br. Matías Fabregat, B.S. Joaquina Farías, MSc. Mariana Fernández, B.S. Ana Laura Reyes, Br. Jorge Souto, MSc. Pilar Zorrilla.

8. References

ADA (2004). American Diabetes Association. Diagnosis and Classification of Diabetes Mellitus, American Diabetes Association. *Diabetes Care* Vol. 27 (s1), (January, 2004), pp.55-60, ISSN 0149-5992

ADA (2010). American Diabetes Association (2010). Diagnosis and Classification of Diabetes Mellitus. *Diabetes Care*, Vol.33, (January, 2010), pp.S62-S69; doi:10.2337/dc10-S062, ISSN 0149-5992.

ALAD (2010). Asociación Latinoamericana de Diabetes. Guías ALAD de diagnóstico control y tratamiento de la Diabetes Mellitus Tipo 2. pp 1-78
    http://www.revistaalad.com.ar/guias/GuiasALAD_DMTipo2_v3.pdf.

Alberti, K.G. & Zimmet, P.Z. (1998). For the WHO Consultation: Definition, diagnosis and classification of diabetes mellitus and its complications. I. Diagnosis and classification of diabetes mellitus: provisional report of a WHO Consultation. *Diabetes Medicine*, Vol.15, N°7, (July 1998), pp.539 –553, ISSN 1464-5491.

Almind, K.; Bjorbaek, C.; Vestergaard, H.; Hansen, T.; Echwald, S. & Pedersen, O. (1993) Amino-acid polymorphisms of insulin-receptor substrate-1 in non-insulin-dependent diabetes-mellitus. *Lancet*, Vol.342, N° 8875, (October 1993), pp.828-832, ISSN 1474-4422.

Almind, K.; Inoue, G.; Pedersen, O. & Kahn, C.R. (1996) A common amino acid polymorphism in insulin-receptor substrate-1 causes impaired insulin signalling evidence from transfection studies. *Journal Clinical Investigation*, Vol.97, N°11, (Jun 1996), pp.2569-2575, ISSN 1365-2362

Altshuler, D.; Hirschhorn, J.N.; Klannemark, M.; lindgren C.M.; Vohl, M.C.; Nemesh, J.; Lane, C.R.; Schaffner, S.F.; Bolk, S.; Brewer, C.; Tuomi, T.; Gaudet, D.; Hudson, T.J.;

Daly, M.; Groop, L. & Lander, L.S. (2000). The common PPARgamma Pro12Ala polymorphism is associated with decreased risk of type 2 diabetes. *Nature Genetics* Vol.26, N°.1, (September 2000), pp.76-80. ISSN 1061-4036.

Aubert, J.; Champigny, O.; Saint-Marc P.; Negrel, R.; Collins, S.; Ricquier, D. & Ailhaud, G. (1997). Up-regulation of UCP-2 gene expression by PPAR agonists in preadispose and adipose cell. *Biochemical Biophysical Research Communications*, Vol.238, N°2, (September 1997), pp.606-611, ISSN. 1090-2104.

Auwerx, J. (1999). PPARgamma, the ultimate thrfty gene. *Diabetologia*, Vol. 42, N°.9, (September 1999), pp.1033-1049, ISSN 0012-186X

Banting, F.G.; Best, C.H.; Collip, J.B.; Campbell, W.R. & Fletcher, A.A. (1922). Pancreatic extract in the treatment of diabetes mellitus. *Canadian Medical Association Journal*, Vol. 12, N°3, (March 1922), pp.141–146, ISSN. 0008-4409

Barreiro, L.B.; Patin, E.; Neyrolles, O.; Cann, H.M.; Gicquel, B. & Quintana-Murci, L. (2005). The heritage of pathogen pressures and ancient demography in the human innate immunity *CD209/CD209L* region. *American Journal of Human Genetic*, Vol.77, N°5, (August 2005), pp. 869-886, ISSN 1537-6605.

Barreiro, L.B.; Laval, G.; Quach, H.; Patin, E. & Quintana Murci, L. (2008). Natural selection has driven population differentiation in modern humans *Nature genetics*, Vol.40, N°.3, (February 2008), pp.340-345, ISSN 1061-4036.

Bell, Ch.G.; Walley, A.J. & Froguel Ph. (2005). The genetics of human obesity. *Nature Reviews Genetics*, Vol. 6, N°.3, (March 2005), pp.221-234, doi:10.1038/nrg1556, ISSN 1061-4036

Cardoso, H.; Crispino, B.; Mimbacas, A. & Cardoso, E. (2004). A low prevalence of cystic fibrosis in Uruguayans of mainly European descent. *Genetics Molecular Research* Vol.3, N°.2, (March 2004) pp.258-263 ISSN 1676-5680.

Carmona, M.C.; Valmaseda, A.; Iglesias, R.; Mampel, T.; Viñas, O.; Giralt, M. & Villaroya, F. (1998). 9-cis retinoic acid induces the expression of uncoupling protein-2 gene in brown adipocytes. *Federation of European Biochemical Societies*, Vol.441, N°.3, (December 1998), pp.447-450, ISSN 1873-3468.

Chawla, A.; Schwarz, E.J.; Dimaculangan, D.D. & Lazar, M.A. (1994) Peroxisome proliferator-activated receptor (PPAR) gamma: adipose-predominant expression and induction early in adipocyte differentiation. *Endocrinology*, Vol. 135, N°2, (August 1994), pp.798-800, ISSN. 0013-7227.

Clausen, J.; Hansen, T.; Bjoerbaek, C.; Echwald, S.; Urhammer, S.; Rasmussen, S.; Andersen, C.; Hansen, L.; Almind, K.; Winther, K.; Haraldsdottir, J.; Borch-Johnsen, K. & Pedersen, O. (1995). Insulin resistance: Interactions between obesity and a common variant of the insulin receptor substrate-1. *Lancet*, Vol.346, N°8972, (August 1995), pp.397-402, ISSN 0140-6736.

Dabelea, D.; Hanson, R.; Bennett, P.H.; Roumain, J.; Knowler, W.C. & Pettitt, D.J. (1998). Increasing prevalence of type 2 diabetes in American Indian children. *Diabetologia*, Vol.41, N°8, (August 1998), pp. 904 – 910, ISSN 0012-186X.

Das, S.K. & Elbein, S.C. (2006). The Genetic Basis of Type 2 Diabetes. *Cellscience*, Vol.2, No.4, (August 1994), pp.100–131, ISSN 1742-8130.

De Dios A. & Frechtel G. Ruiz M. (2011). Genética molecular de la diabetes y sus complicaciones. In: *Diabetes mellitus*, M. Ruiz & M.L. Ruiz Morosini, pp.27-31, Acadia, ISBN 978-987-570-153-3, Buenos Aires, Argentina.

Deeb, S.S.; Fajas, L.; Nemoto, M.; Pihlajamäki, J.; Mykkänen, L.; Kuusisto, J.; Laakso, M.; Fujimoto, W & Auwerx, J. (1998). A Pro12Ala substitution in PPARgamma2 associated with decreased receptor activity, lower body mass index and improved insulin sensitivity. *Nature Genetics*, Vol.20, No.3, (November 1998), pp. 284-287, ISSN 1061-4036.

Dobson, M. Nature of the urine in diabetes. Medical Observations and Inquiries, 1776, Vol.5. pp.298–310 In: Goldfine ID & Youngre JF. (1998). Contributions of the American Journal of Physiology to the discovery of insulin. *Endocrinology Metabolism* Vol.37, (February 1998), E207–E209, 1998, ISSN 94143-161

DPP   (Clinical Trils.gov ID n°: NCT00004992). NIH Publication No. 06–5099 http://ndep.nih.gov/media/DPP_FactSheet.pdf, July 2008, http://diabetes.niddk.nih.gov/dm/pubs/preventionprogram/

Fabregat, M.; Javiel, G.; Vitarella, G. & Mimbacas, A. (2010). Estudio de frecuencias génicas del SNP -23Hph1 como segundo loci de susceptibilidad en la población con diabetes en el Uruguay. XIV Congreso de la Asociación Latinoamericana de Diabetes (ALAD), Santiago de Chile, Chile, 7-11 Noviembre http://www.congresoaladchile2010.com/pdfs/trabajos_modalidad_oral.pdf .

Farias, J.; Fabregat, M.; Reyes, A.L.; Souto, J.; Fernandez, M.; Javiel, G.; Vitarella, G. & Mimbacas, A. (2010). El perfil genético como herramienta en la identificación de pacientes con Doble Diabetes. V Congreso Uruguayo de Endocrinología y Metabolismo (SUEM) Montevideo 2-4 de Setiembre, Montevideo, Uruguay http://www.congresoaladchile2010.com/pdfs/trabajos_modalidad_poster.pdf

Federici, M.; Pertrone, A.; Porzio, O.; Bizzarri, C.; Lauro, D.; Alfonso, R.; Patera, I.; Cappa, M.; Nistico, L.; Baroni, M.; Sesti, G.; Di Mario, U.; Lauro, R. & Buzzetti, R. (2003) The Gly9723Arg IRS-1 Variant Is Associated with Type 1 Diabetes in Continental Italy. *Diabetes*,Vol.52, N°3, (March 2003), pp.887–890, ISSN. 0012-1797

Fernández, M.; Acosta, M.; Airaudo, C.; Fernández, J.; Ferrero, R.; Javiel, G.; Pena, A.; Simonelli, B.; Soto, E.; Vitarella, G. & Mimbacas. A. (2009). Estudio comparativo de prevalencia del gen de la ECA en muestras de diabéticos y población general. Revista Médica del Uruguay, Vol.25, N°2 (June 2009), pp. 110-115, ISSN 1688-0390.

Fernández, M.; Javiel, G.; Vitarella, G. & Mimbacas, A. (2010) Estudio preliminar de test genético moleculares sencillos que permitan determinar si el paciente tendrá una buena respuesta al tratamiento inicial con metformina. XIV Congreso de la Asociación Latinoamericana de Diabetes (ALAD), Santiago de Chile, Chile, 7-11 Noviembre http://www.congresoaladchile2010.com/pdfs/trabajos_modalidad_poster.pdf.

Freeman, H. & Cox, R.D. (2006). Type-2 diabetes: a cocktail of genetic discovery. *Human Molecular Genetics*, Vol. 15, N°2, (July 2006), pp. R202–R209, ISSN 1460-2083.

Gascue, C.; Mimbacas, A.; Sans, M.; Gallino, J.P.; Bertoni, B.; Hidalgo, P. & Cardoso, H. (2005). Frequencies of the four major Amerindian mtDNA haplogroups in the population of Montevideo, Uruguay. *Human Biology*, Vol.77, N°.6, (December 2005), pp. 873-878, ISSN 0018-7143, Copyright 48201-1309

Gibson, G. (2009). Decanalization and the origin of complex disease. *Nature Review Genetic*, Vol.10, N°2, (February 2009), pp.134-140, ISSN 1471-0056.

Hansen, L.; Ekstrøm C.T.; Tabanera y Palacios, R.; Anant, M.; Wassermann, K. & Reinhardt, R.R. (2006). The Pro12Ala variant of the PPARG gene is a risk factor for Peroxisome Proliferator-Activated Receptor Agonist-Induced edema in type 2 diabetic patients. *The Journal of Clinical Endocrinology & Metabolism*, Vol.91, N°.9, (September 2996), pp.3446–3450, ISNN 1945-7197

Harris, M. (2002). *Buenos para comer. Enigmas de la Alimentación*, Alianza Editorial S.A., pp.1-336, ISBN: 84-206-3977-X

Hathout, E.H.; Thomas, W.; El-Shahawy, M.; Nahab, F. & Mace, J.W. (2001). Diabetic autoimmune markers in children and adolescents with type 2 diabetes. *Pediatrics*, Vol. 107, N°.6, (June 2001), pp. 1-4, ISSN 1098-4275

Himsworth, A. (1936) Diabetes mellitus: its differentiation into insulin-sensitive and insulin-insensitive types. *Lancet* Vol.227, N°5864, (January 1936), pp.127-130, ISSN 1474-4465

Howard, G.; O'Leary, D.; Zaccaro, D.; Haffner, S.; Rewers, M.; Hamman, R.; Selby J.V.; Saad, M.F.; Savage, P. & Bergman,R. (1996). Insulin sensitivity and atherosclerosis. *Circulation*, Vol.93, N°10, (May 1996), pp.1809-1817, ISSN 1524-4539

Imait, Y.; Fusco, A.; Suzuki, Y.; Lesniak, M.A.; D'Alfonso, R.; Sesti, G.; Bertoli, A.; Lauro, R.; Accili, D. & Taylor; S.I. (1994). Variant sequences of Insulin Receptor Substrate-1 in patients with noninsulin-dependent Diabetes Mellitus. *Journal of Clinical Endocrinology and Metabolism*, Vol.79, N°.6, (December 1994), pp.1655-1658, ISSN 1945-7197

Insúa, M.F. & Fuks, K. (2011). Evolución humana y dieta Introducción: Paradoja evolutiva Nutriinfo.com.ar http://nutrinfo.com/pagina/info/evolucio.html (14/2/2011).

Ito, E.; Ozawa, S.; Takahashi, K.; Tanaka, T.; Katsuta, H.; Yamaguchi, S.; Maruyama, M.; Takizawa, M.; Katahira, H.; Yoshimoto, K.; Nagamatsu, S. & Ishida, H. (2004). PPAR-gamma overexpression selectively suppresses insulin secretory capacity in isolated pancreatic islet through induction of UCP-2 protein. Biochemical and *Biophysical Research Communications* Vol.324, N°22, (November 2004), pp.810-814. ISSN 1090-2104

Kang, E.S.; Park, S. Y.; kim, H.J.; Ahn, C.W.; Cha, B.S.; Lim, S.K.; Nam. C.M. & Lee, H.C. (2005). Effects of Pro12Ala polymorphism of peroxisome proliferator-activated receptor γ 2 gene on rosiglitazone response in type 2 diabetes. *Clinical Pharmacology and Therapeutics*, Vol.78, N°2, (August 2005), pp.202-208, ISSN 1532-6535

Kolb, T. & Mandrup-Poulsen, T. (2005)An immune origen of type 2 diabetes? Diabetologia, Vol.48, (March 2005), pp.1038–1050. DOI 10.1007/s00125-005-1764-9n

Libman, I.M. & Becker, D.J. (2003). Coexistence of type 1 and type 2 diabetes mellitus: double diabetes? *Pediatric Diabetes*, Vol.4, (March 2003), pp. 110-113. ISSN 1399-543X

Marchetti, P.; Lupi, R.; Federici, M.; Marselli, L.; Masini, M.; Boggi, U.; Del Guerra, S.; Patanè, G.; Piro, S.; Anello, M., Bergamini, E.; Purrello, F.; Lauro, R. & Mosca, F. (2002) Insulin secretory function is impaired in isolated human islets carrying the Gly9723Arg IRS-1 polymorphism. *Diabetes*, Vol.51, N°5, (May 2002), pp.1419–1424, ISSN 1939-327X

Marrodán, M.D. (2000). La alimentación en el contexto de la evolución biocultural de los grupos humanos. *Zairak*, Vol.20, pp.109-121 ISSN 1137-439X.

Mercado, M.M.; McLenithan, J.C.; Silver, K.D. & Shuldiner, A.R. (2002). Genetics of Insulin Resistance. *Current Diabetes Reports*, Vol.2, N°1, (February 2002), pp.83–95, ISSN 1539-0829

Mimbacas, A.; Pérez-Bravo, F.; Hidalgo, P.C.; Javiel, G.; Pisciottano, C.; Grignola, R.; Jorge, A.M., Gallino, J.; Gasagoite, J. & Cardoso, H. (2003). Association between type 1 diabetes and DQB1* alleles in a case-control study conducted in Montevideo, Uruguay. *Genetics and Molecular Research*, Vol.2, N°1, (September 2002), pp. 29-35, ISSN 1676-5680.

Mimbacas, A.; Pérez-Bravo, F.; Santos, J.L.; Pisciottano, C.; Grignola, R.; Javiel, G.; Jorge, A.M. & Cardoso, H. (2004). The association between HLA-DQ genetic polymorphism and type 1 diabetes in a case-parent study conducted in an admixed population. *European Journal of Epidemiology*, Vol.19, N°10, (March 2004), pp. 931-934, ISSN 0393-2990

Mimbacas, A.; Trujillo, J.; Gascue, C.; Javiel, G. & Cardoso, H. (2007). Prevalence of vitamin D receptor gene polymorphism in a Uruguayan population and its relation to type 1 diabetes mellitus. *Genetics and Molecular Research*, Vol. 6, N°3, (July 2007), pp. 534-542, ISSN 1676-5680.

Mimbacas, A.; García, L.; Zorrilla, P.; Acosta, M.; Airaudo, C.; Ferrero, R.; Pena, A.; Simonelli, B.; Soto, E.; Vitarella, G.; Fernández, J. & Javiel, G. (2009). Genotype and phenotype correlations in diabetic patients in Uruguay. *Genetics and Molecular Research*, Vol.8, N°4, (September 2009), pp. 1352-1358, ISSN 1676-5680.

Mimbacas, A.; Fernández M.; Souto, J.; Farias, J.; Reyes, A.; García, L.; Acosta, M.; Airaudo, C.; Ferrero, R.; Simonelli, B.; Soto, E.; Vitarella, G.; Fernández, J. & Javiel, G. (2010). Genotype and phenotype correlations in diabetic patients in Uruguay. The 1st Latin American Congress: Controversies to Consensus in Diabetes, Obesity and Hypertension (CODHy). Hilton Hotel, Buenos Aires, Argentina, March 11-14.

Mimbacas, A.; Vitarella G.; Souto, J.; Reyes, AL.; Farías, J.; Fernández, M.; Fabregatm M. & Javiel G. (2011). The phenotype mask the genotype: a posible new diabetes expression. Journal of Pediatric Genetic. In press.

Neel, J.V. (1962). Diabetes mellitus: a "thrifty" genotype rendered detrimental by 'progress'? *American Journal of Human Genetics*, Vol.14, N° 4, (December 1962), pp.353-362. ISSN 1537-6605.

Neufeld, N.; Raffael, L.; Landon, C.; Chen, Y. & Valdheim, C. (1998). Early presentation of type 2 diabetes in Mexican-American youth. *Diabetes Care* Vol.21, N°1, (January 1998), pp. 80-86, ISSN 1935-5548

Nolan J.J. & Murphy E. (2001). ¿Existe la intolerancia oral a la glucosa y, en tal caso, qué hay que hacer?. In: *Diabetes Aspectos difíciles y controvertidos*. G. V. Gill, J.C. Pickup & G. Williams, pp.25-39, Ars Médica, Barcelona, ISBN 0-632-05324-0, España.

Patlak, M. (2002). Combating diabetes. *Federation of American Societies for Experimental Biology Journal (FASEB)*, Vol. 16, N°.14,(December 2002), pp.1853, ISSN 1530-6860.

Patlak, M. (2002). New weapons to combat an ancient disease: treating diabetes. Breakthroughs in Bioscience, *Federation of American Societies for Experimental Biology Journal (FASEB)*, (December 2002), pp. 1-13, ISSN 1530-6860

Pinhas-Hamiel, O.; Dolan, L.M.; Daniels, S.R.; Standiford, D.; Khoury, R. & Zitler, P. (1996) Increased incidence of non-insulin dependent diabetes mellitus among adolescents. *The Journal of Pediatric*, Vol.128, N°5, (May 1996), pp. 608-615, ISSN 1097-6833.

Pinhas-Hamiel, O. & Zeitler, P. (1999). The importance of a name. *The New England Journal of Medicine*, Vol.340, (May 1999), pp. 1418-1421, ISSN 0028-4793

Pinhas-Hamiel, O.; Dolan, L.M. & Zeitler, P. (1997). Diabetic ketoacidosis among obese African-American adolescents with NIDDM. *Diabetes Care*, Vol.20, N°4, (April 1997), pp. 484-486, ISSN 0149-5992

Porzio, O.; Federici, M.; Hribal, M.L.; Lauro, D.; Accili, D.; Lauro, R.; Borboni, P. & Sesti, G. (1999). The Gly972Arg amino acid polymorphism in IRS-1 impairs insulin secretion in pancreatic β cells. The *Journal Clinical Investigation*, Vol.104, N°3, (August 1999), pp.357–364, ISSN 1558-8238 (

Pozzilli, P. & Buzzetti, R. (2007). A new expression of diabetes: double diabetes *Trends in Endocrinology and Metabolism*, Vol.18, N°.2, (January 2007), pp.52-57, ISSN 1879-3061

Pozzilli, P.; Guglielmi, C.; Pronina, E.; Petraikina, E. (2007). Double or hybrid diabetes associated with an increase in type 1 and type 2 diabetes in children and youths. *Pediatric Diabetes*, Vol.8, N°.S9, (December 2007), pp.88-95. ISSN 1399-5448

Pozzilli, P. & Guglielmi C. (2009). Double Diabetes: A Mixture of Type 1 andType 2 Diabetes in Youth. Endocr Dev. Basel, Karger, 2009, vol 14, pp 151-166 In *Endocrine Involvement in Developmental Syndromes*, Cappa M, Maghnie M, Loche S, Bottazzo GF ISBN: 978-3-8055-9042-6 retrieved from http://content.karger.com/

Quintana-Murci, L.; Alcaïs, A.; Abel, L. & Casanova, J.L. (2007). Immunology in natura: clinical, epidemiological and evolutionary genetics of infectious diseases. *Nature Immunology*, Vol.8, N°11, (November 2007), pp.1165-1171, ISSN 1529-2908

Reyes, A.L.; Farias, J.; Fernández, M.; Souto, J.; Fabregat, M.; Javiel, G.; Vitarella, G. & Mimbacas, A. (2010). La genética como potente herramienta para el diagnóstico y clasificación de pacientes diabéticos de clínica compleja. XIV Congreso de la Asociación Latinoamericana de Diabetes (ALAD), Santiago de Chile, Chile, 7-11 Noviembre http://www.congresoaladchile2010.com/pdfs/trabajos_modalidad_poster.pdf

Rotimi, C.N. & Jorde, L.B. (2010). Ancestry and disease in the age of genome medicine. New England Journal of Medicine, Vol.363, N°16, (October 2010), pp.1551-1558, ISSN 0028-4793.

Ruiz M. (2011). Etiopatogenia de la diabetes tipo 2. In: Diabetes mellitus, M. Ruiz & M.L. Ruiz Morosini, 27-31, Acadia, ISBN 978-987-570-153-3, Buenos Aires, Argentina

Sans, M.; Figueiro, G.; Ackermann, E.; Barreto, I.; Egaña, A.; Bertoni, B.; PoittevinGilmet, E.; Maytia, D. & Hidalgo, P.C. (2011). Mitochondrial DNA in Basque-descendants from the city of Trinidad, Uruguay: Uruguayan- or Basque-like population?. Human Biology, Vol.83, No1, (in press)

Scott, C.; Smith, J.; Cradock, M. & Pihoker, C. (1997). Characteristics of youth-onset non-insulin dependent diabetes mellitus and insulin-dependent diabetes mellitus at diagnosis. Pediatrics, Vol.100, N°1, (July 1997), pp.84-91, ISSN 0031-4005

Serrano Ríos M. (2009). Etiopatogenia de la diabetes mellitus tipo 1. In: La diabetes mellitus en la práctica clínica, F.J. Tébar Massó & F. Escobar Jiménez, pp.31-45, Editorial Panamericana, ISBN978-84-7903-450-4, Madrid.

Sesti, G.; Federici, M.; Hribal, M.L.; Lauro, D.; Sbraccia, P. & Lauro, R. (2001). Defects of the insulin receptor substrate (IRS) system in human metabolic disorders. The Federation of American Societies for Experimental Biology Vol.15, N°12, (October 2001), pp.2099-2111, ISSN 1530-6860

Sigal, R.J.; Doria, A.;Warram J.H. & Krolewski, A.S. (1996) Codon 972 polymorphism in the insulin receptor substrate-1 gene, obesity, and risk of noninsulin-dependent diabetes mellitus. Journal Clinical Endocrinoly and Metabolism, Vol.81, N°.4, (April, 1996), pp. 1657-1659, ISSN 1945-7197

Soto, E.; Mimbacas, A.; Gascue, C.; Javiel, G.; Ferrero, R.; Vitarella, G. & Cardoso, H. (2004). Asociación entre hiperhomocisteinemia, cardiopatía isquémica y diabetes tipo 2. Revista Uruguaya de Cardiología, Vol.19, pp.101-106, ISSN 0797-0048

Souto,J.; Javiel, G.; Fernández, J. & Mimbacas A. (2010). Contribución de la Genética en la toma de decisiones terapéuticas, a propósito de 2 casos clínicos. XIV Congreso de la Asociación Latinoamericana de Diabetes (ALAD), Santiago de Chile, Chile, 7-11

Noviembre
http://www.congresoaladchile2010.com/pdfs/trabajos_modalidad_poster.pdf
Stumvoll, M.; Wahl, H.G.; Löblein, K.; Becker, R.; Machicao, F.; Jacob, S. & Häring H. (2001) Pro12Ala Polymorphism in the Peroxisome Proliferator–Activated Receptor-g2 gene is associated with increased antilipolytic insulin sensitivity. Diabetes Vol.50, N°4, (April 2001), pp.876–881, ISSN 0012-1797
Tuomi, T. (2005). Type 1 and Type 2 Diabetes What do they have in common? Diabetes, Vol. 54, NoS2, (December 2005), pp.S40-S45, ISSN 0012-1797
Villaroya, F.; Iglesisas, R. & Giralt, M. (2007), PPARs in the control of Uncoupling Gene expression. Hindawi Publishing Corporation Peroxsimone proliferator-activated receptors research, Vol. 2007, (October 2006), pp74364-74376, ISSN 1637-4765.
Wendorf, M. & Goldfine, I.D. (1991). Archaeology of NIDDM: excavation of the "thrifty" genotype. Diabetes, Vol.40, N°2, (February 1991), pp.161-165, ISSN 0012-1797
Wendorf, M. (1992). Archaeology and the "Thrifty" Non Insulin Dependent Diabetes Mellitus (NIDDM) Genotype. Advances in peritoneal dialysis. Vol.992, N°8, pp.201-2077, ISSN. 1197-8554
Wilkin, T.J. (2009). The accelerator hypothesis: a review of the evidence for insulin resistance as the basis for type I as well as type II diabetes. International Journal of Obesity, Vol.33, N°7, (July 2009), pp.716-726, ISSN 1476-5497
Yen, C.J.; Beamer, B.A.; Negri, C.; Silver, K.; Brown, K.A.; Yarnall, D.P.; Burns D.K., Roth, J. & Shuldiner, A.R. (1997). Molecular scanning of the human peroxisome proliferator activated receptor gamma (hPPAR gamma) gene in diabetic Caucasians: identification of a Pro12Ala PPAR gamma 2 missense mutation. Biochemical Biophysical Research Community. Vol.18, N°2, (December 1997), pp.270-274, ISSN 1090-2104
Yip, J.; Facchini, F.S. & Reaven, G.M. (1998). Resistance to insulin-mediated glucose disposal as a predictor of cardiovascular disease. Journal Clinical Endocrinology Metabolism, Vol.83, N°.8, (August 1998), pp.2773-2776, ISSN 1945-7197
Zhang, Y.; Wat, N.; Stratton, I.M.; Warren-Perry, M.G.; Orho, M.; Groop, L. & Turner, R.C. (1996). UKPDS 19: heterogeneity in NIDDM: separate contributions of IRS-1 and beta 3-adrenergic-receptor mutations to insulin resistance and obesity respectively with no evidence for glycogen synthase gene mutations. UK Prospective Diabetes Study. Diabetologia, Vol.39, N°12, (December 1996), pp.1505-1511, ISSN 0012-180X
Zhang, F.; Lavan, B.E. & Gregoire, F.M. (2007). Selective Modulators of PPAR-γ Activity: Molecular Aspects Related to Obesity and Side-Effects. Peroxsimone proliferator-activated receptors research, (2007), pp.1-7, doi:10.1155, ISSN 1687-4765
Zimmet, P.; Dowse, G. & Finch, C. (1990). The Epidemiology and natural history of NIDDM -lessons from the South Pacific. Diabetes Metabolism Reviews, Vol.6, N°2, (March 1990), pp.91-124, ISSN 0742-4221
Zorrilla, P.; Mimbacas, A.; Gascue, C.; Javiel, G. & Cardoso, H. (2006). Prevalencia del polimorfismo I/D del gen de la enzima convertidora de angiotensina (ECA) en la población de Montevideo. Revista Médica del Uruguay, Vol.12, N°.1, (Octubre 2005), pp.17-21 ISSN 1688-0390.

5

Genetic Testing of Newborns for Type 1 Diabetes Susceptibility – The MIDIA Study

Kjersti S. Rønningen
Department of Pediatric Research
Oslo University Hospital, Rikshospitalet, Oslo
Norway

1. Introduction

Type 1 Diabetes (T1D) is one of the most common chronic diseases with childhood onset, and the disease has increased two to threefold over the past half century by yet unknown means. Recently it was showed that if the present trend continues, the prevalence of cases younger than 5 years of age will rise by 70% within year 2020 (Patterson et al., 2009).

1.1 Background and status of knowledge

Type 1 Diabetes (T1D) is a T-cell mediated autoimmune disease that develops in genetically susceptible individuals whose immune system destroys the majority of insulin-secreting β-cells in pancreatic islets (Eizirik et al., 2009). The incidence of T1D has increased more than two- to threefold over the past half century, the most striking example being Finland where it has risen from 12 to 63/100,000 (Knip & Siljander, 2008; Patterson et al., 2009). This increase in incidence has not been paralleled by an increase in the frequency of major risk genes, including HLA class II, insulin, PTPN22, CTLA-4 and IL2RA (Barrett et al., 2009). Indeed, the prevalence of the classical HLA class II genes, which account for approximately 40% of genetic risk, appears to be decreasing (Gillespie et al., 2004; Fourlanos et al., 2008). There are now more than 40 risk loci associated with T1D with the majority of non-HLA genes displaying odds ratio <1.2. (Barrett et al., 2009). Moreover, most individuals who possess T1D risk genes do not develop the disease. Importantly, the concordance rate among monozygotic twins ranges from as low as 25 to 65% (Redendo et al., 1999, 2008; Hyttinen et al., 2003) and is approximately 6% in siblings. A common explanation has been that changes in environment must contribute to the increase in the disease. In particular, environmental exposures to dietary antigens and microbes have been implicated (Knip et al., 2005; Lefebvre et al., 2006). However, no single pathogenic environmental agent has been identified that explain all cases. In all likelihood, T1D develops by various combinations of pathways in response to commonly encountered environmental exposures.

1.2 Nutritional related factors and type 1 diabetes risk

The Norwegian Institute of Public Health is currently running two large prospective cohort studies; "Environmental Triggers of Type 1 Diabetes" (MIDIA) (www.fhi.no/midia) and "The Norwegian Mother and Child Cohort Study" (MoBa) (www.fhi.no/morogbarn). In MIDIA we will be able to study the impact of the dietary intake in children as well as mothers during the breast-feeding period and in MoBa we will be able to study the dietary intake of the mother during pregnancy for development of T1D in the child. These two studies will be linked to allow several approaches to be tested in the role of early diet and development of T1D. In the MIDIA study newborns have been identified by testing for the high-risk genotype (DRB1*03-DQA1*05-DQB1*02/ DRB1*04:01-DQA1*03-DQB1*03:02) in the HLA-system (Cinek et al., 2000). The MIDIA study is unique compared to the few other ongoing worldwide cohorts because of pregnancy data from the Norwegian Mother and Child Cohort Study (MoBa). Information from questionnaires, public records as well as blood samples from mothers (twice during pregnancy) and children (cord blood) have been collected from 107,000 pregnancies (Magnus et al., 2006; Rønningen et al., 2006). 50% of the children participating in MIDIA have a mother who also participates in MoBa, and consent has been given for linking information from the two studies and using biological specimens (Stene et al., 2007).

1.2.1 Foetal exposure and early life exposure to nutritional factors
Many nutritional factors may operate in uteri (measured as the mother's exposure during pregnancy), and also during postnatal life, and the status of the child is often influenced both by the maternal intake during pregnancy and postnatal exposures. Because the most relevant timing of exposure and possible induction times are unknown for T1D, an approach addressing both intrauterine and postnatal exposure to hypothetical risk factors or protective factors is most sensible.

1.2.2 Breast-feeding and cow's milk
Several epidemiological studies indicate that the risk of T1D is lower in children that have been breast-fed compared to children given breast-milk substitute produced from cow's milk (Norris & Scott., 1996), and recent data also indicate that for avoiding early autoimmunity the duration of breastfeeding is of importance (Rosenbauer et al., 2008). But most case-control studies suffer from potential recall bias, and prospective studies up to now have been few and very small. Case-control studies have also found associations between cow's milk antibodies and T1D see e.g. (Sarugeri et al., 1999; Monetini et al., 2002), but some form of reverse causality cannot be excluded as alternative explanations for the association described in these studies. Although an early study indicated a role of so-called molecular mimicry between a protein in cow's milk and a β-cell antigen (Karjalainen et al., 1992), it was subsequently refuted (Rønningen et al., 1998). Multiple other biologically plausible mechanisms have also been proposed for the possible relation between short duration of breast-feeding or early introduction of cow's milk.

1.2.3 Introduction of solid food
Studies indicate that the time point for introduction of solid food, especially with regard to cereal products, may have an influence on the development of autoimmunity (Norris et al., 2003; Ziegler et al., 2003). Early exposure to cereals is against generally accepted recommendations on infant nutrition in all developed countries and occurs infrequently. For example, Scandinavian babies are rarely exposed to cereals before the age of 4 months. A prospective analysis of data from the Finnish Diabetes Prediction and Prevention (DIPP) study showed no relation between early or late introduction of cereals and emergence of advanced β-cell autoimmunity. Another study from Finland suggests that an early introduction of fruit, berries and roots associated independently with β-cell autoimmunity

(Virtanen et al., 2006). While a recent study found that higher maternal intake of potatoes in the last trimester of pregnancy was associated with delayed onset of autoimmunity in the offspring (Lamb et al., 2008). Inconsistencies between the studies indicate that additional studies are required, including resolving the question of what aspects of cereals or other solid food items which are involved.

1.2.4 Cod liver oil, vitamin D and omega-3 fatty acids

A Norwegian study found intake of cod liver oil by the mothers during pregnancy or possibly by the child during the first year of life to be associated with lower risk of T1D in the child (Stene et al., 2000), but a subsequent larger study indicated that the child's intake was most important (Stene & Joner, 2003). Other vitamin D supplements were not associated in the Norwegian studies, pointing towards a possible effect of long-chain omega-3 fatty acids. Such fatty acids (e.g. EPA, DHA) have anti-inflammatory effects and potentially preventive effects for T1D (Chase et al., 1979). Results from a case-control study indicated, however, that vitamin D supplementation in early childhood could protect against T1D , and this has also been supported both from an European collaborative study (EURODIAB, 1999) as well as in a prospective study of children born in 1965 in Finland (Hyppönen et al., 2001). The longitudinal, observational study, the Diabetes Study in the Young (DAISY), conducted in Denver, Colorado, between January 1994 and November 2006, suggested that higher consumption of total omega-3 fatty acids, which was reported by a food frequency questionnaire, was associated with a lower risk of autoimmunity in children at increased genetic risk for type 1 diabetes. This association was further sustained by the observation of a higher proportion of omega-3 fatty acids found in the erythrocyte membranes in a subset of the children. Given that fish are a source of both omega-3 fatty acids and vitamin D, vitamin D was initially included in the analysis, but no association was found (Norris et al., 2007). Neither was it support for an effect of marine omega-3 fatty acids analysed separately. Pilot data from the MIDIA study do, however, indicate a protective effect against progression from autoimmunity to development of T1D (unpublished data). Although epidemiological studies can suggest possible associations, randomized clinical trials are necessary to prove a cause and effect. The pilot trial Nutritional Intervention to Prevent (NIP) T1D among babies with high genetic risk was therefore recently initiated (Chase et al., 2009).

1.2.5 Vitamin E

Hypothesising that antioxidants may protect against destruction of β-cells, Finnish researchers measured serum α-tocopherol concentration in frozen sera from 19 cases who developed T1D and in about 60 individually matched controls from a prospective cohort of individuals aged above 20 years (Knekt et al., 1999). Higher α-tocopherol was associated with a significantly lower risk of T1D. Another study from Finland, attempted to replicate this finding in siblings of persons with T1D, and found partial support, although the results were not significant (Uusitalo et al., 2005). Recently both concentration of α- and γ-tocopherol were studied in the Type 1 Diabetes Prediction and Prevention project (DIPP). Although it seemed unlikely that high concentration of α- or γ-tocopherol protect against advanced β–cell autoimmunity in young children, there was a suggestive protective effect of high levels of γ-tocopherol at the age of 1 year on development of autoimmunity, which needs to be replicated (Uusitalo et al., 2008).

1.2.6 Sugar

A Norwegian study shows that children receive from 9% to 24% of their energy from added sugar in the diet, where a major part comes from soft drinks (Øverby et al., 2004). Despite the fact that the increase in intake of simple sugar (in the form of sweets and drinks) in ecological studies correlate with increasing incidence of T1D, only a couple of studies have attempted to investigate this at the individual level. In one study an association between sugar intake and T1D incidence was not found (Dahlquist et al., 1990), but in two more recent studies a correlation was found (Pundziute-Lycka et al., 2004; Benson et al., 2008). Both studies used a case-control design which is likely to suffer from recall bias. Prospective studies with proper registration of dietary habits are therefore needed. The role of diet at different ages in a child's life may also be important.

1.2.7 Overweight

A few studies have observed an association between high birth weight and increased risk of T1D (Stene et al., 2001), although the relation is not very strong, but overweight and obesity are increasing. Gestational diabetes in the mother is a risk factor for a high birth weight and gestational diabetes has increased the last decades. Today a considerable proportion of pregnant women have gestational diabetes. Gestational diabetes may be a consequence of increased body weight in connection with the increased insulin resistance following pregnancies in general. Data from the MIDIA study indicate that both the mothers Body Mass Index (BMI) before getting pregnant as well as high weight gain during pregnancy increase the risk for autoimmunity at an early age for the offspring (Rasmussen et al., 2009). Obesity during childhood is emerging as a possible risk factor for T1D (EURODIAB, 2002; Pundziute-Lycka et al., 2004), but further studies are needed, including to find what particular aspects of body size/obesity (such as inflammatory cytokines or other markers) are most relevant in this relation. Since all the potential relations described above have very important public health implications, the different factors need to be investigated in larger well-designed prospective studies.

1.3 The hygiene hypothesis

The hygiene hypothesis states that the lack of exposure to parasites, symbiotic organisms and infectious agents in early childhood increases the susceptibility to allergic and autoimmune diseases (Zazdanbakhsh et al., 2001). Since humans have evolved coexisting in a shared environment with microbial agents throughout much of our evolutionary history, these agents might be necessary for the development of a balanced and regulated immune system (Stoll, 1947). The decline in non-specific infectious and microbial exposure in many populations is thus proposed to be the cause of the concomitant increase in atopic disorder over the past few decades (Bachlin & Degremont, 1997), and this hypothesis has been extended to autoimmune diseases such as T1D (Kyronseppa, 1993).

1.3.1 The hygiene hypothesis and epidemiology

The hygiene hypothesis is supported by epidemiological studies that show higher prevalence of autoimmune diseases in North America and Europe compared to South America and Africa, higher incidence associated with increased material wealth and higher risk for autoimmune diseases for third world immigrants to the industrialized countries (Herrström et al., 2001). There are also many studies showing that some infections and microbial agents reduce the incidence of autoimmune diabetes in experimental animals

(Blaser, 1998; Malaty, 1994). There are fewer studies in man suggesting protective effect of childhood infections against T1D (Sepp et al., 1997; Samulsson & Ludvigsson, 2003; Horman et al., 2004).

1.3.2 Intestinal parasites

Since immunomodulatory effects of parasites have been reported (Samulsson & Ludvigsson, 2003), and there is evidence that infections protect against the development of allergic disorders, parasites become obvious and major candidates for the hygiene hypothesis. In 1947 it was reported that 40-60% of European children were positive for helminths (Horman et al., 2004), while in recent years only 5-23% are found positive (Strachan, 1989; Jones et al., 2000; Yazdanbakhsh et al., 2002; Cooke, 2009; Bach, 2002; Honeyman, 2005; van der Werf et al., 2007; Gibbon et al., 1997; Parslow et al., 2001; Pundziute-Lycka et al., 2003; Round & Mazmanian, 2009). The most prevalent of the helminths is Enterobius Vermicularis (pinworm) which is usually asymptomatic and each bout is self-limiting since the worms cannot reproduce within the gut. Most common of the water borne parasites are Cryptosporium and Giardia. While the genus Giardia comprises six species, more than 20 variants of Cryptosporium are known (Nygard et al., 2003).

1.3.3 Bacterial colonization and virus infection in the intestines

Another interesting possibility is that the age at infection makes a difference in the pathology. In a similar fashion, it has been shown that colonization of the gut and intestines in early infancy by bacteria plays a role in the development of the adaptive immune system and structural development of the gut (Strachan, 1989). It is well known that due to improved hygiene some viral infections that would normally occur in early life are encountered for the first time at a later stage. For example, mononucleosis is associated with late infection of Epstein-Barr virus (EBV) (Pohl, 2009). Mononucleosis is rare in third world countries. Similarly, hepatitis A and B are less likely to cause disease if exposed to at an early age, and chickenpox (caused by varicella-zoster virus) is more severe in adults. Apparently, late infections typically give rise to a more severe pathology and concomitant increased activation of the immune system. The increased activation of the immune system may dispose for the establishment of an autoimmune condition. This hypothesis would explain the apparent conflict in data indicating that viral infections may confer protection and susceptibility. The MIDIA study offers a unique possibility to test this hypothesis.

1.4 Viral infections as triggers of type 1 diabetes

Viral infections have long been considered as triggers of T1D, and there are several lines of evidence implying virus infections in utero or early life in the aetiology of T1D . The high frequency of T1D in children with congenital rubella syndrome was the first indication of a viral involvement, and hinted towards the importance of the intra-uterine environment (Menser et al., 1978). Intra-uterine rubella infection is now rare in Scandinavia due to vaccination, but the incidence of T1D is high and continues to rise. Mumps and measles were also suspected of playing a role in T1D (Vuorinen et al., 1992), and a plateau in T1D incidence in Finland was also noted after measles, mumps and rubella vaccine was introduced (Hyöty et al., 1993). Measles vaccination was also suggested to be protective in a Swedish study (Dahlquist et al., 1991). Another interesting observation is that acute viral infections can be associated with disease onset (Elfaitouri et al., 2007; Frisk et al., 1992; Osame et al., 2007). There is also a seasonal correlation between periods of viral infections and onset of T1D (Jun & Yoon, 2003; Richer & Horwitz, 2003). Several viruses have been implicated as having an association with T1D, amongst them members of the picornaviridae and other viruses.

1.4.1 Mechanisms proposed for viral triggering of autoimmunity

There is unfortunately limited data on viral infections in young children (and infection load in early life), but there are several proposed mechanisms for how viruses might be associated with T1D. Viruses can activate polyclonal cells and trigger production of autoantibodies (Hiemstra et al., 2001), viruses can directly infect and lyse cells, viral antigens might mimic self-antigens, inflammatory responses stemming from viral infections might trigger autoimmunity (Horwitz et al., 1998), or as predicted in the hygiene hypothesis, viruses might be needed for proper maturation and regulation of the immune response.

1.4.2 Picornavirus

Picornaviruses are small RNA viruses that replicate mainly in the gut, and are spread by the fecal-oral route. The family has several well-known human and animal pathogens, but also many viruses without any known pathology. Human picornaviruses are known to be mostly asymptomatic and are common in infancy, with a prevalence of 10-12% in stool samples for human enterovirus (Cinek et al., 2006), human parechovirus (Tapia et al., 2008) and cardiovirus (Blinkova et al., 2009). The picornaviridae family currently consists of 8 current genera and 4 proposed genera.

The enterovirus genus consists of ten species, with six of them having human hosts (human enteroviruses A-D, rhinovirus A-B). Human enteroviruses are the most promising candidates, with two case-control studies that have shown an association between maternal enterovirus infection during pregnancy or enterovirus infection in children and risk of T1D (Dahlquist et al., 1995; Viskari et al., 2005). There are also studies that showed no association (Richer & Horwitz, 2009). In particular, Coxsackievirus (a member of human enterovirus B) is suspected of having a role in the development of autoimmunity (reviewed in Graves et al., 2003). In addition, enteroviruses have been shown to be more present in the sera (Elfving et al., 2008; Oikarinen et al., 2008), small intestine (Richardson et al., 2009) and pancreatic islets (Harvala & Simmonds, 2009) of recently diagnosed T1D patients (Clements et al., 1995; Andreoletti et al., 1997). A recent study by our group suggest that there is less enterovirus infections among children with high genetic risk for T1D compared with control children, although the difference is not statistically significant due to the low number of children presently tested (Tapia et al., 2011). Moreover, there appear to be a higher prevalence of enterovirus infections during early life in children who do not develop autoimmunity later, suggesting that enteroviral infections confer a protective effect against the development of autoimmunity (Wolthers et al., 2008). The parechovirus genus consists of two species, the murine virus Ljungan virus (LV) and human parechovirus (HPeV). Human parechovirus 1 and 2 have been known since the 1960s, and were originally classified with the enteroviruses as echovirus 22 and 23. Several new parechoviruses have recently been reported, with HPeV3-8 being described from 2004 to 2009 and HPeV9-14 recently announced. They are common in children, uncommon in adults and are present worldwide. Our previous data show that human parechoviruses are present in approximately 12% of stool samples from infants without causing symptoms (Tapia et al., 2008). There are, however, studies linking them to several serious conditions. Our most recent case-control study shows no difference in positivity for human parechovirus infections in stool samples (Tapia et al., 2010). Ljungan virus has earlier been shown to cause diabetes-like condition in rodents (Niklasson et al., 2006), but was not identified in samples from children in our studies (Tapia et al., 2008, Tapia et al., 2010). HPeV1 has been reported to show no association with T1D (Tauriainen et al., 2007), but there is no data on the other types of HPeVs. However, sequencing should be done to see if there is any difference in strains, and to test for all the new human Parechoviruses. Human parechoviruses seem to be asymptomatic, common viruses in childhood, and data on their epidemiology (and of other common asymptomatic viruses) will be used to test the hygiene hypothesis.

1.4.3 Cardiovirus

The genus Cardiovirus consists of 2 species, encephalomyocarditis virus and theliovirus (Liang et al., 2008). Until recently only rodent cardioviruses have been known. Encephalomyocarditis virus has been shown to induce diabetes in mice, and thelioviruses have been associated with myocarditis, and MS like symptoms in mice (Chiu et al., 2008). Recently, human thelioviruses, termed Saffold virus 1-8, have been discovered (Drexler et al., 2008). There is little known about them, but a serological study shows that SAFV3 are ubiquitous and cause infection early in life (Zoll et al., 2009), but are apparently asymptomatic. Being a recently discovered virus, only a few studies have detected it with molecular methods (Abed & Boivin, 2008; Jones et al., 2007; Day, 2009; Coulson et al., 2002), so making assumptions about its epidemiology may be premature. Being in the picornaviridae family, and being closely related to rodent pathogens suggest they might be unknown human pathogens, and they should be studied both to get a clear picture of infections in early childhood and if there is any association with T1D in humans. The MIDIA study offers an excellent opportunity to study these viruses.

1.4.4 Reovirus

The family reovirus consists of six genera. Two of these genera, rotavirus and reovirus, have been shown to infect β-cells, and are of interest to the project. They are double-stranded RNA viruses, also known to be common and ubiquitous (Honeyman et al., 1998). Rotaviruses are the single most important cause of severe diarrheal illness in infancy in both the developed and undeveloped world. They are spread through the fecal-oral route. Studies in mice have shown infection of β-cells (Comins et al., 2008) indicating molecular mimicry (Toniolo et al., 1980). These viruses are being studied by a post doc. in the MIDIA project, and we will pool our data to study the infections in childhood.

The name reovirus is a derivation of respiratory enteric orphan viruses, acknowledging that they can infect the respiratory and gastrointestinal system, but are not associated with any known disease (Wetzel et al., 2006). They are generally regarded as benign, but have also been associated with symptoms. In mice, they have been shown to infect β-cells, but have also been shown to delay overt diabetes in mice. Screening longitudinally collected stool samples for these viruses will show whether they are associated with any disease in human infants, and also be used to test the hygiene hypothesis.

1.4.5 Other viruses

Our results show that infections in early life are much more prevalent and asymptomatic than previously known, but also highlight the need for more studies on viral infections in children. There are several viruses that are considered common in childhood that should be studied to test the hygiene hypothesis, and viruses that have been implicated with T1D, or human strains of animal viruses associated with T1D, should be studied. In addition, newly discovered viruses will also be evaluated as candidates for testing. However, these viruses will have a lower priority than the candidates listed above.

1.5 Psychosocial effects of risk information
We are all born with variants in our genes which make us susceptible to diseases. With the developments in biotechnology and increasing knowledge about the relation between genes and diseases, we are faced with both new opportunities and new dilemmas. The use of tests that provide knowledge about risks and possibilities for illness in the future raises many fundamental questions of ethical, legal and psychosocial character.

1.5.1 Cohort studies giving risk information
In the MIDIA study parents were informed about that their child had the high-risk genotype for T1D (babies carrying HLA-DRB1*03-DQA1*05-DQB1*02/ DRB1*04:01-DQA1*03-DQB1*0302) or not. 2.1% of Norwegian newborns carry the high-risk genotype, and this group represents approximately 34% of future cases of T1D. Children with the high-risk genotype have 7% risk for getting T1D before 15 years of age and a lifetime risk at 20% (Rønningen et al., 1991; Undlien et al., 1997; Joner & Søvik, 1982, 1989; Mølbak et al., 1994).
Several other studies have used predictive genetic testing of newborns as a strategy to solve research questions about environmental factors contributing to T1D, including BABYDIAB in Germany (Ziegler et al.; 2011, Schatz et al.; 2000), DIPP in Finland (Kimpimaki et al.; 2001), PANDA in Florida (Carmichael et al., 2003, Krischer, 2007), DiPiS in Sweden (Lernmark et al., 2004), DAISY in Colorado (Rewers et al., 1996), and the multinational TEDDY study in the USA and Europe (Kiviniemi et al.; 2007, TEDDY study group; 2008). The main advantage for study participants identified as having increased risk for T1D is the possibility of early detection of the destruction of the insulin producing cells by autoantibodies, resulting in a milder disease onset having parents who are prepared in advance for the possibility of T1D onset, and therefore will handle the new life situation with a child with T1D better than other parents. In addition children with known increased genetic risk for T1D who also have developed autoantibodies will be the first to participate in intervention studies when possible preventive get available. However, there may be disadvantages of living with the knowledge of an increased susceptibility to a disease with no prevention. Thus, even though predictive testing is highly acknowledged as a valuable research method per se, the predictive testing has given rise to concerned debate.

1.5.2 Particular aspects for the Norwegian MIDIA and MoBa studies
With the widespread and increasing use of genetic tests, assessing the adverse effects of information about susceptibility genes for disease on the tested subject is important. The MIDIA study aimed to estimate the effect on maternal mental health from receiving genetic risk information about their newborns. Outcome measurements were maternal self-reported scores of anxiety and depression symptoms, satisfactory with life, self-esteem, and serious worry about their child. A number of previous studies (Hood et al., 2005; Johnson et al., 2004; Kerrush et al., 2007) have examined maternal reactions after being informed about their children having elevated genetic risk for T1D. None of these studies have shown a

significant effect on symptoms of anxiety or other mental health disorders as result of the testing, though a few mothers did seem to react strongly. Previous studies were conducted in a setting in which the mothers were asked questions about it in connection with the genetic testing project. The MIDIA study was designed differently. When completing the questionnaire the mothers were not aware that their answers were going to be used for any particular comparisons, though they were rightfully informed that the personal data would be used for multiple research purposes. Thus, our results were not affected by reporting bias associated with maternal attitudes towards genetic risk information or other factors motivating to under- or over-report poor mental health. Since 50% of mothers who got their child tested for genetic high-risk for T1D also participated in the Norwegian Mother and Child Cohort (MoBa) study, all data used came from MoBa. In MoBa data was available both from the 30th week of pregnancy and when the child was 6 months of age. These data therefore permit to answer the main question to what extent receiving information about a young child having high risk for T1D changes maternal well being and health.

2. Material and methods

2.1 Research design and subjects

The MIDIA study is a longitudinal cohort study with inclusion of children with the high-risk HLA genotype (DRB1*04:01-DQA1*03-DQB1*03:02/DRB1*03-DQA1*05-DQB1*02), with follow-up from three months of age up to 15 years of age. Recruitment to MIDIA started in small scale in the summer of 2001, covered the whole country of Norway from March 2006 (60,000 births per year) and was stopped in December 2007 since it was suddenly found to be against the Norwegian Biotechnology Law. Both approvals from the Regional Medical Committee and the Norwegian Data Inspectorate had been given before recruitment to MIDIA started. In December 2007 close to 48,000 children were recruited to MIDIA. Of those 1,047 were identified with the high-risk genotype. Approval from the government was given for further follow-up of those already identified with the high-risk genotype. At the end of March 2011, 19 of these children had got Type 1 Diabetes, 33 were confirmed positive for two or three autoantibodies and 24 for one. A total of 4,829 blood samples, 18,275 stool samples and 4,412 questionnaires are presently available for analysis in the cohort.

A questionnaire summarizing weekly diaries was filled out at 3, 6, 9 and 12 months of age. Blood samples were taken at the same intervals. After this period, a questionnaire and a blood sample are asked for annually (Stene et al., 2007). For more information on MIDIA, see www.fhi.no/midia. In The Norwegian Mother and Child Cohort Study (MoBa), questionnaires have been asked for at 17th, 22nd and 30th week of pregnancy, and when the child is 6 and 18 months old as well as then the child get 3, 5, 7 years of age (Magnus et al., 2006) . Blood samples were asked for at 17th week of pregnancy and at the time of delivery from the mother and cord blood was taken from the baby (Rønningen et al., 2006). For more information on MoBa, see www.fhi.no/morogbarn.

2.2 Outcome measurements

The incoming blood samples in the MIDIA study are immediately tested at the Hormone Laboratory, Aker Hospital, for diabetes associated autoantibodies as marker of β-cell autoimmunity, autoantibodies against insulin, anti-glutamic acid decarboxylase (GAD), and against the protein tyrosine kinase related protein IA-2 (Petersen et al., 1994; Bingley et al., 2001). High titres of one autoantibody or titres above the cut-off for two or three autoantibodies on at least two consecutive time periods (3-6 months apart) is defined as islet autoimmunity for the purpose of data analysis, and will be used as the first outcome (optimal cut-off values for the autoantibodies has been defined after participation by the Hormone laboratory in international autoantibody standardisation workshops; DASPs). Clinical diagnosis of T1D will also be used as outcome, and analysis will be performed when a sufficient number of children have developed either autoimmunity or T1D.

2.3 Measurement of nutrition-related factors ("exposures")
2.3.1 Questionnaires
A questionnaire summarising weekly diaries were filled out when the children were 3, 6, 9 and 12 months old, and annually thereafter. The questionnaires include for examples detailed information about dietary habits of the mother and the child (detailed information about diet for the mother as long as she breast-fed and intake of specific food items, etc.). Since few studies have been conducted on children's diet in Norway, new dietary questions had to be developed for both the MIDIA and the MoBa study. Validation of various aspects of dietary habits of pregnant women has recently been undertaken within the MoBa study. Blood samples and questionnaires from MIDIA can be used to assess validity of relevant information in childhood (Brantsæter et al., 2007a, 2007b, 2008, 2009; Willett, 1998; Serdula et al., 2001).

2.3.2 Biomarkers: Fatty acids, vitamin D and E
The distribution of fatty acids in the plasma phospholipid fraction as well as Vit D and Vit E will be analyzed in plasma samples from the same aliquots at a commercial laboratory in Oslo (AS Vitas; http://www.vitas.no/) using solid phase extraction and gas chromatography.

2.4 Measurement of exposure to virus (viral infections)
2.4.1 Real-time PCR
The real-time PCR have been run on ABI7300 real times machines according to earlier publications (Cinek et al., 2006). Primers were first designed for main type of virus and thereafter for subtypes (serotypes) and optimalisation was performed for each of the reactions.

2.4.2 Sequencing
Sequencing for enterovirus, picornavirus and E.coli as well as other bacterial species will be done as earlier published (Tapia et al., 2011; Witsø et al., 2006, 2007; Muinck et al., 2011). Deep sequencing will be performed on at 454 machines at the Centre for Ethological and Evolutional Sciences (CEES), Institute of Biology, University of Oslo according to the manufacture instructions.

2.4.3 Questionnaires
Data from questionnaires will be used to test association between viral RNA/DNA in stool and symptoms reported by the parents (coughing, diarrhea, vomiting), and will be used to search for risk factors of viral infection, such as breastfeeding, number of siblings and socioeconomic status.

2.5 Identification of eggs from enterobius vermicularis

Parents of children participating in MIDIA have been asked to collect tape samples touching the anal region on three following mornings. They have then sent the samples in specially designed containers for tape sampling to the central laboratory in Oslo. Here all the tape samples have been examined by two scientists at different times. A child has been regarded as positive if down to one egg have been identified on one of the tapes.

3. Results

3.1 Psychosocial effects of risk information

3.1.1 Effects of genetic risk information on mental health variables among MIDIA mothers

In the study of mothers who had participated in both MIDIA and MoBa (N=166 for those having a child with high genetic risk for T1D and N=7,224 for those who had been told that their child did not have the high-risk genotype) there were no sosiodemographic characteristics differences between those who had got the risk-information and those who had let their child be genotyped in MIDIA, but had been told that their child did not carry the high-risk genotype. Information on genetic risk in newborns was found to have no significant impact on maternal symptoms of anxiety and depression, self-esteem, satisfaction with life, or serious worry about their child. Mental health before birth was strongly associated with mental health after birth, see Table 1. Maternal symptoms of anxiety and depression were assed using a short version of SCL-25, including 4 question for anxiety and 4 for depression (Aas et al., 2010). The five-item Satisfaction With Life (SWLS) was developed to measure the cognitive component of subjective well-being. The short-form of the Rosenberg Self-Esteem Scale (RSES) used in the MoBa study includes four items. Maternal worry about their child was one of the items in an 11-item checklist of life events experienced during the last year, given in the 6 month questionnaire. The question was phased "Have you been serious worried that there is something wrong with your child?" Responses were coded as "yes" or "no". A dichotous variable was constructed to indicate the presence of maternal T1D. The variable was based on health questions from both The Medical Birth Registry of Norway (MBRN) and the MoBa questionnaires. The results from the linear regression analyses of the association between genetic risk information and change in maternal mental health are shown as unstandardized (B) and standard (β) coefficients in Table 1. The upper part of the table shows the results from the regression analysis with symptoms of anxiety and depression (SCL) as the dependent variable. The estimated regression coefficient (B=-0.001, p=0.95) for child's genetic risk indicate no effect of genetic information on changes in maternal mental health from baseline to post-disclosure. The maternal T1D status had neither any effect (B=0.040, p=0.409). However, as expected, the baseline anxiety/depression score was strongly associated with post-disclosure scores (B=0.536, p<0.001).

3.1.2 How often do parents think on that they have a child with high genetic risk for T1D

Although 5% of mothers and 2% of fathers did think of their child's high genetic risk for T1D when they filled out the 3 month questionnaire, usually just 2 week after they had got the information, very few parents continued to think often about their child's high genetic risk for T1D. To answer the questionnaire with the same questions each time needs that you sometimes think about having a high-risk child for T1D, see Figure 1 and 2.

Effects of maternal diabetes and genetic risk information on mental health variables

	B (95% CI)	β	p	Adjusted R²
Symptoms of anxiety and depression				
Child's genetic risk	-0.001 (-0.047 - 0.044)	-0.001	0.953	
Maternal type 1 diabetes	0.040 (-0.055 - 0.135)	0.008	0.409	
Baseline anxiety/depression	0.536 (0.517 - 0.555)	0.544	< 0.001	
				0.296
Self esteem				
Child's genetic risk	0.037 (-0.022 - 0.097)	0.011	0.218	
Maternal type 1 diabetes	-0.040 (-0.164 - 0.083)	-0.006	0.521	
Baseline self esteem	0.682 (0.664 - 0.700)	0.651	< 0.001	
				0.423
Satisfaction with life scale				
Child's genetic risk	-0.080 (-0.198 - 0.039)	-0.013	0.187	
Maternal type 1 diabetes	0.016 (-0.231 - 0.263)	0.001	0.902	
Baseline SWLS	0.609 (0.590 - 0.628)	0.587	< 0.001	
				0.345

Table 1.

3.2 Nutrition-related factors

Cohort design was used for assessing whether BMI before pregnancy and weight gain during pregnancy predicted the risk of islet autoimmunity in 885 children who were followed with serial blood samples and questionnaires. 36 of the children developed autoimmunity, of whom 10 developed Type 1 Diabetes. Both maternal BMI before pregnancy and weight gain < or = 15 kg predicted increased risk for islet autoimmunity, significant hazard ratio at 2.5 for both situations (Rasmussen et al., 2009).

3.3 Virus in stool samples

Among 911 children, were stool samples were available, 27 had developed autoimmunity in two or more consecutive samples (case children) in December 2008. In the pilot study based on these cases two control children per case were matched by follow-up time, day of birth, and county of residence. The frequency of human enterovirus RNA in stool samples from cases before seroconversion (43 of 339, 12.7%) did not differ from the frequency in control subjects (94 of 692, 13.2%) (Tapia et al., 2011a). There was neither any difference in the prevalence of human parechovirus when cases and controls were compared: 13.0% and 11.1%, respectively (Tapia et al., 2011b). None of the 3,803 samples analysed were positive for rodent parechovirus-Ljungan virus (Tapia et al., 2008, Tapia et al., 2010). Indicating that Ljungan virus is rare among Norwegian children, and in contract to what have been reported earlier does not seem to be involved in T1D susceptibility.

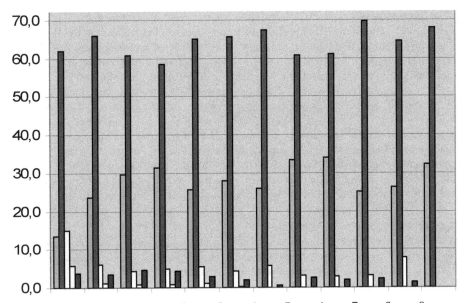

Fig. 1. Mothers thoughts about having a child with high genetic risk of T1D

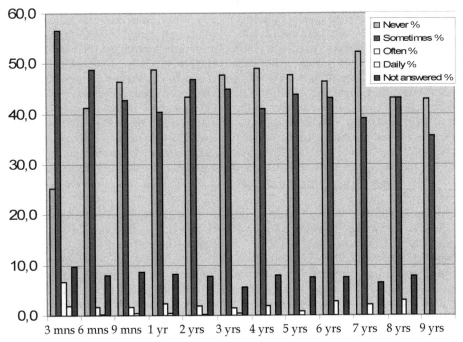

Fig. 2. Fathers thoughts about having a child with high genetic risk of T1D

3.4 The frequency of enterobius vermicularis among MIDIA children

During the last generation T1D has shown a strong increase in incidence in the Western part of the world. During the same period also the number of children suffering of allergic diseases has increased. In countries in Africa both T1D and allergic diseases are rare. The aim of this study was to examine if this had to do with the decrease in children having enterobius vermicularis (pinworm). Data has shown that intestinal worms are involved in development of intestinal immunity. The prevalence of pinworm has decreased in all European countries. While 40-60% was infected in 1947, only 5-23% has been shown positive in recent reports (Herrström et al., 1997). In MIDIA all who still participated in the project (N=943), was in the period January-June in 2010 invited to send in anal tape samples taken 3 following mornings. Of the 397 who participated, 18% did have pinworm egg on at least one of the tapes. This was a much higher frequency than expected, but more analysis will be performed, including analysis of the particular questionnaires developed for this project.

3.5 Lower respiratory tract infections

A MIDIA cohort study was most recently able to study 42 cases and 843 non-cases, which showed that self-reported "pneumonia, bronchitis or RS-virus" gave a hazard ration at 3.5, p=0.001 for developing for islet autoimmunity before 4 years of age.

4. Discussion

4.1 Data from the MIDIA project

The first nested case-control study in MIDIA on intestinal virus as triggers for Type 1 Diabetes did not support the hypothesis that faecal shedding of enteroviral RNA is a major predictor of advanced islet autoimmunity. Neither was there any association between human parechovirus and islet autoimmunity. Although also the rodent parechovirus, Ljungan virus, has been proposed as a potential environmental trigger for Type 1 Diabetes, the results from the MIDIA study indicate that Ljungan virus is rare in young children since it was not found neither in controls or cases. The two cohort studies performed in MIDIA do, however, show that both maternal weight and self reported lower respiratory tract infections predict risk of islet autoimmunity, and particularly in the youngest age group. The MIDIA study did not find any evidence supporting the notion that genetic risk information about newborns has a negative impact on the mental health of Norwegian mothers. All recruitment to the MIDIA study had, however, to be stopped in December 2007. The following part of the discussion will focus on the reason and the consequences for further research on environmental triggers of T1D.

4.1.1 Stopping of an ongoing T1D study based on the Norwegian Biotechnology Law

The MIDIA study had the needed approvals for research studies in Norway (from the Regional Ethic Committee and the Data Inspectorate) before recruitment started in the summer of 2001. Since all recruitment was based on special teaching of Norwegian public health care nurses given by the principal investigator and a study coordinator, the recruitment started in small scale. Most of the public health care nurses in Norway started after they had got the needed information and education to voluntary recruit to MIDIA as well as being responsible for most of the blood samples taken. From 2006 the recruitment covered the whole country. In June 2007, one of the mothers of a participating baby was, however, interviewed in the biggest newspaper in Norway. She here complained about not haven received good enough information about MIDIA before she and her husband had consented to participate. The Directorate for Health and Social Affairs then immediately decided that recruitment to MIDIA had to be stopped. Some days later it was, however, decided that new evaluation of the project had to take place according to the Norwegian Biotechnology Law, which tells that genotyping of children under the age of 18 years can only take place if there are a clear health benefit for a certain disease to get knowledge about genetics. During the fall of 2007 both the Biotechnology Board, the Ethical Committee for the Norwegian Medical Association, the National Committee for Medical Ethics as well as several experts contacted by the Directorate of Social and Health Affairs evaluated the MIDIA project. All these boards had earlier evaluated the MIDIA study; e.g. during the time of recruitment to the study. In addition the Health Department had clearly told that children who also had developed autoantibodies in MIDIA could get health insurance. The last aspect was based on the Biotechnology Law, which Norway has had since 1994, where it is clearly told that genetic risk for a disease cannot be used by the health insurance companies. The Directorate of Social and Health Affairs found, however, genotyping in MIDIA illegal December 10, 2007. A few days after the Norwegian Data Inspectorate said in newspapers that all data already collected from participants in MIDIA had to be thrown away. All ended luckily up with voting in the Norwegian Parliament in June 2008. As long as the Medical Regional Committee and the Norwegian Data Inspectorate approved the MIDIA study ones more, and all parents of children who already had been identified as high-risk children, gave a new informed consent , research in MIDIA could continue. In this respect Norway is different from Sweden, Finland, Germany and five states in USA were no similar Biotechnology Law Has given problems with genotyping of 350,000 children for the TEDDY study.

4.1.2 Ethics and data protection in human biomarker studies

The Norwegian Biotechnology Law tells: "Genetic testing of a child under the age of 18 years is not allowed if circumstances cannot be detected that can reduce or prevent health disadvantages for the child." Since the law came in 1994 it had only counted for clinical practice, the MIDIA project had been run for 6 ½ year before it was stopped December 10, 2007. In the work performed before the law got in use, science was never mentioned. Important questions in this context are:

1. Do important scientific T1D projects involving genotyping of children have to be performed elsewhere in the word? Should not Norway as one of the riches countries in the word has a certain responsibility?
2. Are not the parents able to give informed consent of behalf of their child?
3. How should health benefit be defined?
4. Is it not so that if clear health benefit has been shown, it is no longer research but part of general recommendation for public health or part of the health care system?

The year after recruitment to MIDIA was stopped funding was given from the Norwegian Research Council to the study "Nutritional Intervention to Prevent Type 1 Diabetes". The project was based on that the incidence of T1D is increasing, particularly in very young children. The hypothesis was that the Decrease of omega-3 fatty acids in the diet has contributed to this increase. One case-control study from Norway reported that children with T1D less often than the control children had a mother who had taken cod liver oil during pregnancy, while a newer study from Norway indicated a protective effect of cod liver oil during infancy (Stene et al., 2000; Stene & Joner, 2003). In the longitudinal, observational study, the Diabetes Autoimmunity Study in the Young (DAISY), conducted in

Denver, Colorado, between January 1994 and November 2006, 1770 children at increased genetic risk were followed. Islet autoimmunity was assessed in association with reported daily intake of polyunsaturated fatty acids. The data strongly indicated that dietary intake of omega-3 fatty acids is associated with reduced risk for autoimmunity in children at increased risk for T1D (Norris et al., 2007). We therefore proposed to conduct a prospective double blinded dietary intervention trial using high dosage of the omega-3 fatty acid DHA or "placebo" (containing the same amount of DHA found in the recommended daily dosage of cod liver oil). The reason for choosing 1,8 g DHA daily was to be able to be included in a multi-centre study since a pilot study in USA already have been performed as a feasibility study using exactly this dosage. But in USA they use plant oil as placebo (Chase et al, 2009). In Norway this cannot be given since mother of babies in Norway get recommended from their public health care nurse to give cod liver oil. But they are told to start with one tea spoon and to increase the daily intake to 5 ml within the child is 6 months. But at this stage babies start spotting. Indeed very few parents continue to give their infant cod liver oil. The Directorate for Health decided, however, that "Nutritional Intervention to Prevent Type 1 Diabetes" was illegal, and could therefore never be started based on the Norwegian Biotechnology Law.

4.1.3 Need for trans-national studies

Most recently two big NIH funded studies are going on. In the Type 1 Diabetes Genomics Consortium forces worldwide have been working together. All genotyping has been based on linkage studies (two siblings with Type 1 diabetes and parents without the disease is needed). Getting all who earlier was competing in identifying new T1D susceptibility genes to collaborate gave access to all available multiplex families. All genes that earlier was indicated to be of importance for T1D were confirmed, and 40 genes conferring susceptibility to T1D has now been identified (Barrett et al, 2009). In addition genome wide association studies have been performed by the same group (Welcome Trust Case Control Consortium, 2010).

In TEDDY (The Environmental Determinants for Type 1 Diabetes in the Young), another NIH funded study, centres in Denver, Colorado, Seattle, Washington, parts of Georgia and Florida, parts of Finland, Sweden and Germany have recruited and genotyped 350,000 new-borns and inform the parents about the high genetic risk. The protocol is the same everywhere, and all collected samples are sent to the coordinating centre in Florida. The follow-up is more intense than in MIDIA. Here all who participate, both scientists and parents know that it is an observational study where any intervention never can be given. The children Will be followed-up for 15 years.

5. Conclusions

The first nested case-control study in MIDIA on intestinal virus as triggers for Type 1 Diabetes did not support the hypothesis that faecal shedding of enteroviral RNA is a major predictor of advanced islet autoimmunity. Neither was there any association between human parechovirus and islet autoimmunity. Although also the rodent parechovirus, Ljungan virus, has been proposed as a potential environmental factor for Type 1 Diabetes, the results from the MIDIA study indicate that Ljungan virus is rare in young children since it was not found neither in controls or cases. The two cohort studies performed in MIDIA do, however, show that both maternal weight and self reported lower respiratory tract infections predict risk of islet autoimmunity, and particularly in the youngest age group. The MIDIA study did not find any evidence supporting the notion that genetic risk information about newborns has a negative impact on the mental health of Norwegian Mothers. Recruitment to MIDIA was stopped based on the Norwegian Biotechnology Law. It is therefore needed to extend international collaboration to identify the environmental triggers of type 1 diabetes. With the estimated increase of children with 50% having Type 1 Diabetes in 2020, and that the increase will be highest among children younger than 5 years (increase in prevalence with 70%) it is really important to extend collaborative efforts.

6. Acknowledgement

The MIDIA study was funded by the Norwegian Research Council (grants 135893/330, 155300/320, 156477/730, 166515/V50), The Norwegian Organisational for Help and Rehabilitation (EkstraStiftelsen), Norwegian Diabetes Association, New Generis (EU Grant Food-CT-2005-016320). The Norwegian Mother and Child Cohort Study Was supported by the Norwegian Ministry of Health, NIH-NIEHS (grant no. N01-ES-85433), NIH-NINDS (grant no. 1 UO1 NS 047537-01), and the Norwegian Research Council/FUGE (grant no. 151918/S10). I am very grateful for all the help I got from Trond Rasmussen in writing this book chapter.

7. References

Abed, Y. & Boivin, G. (2008). New Saffold cardioviruses in 3 children, Canada. *Emerg Infect Dis,* 14, 834-6.

Andreoletti, L. et al. (1997). Detection of coxsackie B virus RNA sequences in whole blood samples from adult patients at the onset of type I diabetes mellitus. *J Med Virol,* 52, 121-7.

Bach, J. F. (2002). The effect of infections on susceptibility to autoimmune and allergic diseases. *N Engl J Med,* 347, 911-20.

Bachlin A, Degremont A. (1997). Pinworm infection in kindergartens of Basel. *Schweiz Rundsch med Prax,*11, 1183-1185.

Barrett JC, Clayton DG, Concannon P, Akolkar B, Cooper JD et al. (2009). Genome-wide associationstudy and meta-analysis find over 40 loci affect risk of type 1 diabetes. *Nat Genet,* 41, 703-707.

Benson VS, Vanleeuwen Ja, Taylor J, McKinney PA, Van Til l. (2008). Food consumption and the risk of type 1 diabetes in children and youth: a population-based, case-control study in Prince Edward Island, Canada. *J Am Coll Nutr,* 27, 414-20.

Bingley PJ, Bonifacio E, Ziegler AG, Schatz DA, Atkinson MA, Eisenbarth GS. (2001). Proposed guidelines on screening for risk of type 1 diabetes. *Diabetes Care,* 24, 398.

Blaser MJ. (1998). Helicobacters are indigenous to the human stomac; duodenal ulceration is due to changes in gastric microecology in modern era. *Gut,* 43, 721-727.

Blinkova, O. et al. (2009). Cardioviruses are genetically diverse and cause common enteric infections in South Asian children. *J Virol,* 83, 4631-41

Brantsæter AL, Haugen M, Rasmussen S, Alexander J, Samuelsen SO, Meltzer HM. (2007a). Urinary flavonoids and plasma carotenoids in the validation of fruit, vegetable and tea intake during pregnancy in the Norwegian Mother and Child Cohort Study (MoBa). *Public Health Nutrition*, 10, 274-283.

Brantsæter AL, Haugen M, Hagve T-A, Aksnes, Rasmussen SA, Julshamn K, Alexander J, Meltzer. HM. (2007b). Self-reported dietary supplement use is confirmed by biological markers in the Norwegian Mother and Child Cohort Study. *Ann Nutr Metab*, 51, 146-154.

Brantsæter AL, Haugen M, Alexander J, Meltzer HM. (2008). Validity of a new Food frequency questionnaire for pregnant women in the Norwegian Mother and Child Cohort Study. *Maternal and Child Nutrition*, 4, 14-27.

Brantsæter AL, Haugen M, Julshamn K, Alexander J, Meltzer HM. (2009). Evaluation of urinary iodine excretion as a biomarker for intake of milk and dairy products in pregnant women in the Norwegian Mother and Child Cohort Study (MoBa). *Eur J Clin Nutr*, 63, 347-54.

Carmichael SK, Johnson SB, Baughcum et al. (2003). Prospective assessment in newborns of diabetes autoimmunity (PANDA): Maternal understanding of infant diabetes risk. *Genetic in Medicine* 5, 77-83.

Chase HP, Williams RL, Dupont J. (1979). Increased prostaglandin synthesis in childhood diabetes mellitus. *J Pediatr*, 94, 185-9.

Chase HP, Lescheck E, Rafkin-Mervis L, Krause-Steinrauf H, Chritton S, Asare SM, Adams S, Skyler JS, Clare-Salzler M, And the Type 1 Diabetes TrialNet NIP Study Group. (2009). Nutritional Intervention to Prevent (NIP) Type 1 Diabetes. A Pilot Trial. ICAV: Infant, Child, & Adolescent Nutrition, E (Pub), 10.1177/1941406409333466, April 14, 98-107.

Chiu, C. Y. et al. (2008). Identification of cardioviruses related to Theiler's murine encephalomyelitis virus in human infections. *Proc Natl Acad Sci U S A*, 105, 14124-9.

Cinek O, Wilkinson E, Paltiel L, Saugstad OD, Magnus P, Rønningen KS. (2000). Screening for the IDDM high-risk genotype. A rapid microtitre plate method using serum as source of DNA. *Tissue Antigens*, 56, 344-9.

Cinek O, Witsø E, Jeansson S, Rasmussen T, Drevinek P, Wetlesen T, Vavrinec J, Grinde B, Rønningen KS. (2006). Longitudinal observation of enterovirus and adenovirus in stool samples from Norwegian infants with the highest genetic risk of type 1 diabetes. *J Clin Virol*, 35(1), 33-40.

Clements, G. B., Galbraith, D. N. & Taylor, K. W. (1995). Coxsackie B virus infection and onset of childhood diabetes. *Lancet*, 346, 221-3.

Comins, C. et al. (2008). Reovirus: viral therapy for cancer 'as nature intended'. *Clin Oncol (R Coll Radiol)* 20, 548-54.

Cooke, A. (2009). Infection and autoimmunity. *Blood Cells Mol Dis*, 42, 105-7.

Coulson, B. S. et al. (2002). Growth of rotaviruses in primary pancreatic cells. *J Virol*, 76, 9537-44.

Dahlquist GG, Blom LG, Persson LA, Sandström AI, Wall SG. (1990). Dietary factors and the risk of developing insulin dependent diabetes in childhood. *BMJ*, 300, 1302-6.

Dahlquist, GG., Blom, L., Lönnberg, G. (1991). The Swedish Childhood Diabetes Study-a multivariate analysis of risk determinants for diabetes in different age groups. *Diabetologia*, 34, 757-62

Dahlquist GG, Ivarsson S, Lindberg B, Forsgren M. (1995). Maternal enteroviral infection during pregnancy as a risk factor for childhood IDDM. A population-based case-control study. *Diabetes*, 44, 408-13.

Day, J. M. (2009). The diversity of the orthoreoviruses: molecular taxonomy and phylogentic divides. *Infect Genet Evol*, 9, 390-400.

Drexler, J. F. et al. (2008). Circulation of 3 lineages of a novel Saffold cardiovirus in humans. *Emerg Infect Dis*, 14, 1398-405.

Eizirik S, Freyer J, Siewert C Baron U, Olek S et al. (2009). The role of inflammation in insulitis and β-cell loss in type 1 diabetes. *Natr Rev Endocrinol*, 219-26.

Elfaitouri, A. et al. (2007). Recent enterovirus infection in type 1 diabetes: evidence with a novel IgM method. *J Med Virol*, 79, 1861-7.

Elfving, M. et al. (2008). Maternal enterovirus infection during pregnancy as a risk factor in offspring diagnosed with type 1 diabetes between 15 and 30 years of age. *Exp Diabetes Res*, 2008, 271958.

EURODIAB Substudy 2 Study Group. (1999). Vitamin D supplement in early childhood and risk for type 1 (insulin-dependent) diabetes mellitus. *Diabetologia*, 42, 51-4.

EURODIAB Substudy 2 Study Group. (2002). Rapid early growth is associated with increased risk of childhood type 1 diabetes in various European populations. *Diabetes Care*, 25, 1755-60.

Fourlanos S, Varney MD, Tait BD, Morrahan, Honeyman MC. (2008). The rising incidence of type 1 diabetes is accounted for by cases with lower-risk human leukocyte antigen genotypes. *Diabetes Care*, 31, 1546-9.

Frisk, G., Friman, G., Tuvemo, T., Fohlman, J. & Diderholm, H. (1992). Coxsackie B virus IgM in children at onset of type 1 (insulin-dependent) diabetes mellitus: evidence for IgM induction by a recent or current infection. *Diabetologia*, 35, 249-53.

Gibbon, C., Smith, T., Egger, P., Betts, P. & Phillips, D. (1997). Early infection and subsequent insulin dependent diabetes. *Arch Dis Child*, 77, 384-5.

Gillespie KM, Bain SC, Barnett AH, Bingley PJ, Christie MR et al. (2004). The rising incidence of childhood type 1 diabetes and reduced contribution of high-risk HLA haplotypes. *Lancet*, 364, 1699-1700.

Graves, P. M. et al. (2003). Prospective study of enteroviral infections and development of β-cell autoimmunity. Diabetes autoimmunity study in the young (DAISY). *Diabetes Res Clin Pract*, 59, 51-61.

Harvala, H. & Simmonds, P. (2009). Human parechoviruses: biology, epidemiology and clinical significance. *J Clin Virol*, 45, 1-9.

Herrström P, Friström A, Karlsson A, Högstedt B. (1997). Enterobius vermicularis and finger sucking in young Swedish children. *Scand J Prim Health Care*, 15(3), 146-8.

Herrström P, Henricson KA, Raberg A, Karlsson A, Hogstedt B. (2001). Allergic disease and the infestation of Enterobius vermicularis in Swedish chldren 4-10 years of age. *J Investg Allergol Clin Immunol*, 11, 157-160.

Hiemstra, H. S. et al. (2001). Cytomegalovirus in autoimmunity: T cell crossreactivity to viral antigen and autoantigen glutamic acid decarboxylase. *Proc Natl Acad Sci U S A*, 98, 3988-91.

Hilner, J.E., Perdue L.H., Sides E.G., Pierces J.J., Wagner A.M. et al. (2010). Designing and implementing samples and data collection for an international genetic study: the Type 1 Diabetes Genetic Consortium (T1DGC). *Clin Trials*, 7, S5-32.

Honeyman, M. C., Stone, N. L. & Harrison, L. C. (1998). T-cell epitopes in type 1 diabetes autoantigen tyrosine phosphatase IA-2: potential for mimicry with rotavirus and other environmental agents. *Mol Med*, 4, 231-9.

Honeyman, M. (2005). How robust is the evidence for viruses in the induction of type 1 diabetes? *Curr Opin Immunol* 17, 616-23.

Hood KK, Johnsen SB, Carmicael SK et al. (2005). Depressive symptoms in mothers of infants identified as genetically at risk for type 1 diabetes. *Diabetes Care*, 28, 1898-1903.

Horman A, Korpela H, Sutinen J, Wedel H, Hanninen M-L. (2004). Meta-analysis in assessment of the prevalence and annual incidence of Giardia spp. And Cryptosporium spp. infections in humans in the Nordic countries. *Inter J for Parasitol*, 34, 1337-1346.

Horwitz, M. S. et al. (1998). Diabetes induced by Coxsackie virus: initiation by bystander damage and not molecular mimicry. *Nat Med*, 4, 781-5.

Hyöty, H. et al. (1993). Decline of mumps antibodies in type 1 (insulin-dependent) diabetic children and a plateau in the rising incidence of type 1 diabetes after introduction of the mumps-measles-rubella vaccine in Finland. Childhood Diabetes in Finland Study Group. *Diabetologia*, 36, 1303-8.

Hyppönen E, Lärä E, Reunanen A, Järvelin MR, Virtanen SM. (2001). Intake of vitamin D and risk of type 1 diabetes: a birth-cohort study. Lancet, 358, 1500-3.

Hyttinen V, Kaprio J, Kinnunen L, Koskenvuo M, Tuomilehto J. (2003). Genetic liability of type 1 diabetes and the age of onset age among 22,650 young Finnish twin pairs: a nationwide follow-up study. *Diabetes*, 52, 1052-5.

Johnson SB, Baughcum AE, Carmicael SK, She JX, Schatz DA. (2004). Maternal anxiety associated with newborn genetic screening for type 1 diabetes. *Diabetes Care*, 27, 392-397.

Joner G & Søvik O. (1989). Increasing evidence of diabetes mellitus in Norwegian children 0-14 years of age 1973-1982. *Diabetologia*, 32, 79-83.

Joner G & Søvik O. (1991). The incidence of type 1 (insulin-dependent) diabetes mellitus 15-29 years in Norway 1978-1982. *Diabetologia*, 34, 271-4.

Jones, M. S., Lukashov, V. V., Ganac, R. D. & Schnurr, D. P. (2007). Discovery of a novel human picornavirus in a stool sample from a pediatric patient presenting with fever of unknown origin. *J Clin Microbiol*, 45, 2144-50.

Jones, P. D., Gibson, P. G. & Henry, R. L. (2000). The prevalence of asthma appears to be inversely related to the incidence of typhoid and tuberculosis; hypothesis to explain the variation in asthma prevalence around the world. *Med Hypotheses*, 55, 40-2.

Julier, C., Akolkar B., Concannon P., Motrahan G., Nierras, C., Pugliese, A. (2009). Type 1 Diabetes Consortium. The Type 1 Diabetes Consortium "Rapid Response" family-based candidate gene study; strategy, gene selection, and main outcome. *Genes Immun*, 10 (Suppl 1), 121-7.

Jun, H. S. & Yoon, J. W. (2003). A new look at viruses in type 1 diabetes. *Diabetes Metab Res Rev*, 19, 8-31.

Karjalainen J, Martin JM, Knip M, Ilonen J, Robinson BH, Savilahti E, Åkerblom HK, Dosch H. (1992). A bovine albumin peptide as a possible trigger of insulin-dependent diabetes mellitus. *N Eng J Med*, 327, 302-7.

Kerrush NJ, Campbell-Stokes PL, Gray A, Marriman TR, Robertson SP, Taylor BJ. (2007). Maternal psychological reactions to newborn screening for type 1 diabetes. *Pediatrics*, 120, 392-7.

Kimpimaki T, Kupila A, Hamalainen AM et. al. (2001). The first sign of β-cell autoimmunity appear in infancy in genetically susceptible children from the general population. The Finnish type 1 diabetes prediction and prevention study. *J of Clin Endocrinol and Metabolism*, 86, 4782-8.

Kiviniemi M, Hermann R, Nurmi J et al. (2007). A high-throughput population screening system for type 1 diabetes: An application for the TEDDY (The environmental determinants in the young) study. *Diabetes technology & therapeutics*, 9, 460-72.

Knekt P, Reunanen A, Marniemi J, Leino A, Aromaa A. (1999). Low vitamin E status is a potential risk factor for insulin-dependent diabetes mellitus. *J Intern Med*, 245, 99-102.

Knip M, Veijola R, Virtanen SM, Hyoty H, Vaarala O et al. (2005). Environmental triggers and determinants of type 1 diabetes. *Diabetes*, 54 (Suppl 2), 125-36.

Knip M & Siljander H. (2008). Autoimmune mechanisms in type 1 diabetes. *Autoimmun Rev*, 7, 550-7.

Krischer J. (2007). The environmental determinants of diabetes in the young (TEDDY) study; study design. *Pediatric Diabetes*, 8, 286-98.

Kyronseppa H. (1993). The occurence of human intestinale parasites in Finland. *Scand J Infect Dis*, 25, 671-673.

Lamb MM, Myers MA, Barriga K, Zimmet PZ, Rewers M, Norris JM. (2008). Maternal diet during pregnancy and islet autoimmunity in offspring. *Pediatric Diabetes*, 9, 135-41.

Lefebvre DE, Powell KL, Strom A, Scott FW. (2006). Dietary proteins as environmental modifiers of type 1 diabetes. *Annu Rev Nutr*, 26, 175-202.

Lernmark B, Elding-Larsson H, Hansson G, et al. (2004). Patient responses to participation in genetic screening for diabetes risk. *Pediatric Diabetes*, 5, 174-81.

Liang, Z., Kumar, A. S., Jones, M. S., Knowles, N. J. & Lipton, H. L. (2008). Phylogenetic analysis of the species Theilovirus; emerging murine and human pathogens. *J Virol*, 82, 11545-54.

Magnus P, Irgens LM, Haug K, Nystad W, Skjærven R, Stoltenberg C and the MoBa Study Group. (2006). Cohort profile: The Norwegian Mother and Child Cohort Study (MoBa). *Int J Epidemiol*, 35, 1146-50.

Malaty HM, Graham DY. (1994). Importance of childhood socioeconomic status on the current prevalence of Helicobacter pylori infections. *Gut*, 35, 742-5.

Menser, M. A., Forrest, J. M. & Bransby, R. D. (1978). Rubella infection and diabetes mellitus. *Lancet*, 1, 57-60.

Monetini L, Cavallo MG, Manfrini S, Stefanini L, Picarelli A, Di Tola M, et al. (2002). Antibodies to bovine β-casein in diabetes and other autoimmune diseases. *Horm Metab Res*, 34, 455-9.

Muinck EJD, Øien T, Storrø O, Johansen R, Stenseth NC, Rønningen KS, Rudi K. (2011). Diversity, transmission and presence of Escherichia coli in a cohort of mothers and their infants. *Environmental Microbiolog Reports*, published online Jan 5.

Mølbak AG, Christau B, Marner B, Borch-Johnsen K, Nerup J. (1994). Incidence of insulin-dependent diabetes mellitus in age groups over 30 years in Denmark. *Diabet Med*, 11, 650-5.

Niklasson, B., Nyholm, E., Feinstein, R. E., Samsioe, A. & Hornfeldt, B. (2006). Diabetes and myocarditis in voles and lemmings at cyclic peak densities-induced by Ljungan virus? *Oecologia*, 150, 1-7.

Norris JM & Scott FW. (1996). A meta-analysis of infant diet and insulin-dependent diabetes mellitus; do bias play a role? *Epidemiology*, 7, 87-92.

Norris JM, Barriga K, Klingensmith G, Hoffman M, Eisenbarth GS, Erlich HA, et al. (2003). Timing of initial cereal exposure in infancy and risk of islet autoimmunity. *JAMA*, 290, 1713-20.

Norris JM, Yin Xiang, Lamb MM, Barriga K, Seifert J, Hoffman M, Orton HD, Baron AE, Clare-Saltzler M, Chase HP, Szabo NJ, Erlich H, Eisenbarth GS, Rewers M. (2007). Omega-3 polyunsaturated fatty acid intake and islet autoimmunity in children at increased risk for type 1 diabetes. *JAMA*, 26, 1420-8.

Nygard k, Vold L, Robertson L, Lassen J. (2003). Are domestic Cryptosporium and Giardia infections in Norway underdiagnosed? *Tidsskr Nor Lægeforen*, 123, 3406-9.

Oikarinen, M. et al. (2008). Detection of enteroviruses in the intestine of type 1 diabetic patients. *Clin Exp Immunol*, 151, 71-5.

Osame, K. et al. (2007). Rapid-onset type 1 diabetes associated with cytomegalovirus infection and islet autoantibody synthesis. *Intern Med*, 46, 873-7.

Parslow, R. C., McKinney, P. A., Law, G. R. & Bodansky, H. J. (2001). Population mixing and childhood diabetes. *Int J Epidemiol*, 30, 533-8; discussion 538-9.

Patterson CC, Dahlquist GG, Gyurus E, Green A, Soltesz G, EURODIAB Study Group. (2009). Incidence trends for childhood type 1 diabetes I Europe during 1989-2003 and predicted new cases 2005-2020, a multicentre prospective registration study. *Lancet*, 373, 2027-33.

Petersen JS, Hejnaes KR, Moody A, Karlsen AE, Marshall MO, Hoier-Madsen M, et al. (1994). Detection of GAD65 antibodies in diabetes and other autoimmune diseases using a simple radioligand assay. *Diabetes*, 43, 459-6.

Pohl, D. (2009). Epstein-Barr virus and multiple sclerosis. *J Neurol Sci*, 286(1-2), 62-4.

Pundziute-Lycka, A., Urbonaite, B., Ostrauskas, R., Zalinkevicius, R. & Dahlquist, G. G. (2003). Incidence of type 1 diabetes in Lithuanians aged 0-39 years varies by the urban-rural setting, and the time change differs for men and women during 1991-2000. *Diabetes Care*, 26, 671-6.

Pundziute-Lycka A, Persson LA, Cedermark G, Jansson-Roth A, Nilsson U, Westin V, et al. (2004). Diet, growth, and the risk for type 1 diabetes in childhood: a matched case-referent study. *Diabetes Care*, 27, 2784-9.

Rasmussen T, Stene LC, Cinek O, Torjusen PA, Wetlesen T, Rønningen KS. (2009). Maternal body mass index before pregnancy and weight gain during pregnancy and risk of persistent diabetes associated autoantibodies in children with the high-risk HLA-genotype: The MIDIA study. *Diabetes Care*, 32(10), 1904-6.

Redendo MJ, Rewers M, Yu L, Garg S, Pilcher CC et al. (1999). Genetic determination of islet cell autoimmunity in monozygotic twin, dizygotic twin, and non-twin siblings of patients with type 1 diabetes: prospective twin study. *BMJ*, 318, 698-702.

Redendo MJ, Jeffrey J, Fain PR, Eisenbarth GS, Orban T. (2008). Concordance for islet autoimmunity among monozygotic twins. *N Engl J Med*, 359, 2849-50.

Rewers M, Bugawan TL, Norris JM et al. (1996). Newborn screening for HLA markers associated with IDDM: Diabetes Autoimmunity Study in the Young (DAISY). *Diabetologia*, 39, 807-12.

Richardson, S. J., Willcox, A., Bone, A. J., Foulis, A. K. & Morgan, N. G. (2009). The prevalence of enteroviral capsid protein vp1 immunostaining in pancreatic islets in human type 1 diabetes. *Diabetologia*, 52, 1143-51.

Richer, M. J. & Horwitz, M. S. (2008). Viral infections in the pathogenesis of autoimmune diseases: focus on type 1 diabetes. *Front Biosci*, 13, 4241-57.

Richer, M. J. & Horwitz, M. S. (2009). Coxsackievirus Infection as an Environmental Factor in the Etiology of Type 1 Diabetes. *Autoimmun Rev*, 8(7), 611-5.

Rosenbauer J, Herzig P, Giani G. (2008). Early infant feeding and risk of type 1 diabetes mellitus – a nationalwide population-based case-control study in pre-school children. *Diabetes Metab Res Rev*, 24, 211-22.

Round, J. L. & Mazmanian, S. K. (2009). The gut microbiota shapes intestinal immune responses during health and disease. *Nat Rev Immunol*, 9, 313-23.

Rønningen KS, Spurkland A, Iwe T, Vartdal F, Thorsby E. (1991). Distribution of HLA-DRB1, -DQA1 and -DQB1 alleles and DQA1-DQB1 genotypes among Norwegian patients with insulin-dependent diabetes mellitus. *Tissue Antigens*, 37, 105-111.

Rønningen KS, Atrazhev A, Luo L, Smith DK, Korbutt G, Rajotte RV, et al. (1998). Anti-BSA antibodies do not cross-react with the 69-kDa islet cell autoantigen ICA69. *J Autoimmun*, 11, 223-31.

Rønningen KS, Paltiel L, Meltzer HM, Nordhagen R, Lie KK, Hovengen R, Haugen M, Nystad W, Magnus P, Hoppin JA. (2006). The biobank of the Norwegian Mother and Child Cohort Study: a resource for the next 100 years. *Eur J Epidemiol*, 21(8), 619-25.

Samulsson U & Ludvigsson J. (2003). The consentrations of short-chain fatty acids and other microflora-associated characteristics in faeces from children with newly diagnosed type 1 diabetes and control children and their family mambers. *Diabetic Medicine*, 21, 64-67.

Sarugeri E, Dozio N, Meschi F, Pastore MR, Bonifacio E. (1999). Cellular and humoral immunity against cow's milk proteins in type 1 diabetes. *J Autoimmun*, 13, 365-73.

Schatz D, Muir A, Fuller K et al. (2000). Prospective assessment in newborn genetic screening program in the general population [Abstract]. *Diabetes*, 49, A69.

Sepp E, Jugle E, Vasar M, Naaber P, Bjørksten B, Mikelsaar M. (1997). Intestinal microflora of Estonian and Swedish infants. *Acta Paediatr*, 86, 956-61.

Serdula MK, Alexander MP, Scanlon KS, Bowman BA. (2001). What are preschool children eating? A review of dietary assessment. *Annu Rev Nutr*, 21, 475-98.

Stene LC, Ulriksen J, Magnus P, Joner G. (2000). Use of cod liver oil during pregnancy associated with lower risk of type I diabetes in the offspring. *Diabetologia*, 43, 1083-92.

Stene LC, Magnus P, Lie RT, Søvik O, Joner G, the Norwegian Childhood Diabetes Study Group. (2001). Birth weight and childhood onset type 1 diabetes: population based cohort study. *BMJ*, 322, 889-92.

Stene LC, Joner G, the Norwegian Childhood Diabetes Study Group. (2003). Use of cod liver oil during the first year of life is associated with lower risk of childhood-onset type 1 diabetes: a large, population based, case-control study. *Am J Clin Nutr*, 78, 1128-34.

Stene LC, Witsø E, Torjesen PA, Rasmussen T, Magnus P, Cinek O, Wetlesen T, Rønningen KS. (2007). Islet autoantibody development during follow-up of high-risk children from the general Norwegian population from three months of age: Design and early results from the MIDIA study. *J of Autoimmun*, 29, 44-51.

Stoll NR. (1947). This wormy world. *J Parasitol*, 33, 1-18.

Strachan, D. P. (1989). Hay fever, hygiene, and household size. *BMJ*, 299, 1259-60.

Tapia G, Cinek O, Witsø E, Kulich M, Rasmussen T, Grinde B, Rønningen KS. (2008). Longitudinal observation of parechovirus in stool samples from Norwegian infants. *J Med Virol*, 80(10), 1835-42.

Tapia G, Cinek O, Rasmussen T, Grinde B, Rønningen KS. (2010). No Ljungan virus RNA in stool samples from the Norwegian environmental triggers of type 1 diabetes (MIDIA) cohort study. *Diabetes Care*, 33(5), 1069-71.

Tapia G, Cinek O, Rasmussen T, Grinde B, Stene LC, Rønningen KS. (2011). Longitudinal study of parechovirus infection in infancy and risk of repeated positivity for multiple islet autoantibodies: The MIDIA study. *Pediatr Diabetes*, 12(1), 58-62.

Tapia G, Cinek O, Rasmussen T, Witsø E, Grinde B, Stene LC, Rønningen KS. (2011). Human enterovirus RNA in monthly fecal samples and islet autoimmunity in Norwegian children with high genetic risk for type 1 diabetes: the MIDIA study. *Diabetes Care*, 34(1), 151-5.

Tauriainen, S. et al. (2007). Human parechovirus 1 infections in young children-no association with type 1 diabetes. *J Med Virol*, 79, 457-62.

TEDDY study group. (2008). The environmental determinants in the young study. *Annals of the New York Academy of Sciences*, 1150, 1-13.

Toniolo, A., Onodera, T., Yoon, J. W. & Notkins, A. L. (1980). Induction of diabetes by cumulative environmental insults from viruses and chemicals. *Nature*, 288, 383-5.

Undlien DE, Friede T, Rammensee H-G, Joner G, Dahl-Jørgensen K, Søvik O, Akselsen HE, Knutsen I, Rønningen KS, Thorsby E. (1997). HLA-encoded genetic predisposition in IDDM. DR4 subtypes may be associated with different degrees of protection. *Diabetes*, 46, 143-9.

Uusitalo L, Knip M, Kenward MG, Alfthan G, Sundvall J, Aro A, Reunanen A, Åkerblom HK, Virtanen SM. (2005). Childhood diabetes in Finland study group. *J Pediatr Endocrinol Metab*, 18, 1409-16.

Uusitalo L, Nevalainen J, Niinisjø S, Alfthan G, Sundvall j, Korhonen T, Kenward MG, Oja H, Veijola R, Simell O, Ilonen J, Knip m, Virtanen SM. (2008). Serum alpha- and gammetocopherol concentration and risk of advanced β cell autoimmunity in children with HLA-conferred susceptibility to type 1 diabetes mellitus. *Diabetologia*, 51, 773-80.

van der Werf, N., Kroese, F. G., Rozing, J. & Hillebrands, J. L. (2007). Viral infections as potential triggers of type 1 diabetes. *Diabetes Metab Res Rev*, 23, 169-83.

Virtanen SM, Kenward MG, Erkkola M et al. (2006). Age at introduction of new food and advanced b-cell autoimmunity in young children withHLA-conferred susceptibility to type 1 diabetes. *Diabetologia*, 49, 1512-21.

Viskari, H. et al. (2005). Relationship between the incidence of type 1 diabetes and maternal enterovirus antibodies: time trends and geographical variation. *Diabetologia*, 48, 1280-7.

Vuorinen, T., Nikolakaros, G., Simell, O., Hyypia, T. & Vainionpaa, R. (1992). Mumps and Coxsackie B3 virus infection of human fetal pancreatic islet-like cell clusters. *Pancreas*, 7, 460-4.

Wetzel, J. D. et al. (2006). Reovirus delays diabetes onset but does not prevent insulitis in nonobese diabetic mice. *J Virol*, 80, 3078-82.

Wellcome Trust Case Control Consortium, Craddock, N., Hurles, M.E., Cardin N., Pearson, R.D., Plagnol, V. et al. (2010). Genome-wide association study of CNVs in 16,000 cases of eight common diseases and 3,000 shared controls. *Nature*, 464, 713-20.

Willett WC. (1998). Food-frequency methods. In: Willett WC, editor. Nutritional Epidemiology. Second edition ed. Oxford: *Oxford University Press*, 74-100.

Witsø E, Palacios G, Cinek O, Stene LC, Grinde B, Janowitz D, Lipkin WI, Rønningen KS. (2006). High prevalence of human enterovirus a infections in natural circulation of human enteroviruses. *J Clin Microbiol*, 44(11), 4095-100.

Witsø E, Palacios G, Rønningen KS, Cinek O, Janowitz D, Rewers M, Grinde B, Lipkin WI. (2007). Asymptomatic circulation of HEV71 in Norway. *Virus Res*, 123(1), 19-29.

Wolthers, K. C. et al. (2008). Human parechoviruses as an important viral cause of sepsislike illness and meningitis in young children. *Clin Infect Dis*, 47, 358-63.

Yazdanbakhsh, M., Kremsner, P. G. & van Ree, R. (2002). Allergy, parasites, and the hygiene hypothesis. *Science*, 296, 490-4.

Zazdanbakhsh M, van den Biggelaar AHJ, Maizels RM. (2001). Th2 responses without atopy: immunregulation in chronic helminth infections and reduced allergic disease. *Trends Immunol*, 22, 372-7.

Ziegler AG, Schmid S, Huber D, Hummel M, Bonifacio E. (2003). Early infant feeding and risk of developing type 1 diabetes-associated autoantibodies. *JAMA*, 290, 1721-8.

Ziegler AG, Pflueger M, Winkler C, Achenbach P, Akolkar B, Krischer JP, Bonifacio E. (2011). Accelerated progression from islet autoimmunity to diabetes is causing the escalating incidence of type 1 diabetes in young children. *J Autoimmun*, Mar 2.

Zoll, J. et al. (2009). Saffold virus, a human Theiler's-like cardiovirus, is ubiquitous and causes infection early in life. *PLoS Pathog*, 5, e1000416.

Øverby NC, Lillegaard IT, Johansson L, Andersen LF. (2004). High intake of added sugar among Norwegian children and adolescents. *Public Health Nutr*, 7, 285-93.

Aas KK, Tambs K, Kise MS, Magnus P, Rønningen KS. (2010). Genetic testing of newborns for type 1 diabetes susceptibility: a prospective cohort study on effects on maternal mental health. *BMC Med Genet*, 11, 112.

Part 2

Alternative Treatments for Diabetes

6

Honey and Type 1 Diabetes Mellitus

Mamdouh Abdulrhman[1], Mohamed El Hefnawy[2],
Rasha Ali[1] and Ahmad Abou El-Goud[1]
[1]Pediatric Department, Faculty of Medicine, Ain Shams University,
Abbasia - Cairo
[2]National Institute of Diabetes, Cairo
Egypt

1. Introduction

Type 1 diabetes mellitus is by far the most common metabolic and endocrinal disease in children (Peters & Schriger, 1997). The major dietary component responsible for fluctuations in blood glucose levels is carbohydrate. The amount, source (Jenkins et al., 1981; Gannon et al., 1989) and type (Brand et al., 1985) of carbohydrate appear to have profound influence on postprandial glucose levels. The chronic hyperglycemia of diabetes is associated with long-term damage, dysfunction and failure of various organs especially the eyes, kidneys, nerves, heart and blood vessels (American Diabetes Association, 2001).

The glycemic effect of any foodstuff is defined as its effect on blood glucose level postprandially. Both the glycemic index (GI) and the peak incremental index (PII) are used to assess the glycemic effect of different food stuffs (Jenkins et al., 1981). Jennie et al (2003) who studied the use of low glycemic index diets in the management of diabetes found that diets with low glycemic indices (GI), compared with conventional or high-GI diets, improved overall glycemic control in individuals with diabetes, as assessed by glycemic index, peak incremental index, reduced HbA1c and fructosamine. They concluded that using low-GI foods in place of conventional or high-GI foods has a clinically useful effect on postprandial hyperglycemia similar to that offered by pharmacological agents that target postprandial hyperglycemia. Similarly, the American Diabetes Association (2002) stated that the use of low-GI foods may reduce postprandial hyperglycemia.

Honey is the substance made when the nectar and sweet deposits from plants are gathered, modified and stored in the honeycomb by honey bees. It is composed primarily of the sugars glucose and fructose; its third greatest component is water. Honey also contains numerous other types of sugars, as well as acids, proteins and minerals (White et al., 1962; White, 1980; White, 1975). The water content of honey ranges between 15 to 20% (average 17.2%). Glucose and fructose, the major constituents of honey, account for about 85% of the honey solids. Besides, about 25 different sugars have been detected. The principal oligosaccharides in blossom honeys are disaccharides: sucrose, maltose, turanose, erlose. Trace amounts of tetra and pentasaccharides have also been isolated (Bogdanov, 2010). The protein and amino acid content of honey varies from 0.05 to 0.3 %. The honey proteins are mainly enzymes (White, 1975). Honey also contains varying amounts of mineral substances ranging from 0.02 to 1.03 g/100 g (White, 1975). Among honey benefits are its anti-inflammatory (Al Waili & Boni, 2003), anti- oxidant (Frankel et al., 1998; Gheldof & Engeseth, 2002; Gross et al., 2004) and anti-microbial effects (Molan, 1992; Steinberg et al., 1996; Molan, 1997; Theunissen et al., 2001). Further-more, several studies have shown that honey produced an attenuated postprandial glycemic response when compared with sucrose in both patients with diabetes and normal subjects (Ionescu-Tirgoviste et al., 1983; Shambaugh et al., 1990; Samanta et al., 1985; Al Waili, 2004; Agrawal et al., 2007).

C-peptide is considered to be a good marker of insulin secretion and has no biologic activity of its own (Ido et al., 1997). Measurement of C-peptide, however, provides a fully validated means of quantifying endogenous insulin secretion. C-peptide is co-secreted with insulin by the pancreatic cells as a by-product of the enzymatic cleavage of proinsulin to insulin. Consequently, serum C-peptide level can be used as a true indicator of any change in the insulin level, which is the main determinant of plasma glucose level.

Several studies were performed in healthy and in type 2 diabetic patients to evaluate the effects of honey on the insulin and C-peptide levels, and the results were controversial (Bornet et al., 1985; Elliott et al., 2002; Watford, 2002; Al-Waili, 2003).

2. Aim of the study

The aim of this work was to compare the effects of honey, sucrose and glucose on plasma glucose and C-peptide levels in children and adolescents with type 1 diabetes mellitus.

3. Subjects and methods

3.1 Subjects

Twenty patients with type 1 diabetes mellitus, aged 3–18 (mean 10.95 years) and ten healthy non-diabetic children and adolescents, aged 1–17 (mean 8.5 years) were studied. All subjects were within 68–118% and 77–125% of their ideal body weight and height, respectively. The mean BMI of patients and controls were 22.60 and 23.15, respectively. All patients with diabetes had a mean glycosylated hemoglobin of 9.9% (range = 7–15%). The sex ratio in patients and controls was 1:1. The patients were recruited from the regular attendants of the children clinic of the National Institute of Diabetes in Cairo, Egypt. The study was approved by the local ethical committee, and an informed written consent was obtained from at least one parent of each subject before the study. All patients were receiving three insulin injections per day, each consisting of a mixture of a medium-acting insulin (isophane NPH) and a short-acting soluble insulin (human Actrapid).

3.2 Methods

All patients were primarily diagnosed with type 1 insulin-dependent diabetes mellitus by measuring the serum level of C-peptide on presentation [the patient was considered suffering from insulin-dependent diabetes mellitus type 1 if the C-peptide level was below 0.4 ng/dl (Connors, 2000)]. All subjects were subjected to the following:

1. Anthropometric measures including weight in kg and height in cm which were plotted against percentiles for age and sex.
2. Oral sugar tolerance tests using glucose, sucrose and honey in three separate sittings: After an overnight fast (8 h) and omission of the morning insulin dose, a calculated amount of each sugar (amount = weight of subject in kg X 1.75 with a maximum of 75 g) (William & Ruchi, 2005) was diluted in 200 ml water and then ingested over 5 min in a

random order, on separate mornings 1 week apart. The honey dose for each patient was calculated based on the fact that each 100 gm of the honey used in this study contained 77.3 gm sugars. So if a patient weighs for example 20 kg, he/she should receive 20 x 1.75 = 35 gm sugar which will be present in (35 x 100) ÷ 77.3 = 45.3 gm honey. Venous blood was sampled just before ingestion and then every 30 min postprandial for 2 h thereafter. Samples were left to clot, centrifuged and glucose assay was performed chemically on the Synchron CX5 autoanalyzer (Beckman instruments Inc.)[1].

3. Measurement of fasting and postprandial serum C- peptide level: Venous blood samples were withdrawn from each subject at 0 (fasting) and 2 h postprandial after ingestion of each individual sugar. The samples were then centrifuged and serum was stored in aliquots at – 20°C. At the end of the study, samples were calibrated for C-peptide using the biosource c-pep-easia[2], which is a solid phase enzyme amplified sensitivity immunoassay performed on a microtiter plate. A fixed amount of C-peptide labeled with horseradish peroxidase (HRP) competes with unlabeled C-peptide present in the calibrators controls and samples for a limited number of binding sites on a specific antibody. After 2 h incubation at room temperature, the microtiter plates were washed to stop the competition reaction. The chromogenic solution (TMB-H2O2) was added and incubated for 30 min. The reaction was stopped with the addition of stop solution, and the microtiter plate was then read at the appropriate wave length. The amount of substrate turnover was determined colorimetrically by measuring the absorbance which was inversely proportionate to the C-peptide concentration. A calibration curve was plotted and C-peptide concentration in samples was determined by interpolation from the calibration curve.

4. Calculation of glycemic and peak incremental indices (see example figure 3.1):

$$\text{Glycemic index of the food } (\text{Jenkins}, 1987) = \frac{\text{Area under glycemic curve of test food}}{\text{Area under glycemic curve of glucose}}$$

*   Area under curve (AUC) refers to the area included between the baseline and incremental blood glucose points when connected by straight lines. The area under each incremental glucose curve is calculated using the trapezoid rule (note: only areas above the baseline are used).
*   Peak incremental index (PII) (Samanta et al., 1985) is defined as the ratio of the maximal increment of plasma glucose produced by sugar to that produced by glucose

$$\text{Peak incremental index } = \frac{\text{Maximal increment produced by the sugar tested}}{\text{Maximal increment produced by glucose}}$$

Maximal increment is the difference between the peak point and the fasting point.

3.3 Statistical analysis

Standard computer program SPSS for Windows, release 13.0 (SPSS Inc., USA) was used for data entry and analysis. All numeric variables were expressed as mean ± standard deviation (SD). Comparison of different variables in various groups was done using student t-test and Mann–Whitney test for normal and non-parametric variables, respectively. Wilcoxon signed

---

[1] Beckman: 2005, kraemerBLW, Brew, CA 92621, USA.

[2] Biosource Europe S.A – Rue de lindustrie, 8-B-1400-Nivelles-Belgium.

rank tests were used to compare multiple readings of the same variables. Chi-square ($\chi2$) test was used to compare frequency of qualitative variables among the different groups (Daniel, 1995).

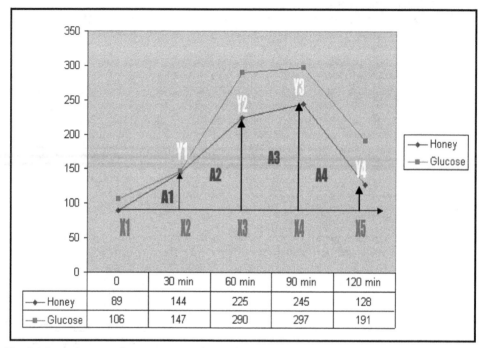

	0	30 min	60 min	90 min	120 min
—◆— Honey	89	144	225	245	128
—■— Glucose	106	147	290	297	191

Fig. 3.1 Oral glucose tolerance curve of one of our patients

For calculation of the area under honey curve (AUC) $= A_1+A_2+A_3+A_4$

A_1 is a triangle $= 1/2$ base x height $= 1/2(X_2 - X_1)$ x $(Y_1 - X_2) = \frac{1}{2}(30)$ x $(144 - 89) = 15$ x $55 = 825$

A_2 is a trapezoid $= 1/2$ sum of the parallel sides (heights) x base

$$= 1/2[(Y_1 - X_2) + (Y_2 - X_3)] \times (X_4 - X_5) = 1/2[(144 - 89) + (225 - 89)] \times 30 = 1/2(55 + 136) \times 30 = 1/2(191) \times 30 = 95.5 \times 30 = 2865$$

A_3 is a trapezoid $= 1/2$ sum of the parallel sides (heights) x base

$$= 1/2[(Y_2 - X_3) + (Y_3 - X_4)] \times (X_4 - X_3) = 1/2[(225 - 89) + (245 - 89)] \times 30 = 1/2(136 + 156) \times 30 = 1/2(292) \times 30 = 146 \times 30 = 4380$$

A_4 is a trapezoid $= 1/2$ sum of the parallel sides (heights) x base

$$= 1/2[(Y_3 - X_4) + (Y_4 - X_5)] \times (X_3 - X_2) = 1/2[(245 - 89) + (128 - 89)] \times 30 = 1/2(156 + 39) \times 30 = 1/2(195) \times 30 = 97.5 \times 30 = 2925$$

$$AUC = A_1 + A_2 + A_3 + A_4 = 825 + 2865 + 4380 + 2925 = 10995$$

4. Results

No significant difference was found between patients (diabetics) and controls (non-diabetics) as regards the age and anthropometric measures (table 4.1). The mean age of subjects in the diabetic and non- diabetic groups was 11.3 and 8.5 years, respectively, with no statistically significant difference between groups (P > 0.05). The mean weight %, height % and body mass index did not also differ significantly between diabetics and non-diabetics (93.6%, 99.2%, 22.6 versus 94%, 98.2%, 23.1, respectively; P > 0.05). The mean plasma glucose level at 0 (fasting) and 30 min postprandial (i.e. 30 min after intake of glucose, sucrose or honey) did not differ significantly between subjects in both groups (diabetics and non-diabetics) (Tables 4.2 - 4.5) (P > 0.05). In non-diabetics (control), as shown in tables 4.2 and 4.3, the mean plasma glucose level 60, 90 and 120 min after intake of honey became significantly lower than after either glucose or sucrose (P< 0.05). Similarly, as shown in tables 4.4 and 4.5, there was a statistically significant decrease of plasma glucose in diabetics at 60, 90 and 120 min after honey intake, when compared with either glucose or sucrose (P< 0.05). The glycemic index (GI) and the peak incremental index (PII) of either sucrose or honey did not differ significantly between patients and controls (P > 0.05). On the other hand, both the GI and PII of honey were significantly lower when compared with sucrose in patients and controls. In non-diabetics, the glycemic index (GI) of honey was 0.69 compared to 1.32 for sucrose, with statistically significant difference (P< 0.05). In diabetics, the GI of honey was also significantly lower than that of sucrose (o.61 versus 1.19, respectively; P< 0.001) (table 4.6; figure 4.1). The PII of honey in non-diabetics was 0.61, compared to 1.25 for sucrose (P< 0.05). In diabetics, the PII of honey was also significantly lower than that of sucrose (0.60 versus 1.10, respectively; P< 0.001) (table 4.7; figure 4.2).

The mean (±SD) fasting C-peptide of patients and controls were 0.15 (±0.13) and 1.91 (±0.77) ng/ml, respectively (P< 0.001). All diabetic patients had a basal C-peptide level less than 0.7 ng/ml. In diabetics, although honey intake resulted in increase in the mean level of C-peptide, yet this increase was not statistically significant when compared with either glucose or sucrose (P> 0.05) (Table 4.8; figure 4.3). On the other hand, in non-diabetics, honey produced a statistically significant higher C-peptide level, when compared with either glucose or sucrose (P< 0.05) (Table 4.8; figure 4.4).

Variable	Diabetics	Non-diabetics	P
Age (yr)	11.30 ± 4.80	8.50 ± 5.38	>0.05
Weight %	93.60 ± 13.82	94.00 ± 14.28	>0.05
Height %	99.20 ± 13.01	98.20 ± 11.14	>0.05
BMI	22.59 ± 5.50	23.14 ± 2.90	>0.05

P > 0.05 is non significant
BMI: Body Mass Index

Table 4.1 Age and anthropometric measures in diabetics and non-diabetic controls (mean ± SD)

Time (min)	Glucose	Honey	P
0	75.20 ± 17.45	72.30 ± 9.09	> 0.05
30	86.00 ± 19.88	83.30 ± 9.52	> 0.05
60	102.90 ± 24.47	88.80 ± 10.04	< 0.05
90	103.60 ± 21.24	88.50 ± 8.64	< 0.05
120	91.10 ± 20.74	81.00 ± 8.30	< 0.05

Table 4.2 Mean plasma glucose (±SD) (mg/dl) in non-diabetics (control) following equivalent amount of glucose or honey (P < 0.05 is significant)

Time (min)	Sucrose	Honey	P
0	68.50 ± 12.59	72.30 ± 9.09	> 0.05
30	83.80 ± 13.56	83.30 ± 9.52	> 0.05
60	101.60 ± 11.45	88.80 ± 10.04	< 0.05
90	105.40 ± 18.03	88.50 ± 8.64	< 0.05
120	93.60 ± 17.25	81.00 ± 8.30	< 0.05

Table 4.3 Mean plasma glucose (±SD) (mg/dl) in non-diabetics (control) following equivalent amount of sucrose or honey (P < 0.05 is significant)

Time (min)	Glucose	Honey	P
0	206.05 ± 95.79	208.10 ± 92.76	> 0.05
30	257.55 ± 92.79	247.75 ± 99.44	> 0.05
60	339.80 ± 96.86	285.50 ± 86.29	< 0.05
90	328.05 ± 99.75	272.25 ± 85.33	< 0.05
120	297.90 ± 106.86	236.75 ± 76.80	< 0.05

Table 4.4 Mean plasma glucose (±SD) (mg/dl) in diabetics following equivalent amount of glucose or honey (P < 0.05 is significant)

Time (min)	Sucrose	Honey	P
0	198.30 ± 77.762	208.10 ± 92.76	> 0.05
30	268.25 ± 78.78	247.75 ± 99.44	> 0.05
60	320.35 ± 67.17	285.50 ± 86.29	< 0.05
90	323.65 ± 71.27	272.25 ± 85.33	< 0.05
120	310.15 ± 92.63	236.75 ± 76.80	< 0.05

Table 4.5 Mean plasma glucose (±SD) (mg/dl) in diabetics following equivalent amount of sucrose or honey (P < 0.05 is significant)

	Sucrose	Honey	
	GI	GI	P
Non- diabetics	1.32 (0.85–1.92)	0.69 (0.43–1.43)	< 0.05
Diabetics	1.19 (0.31–3.08)	0.61 (0.15–1.92)	< 0.001

Table 4.6 Glycemic index (GI) mean (range) of sucrose and honey (glycemic index of glucose = 1) (P < 0.05 is significant; P < 0.001 is highly significant)

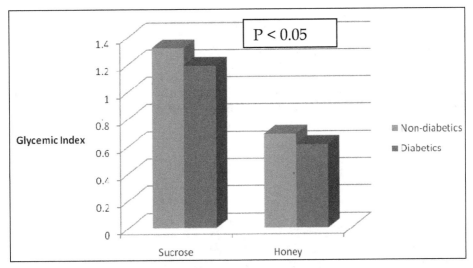

Fig. 4.1 Glycemic index of sucrose and honey

	Sucrose	Honey	P
	PII	PII	
Non- diabetics	1.25 (0.50–1.82)	0.61 (0.30–1.10)	< 0.05
Diabetics	1.10 (0.65–2.98)	0.60 (0.20–1.60)	< 0.001

Table 4.7 Peak incremental index (PII) mean (range) of sucrose and honey (peak incremental index of glucose = 1) (P < 0.05 is significant; P < 0.001 is highly significant)

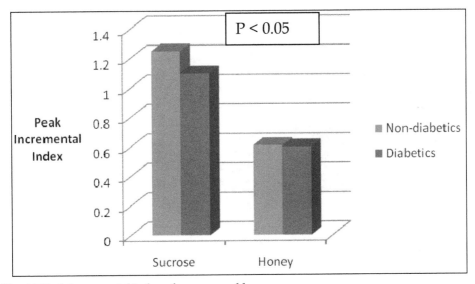

Fig. 4.2 Peak incremental index of sucrose and honey

Group	C-peptide (ng/ml)			P
	After glucose	After sucrose	After honey	
Non-diabetics	3.96 ± 0.84	3.99 ± 1.10	5.50 ± 1.15	P < 0.05
Diabetics	0.29 ± 0.53	0.32 ± 0.53	0.47 ± 1.09	P > 0.05

Table 4.8 Mean C-peptide (±SD) (ng/ml) following equivalent amount of glucose, sucrose or honey in non-diabetics and diabetics (P < 0.05 is significant)

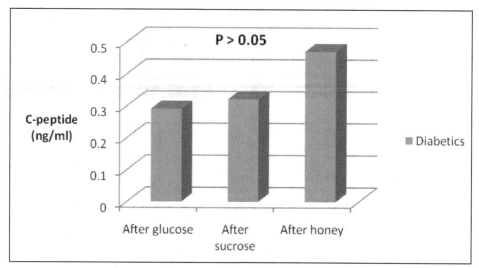

Fig. 4.3 C-peptide following equivalent amount of glucose, sucrose or honey in diabetics

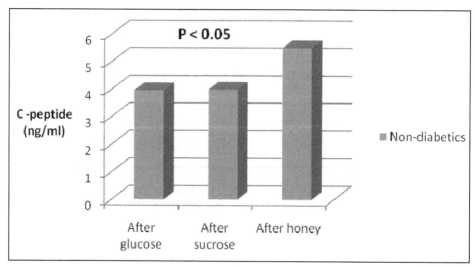

Fig. 4.4 C-peptide following equivalent amount of glucose, sucrose or honey in non-diabetics

5. Discussion

As shown in many studies, sustained hyperglycemia is a risk factor for both micro vascular and macro vascular (as cardiovascular) complications in type 2 diabetes mellitus (Laakso & Lehto, 1997; Bretzel et al., 1998 as cited from Oizumi et al., 2007), while postprandial hyperglycemia has also been considered a risk factor for cardiovascular complications (Tominaga et al., 1999; Risso et al., 2001; Chiasson et al., 2002; Hanefeld et al., 2004; Nakagami et al., 2004 as cited from Oizumi et al., 2007). Many experimental and epidemiological studies have shown that increased postprandial plasma glucose levels may have equally or even more harmful effects than fasting hyperglycemia (Tominaga et al., 1999; Risso et al., 2001; Nakagami et al., 2004 as cited from Oizumi et al., 2007), and the reduction of postprandial plasma glucose levels delays the development of cardiovascular complications (Chiasson et al., 2002; Hanefeld et al., 2004 as cited from Oizumi et al., 2007).

Jenkins (1987) defined the glycemic index as the ratio between the blood glucose areas produced after ingestion of a studied sugar compared to the blood glucose area produced after glucose ingestion itself. He stated that the glycemic response to food affects the insulin response which in turn is also potentiated by other non-glucose dependent factors in this food (Ostman et al., 2001). On the other hand, FAO/WHO (1998) defined the glycemic index as the incremental blood glucose area (0-2 h) following ingestion of 50 g of available carbohydrates (no fibers or resistant starch included), expressed as a percentage of the corresponding area following an equivalent amount of carbohydrate from a standard reference product. Samnata et al (1985) defined the peak incremental index of a certain sugar as the ratio between the maximal increments of the glucose level after ingestion of the sugar compared to the maximal increment produced after ingestion of glucose. He also mentioned that both the glycemic and the peak incremental indices are closely related, highly dependent and positively correlated to the plasma glucose produced after ingestion of any given sugar. Therefore, any change in the plasma glucose level after ingestion of a certain sugar will markedly affect both the glycemic index and the peak incremental index. Hence, the glycemic and the peak incremental indices measure how fast and how much a food raises blood glucose levels. Foods with higher index values raise blood sugar more rapidly than foods with lower index values do in case of the glycemic index and much more in case of peak incremental index.

In our study, no statistically significant differences were found between diabetic patients and non-diabetic controls regarding the glycemic and the peak incremental indices of the studied sugars. Similarly, Samnata et al (1985), who studied the glycemic effect of glucose, sucrose and honey in 12 normal volunteers, eight patients with insulin-dependent diabetes mellitus (IDDM) and six patients with non-insulin-dependent diabetes mellitus (NIDDM), found no significant differences between the normal volunteers and diabetic patients regarding the glycemic and peak incremental indices of both sugars. Since the glycemic index (GI) is the ratio between the area under curve (AUC) of the studied sugar and the AUC of glucose, and the peak incremental index (PII) is the ratio between the maximal blood glucose increment of the studied sugar and that of glucose; it may be expected that both GI and PII will be the same in both diabetics and non-diabetics. Our study showed that honey has statistically significant lower glycemic and peak incremental indices than sucrose and glucose in both patients and controls (< 1 with honey, 1 with glucose being the reference sugar and >1 with sucrose). In agreement, Kaye et al (2002), who published the international table of glycemic index and glycemic load values, found that the GI of honey (0.55 ± 0.05) was lower than that of sucrose (1.10 ± 0.21). Also, Shambaugh et al (1990) found that sucrose caused higher blood sugar readings than honey in normal volunteers. In the study of

Samnata et al (1985), honey ingestion in both diabetics (IDDM) and non-diabetics also resulted in a significantly lower PII compared to the glucose and sucrose. In the study done by Al-Waili (2004), honey compared with dextrose and sucrose caused a lower elevation of plasma glucose levels (PGL) in both diabetics (IDDM) and normal subjects. In an attempt to explain his results, he stated that the mild reduction of plasma glucose levels obtained by honey might be a result of the fructose content of honey which requires metabolic transformation in the liver, a slow process conferring relatively low-GI on these sugars (Jenkins et al., 1981; Wolever et al., 1991). Also, Watford (2002) demonstrated that very small amounts of fructose, which is the main component of honey, could increase hepatic glucose uptake and glycogen storage, as well as reduce peripheral glycemia which could be beneficial in diabetic patients. In the study performed by Agrawal et al (2007), honey was found to produce an attenuated postprandial glycemic response especially in subjects with glucose intolerance. They referred these results to the possibility that the glucose component of honey might be poorly absorbed from the gut epithelium. Also, Tirgoviste et al (1983) studied blood glucose and plasma insulin responses to various carbohydrates in type 2 diabetes, and they found that the increase in plasma glucose was significantly higher after administration of more refined carbohydrates such as glucose than after the complex ones such as honey. Meanwhile, Oizumi et al (2007) and Arai et al (2004) found that consumption of a palatinose (a disaccharide found in honey)-based balanced formula suppressed postprandial hyperglycemia, glycemic and peak incremental indices and produced beneficial effects on the metabolic syndrome–related parameters (namely, the lipid profile and visceral fat accumulation) in diabetic patients. They stated the reason of this observation to be due to the fact that although palatinose is completely absorbed, yet it has the specific characteristics of delayed digestion and absorption as reported by Dahlquist et al (1963) and Lina et al (2002).

Our results showed that honey, compared to glucose and sucrose, caused a significant elevation in the C-peptide levels in non-diabetic subjects. Meanwhile, in diabetic patients, the plasma C-peptide levels did not differ significantly between the three types of sugars. To our knowledge, no similar work was done to study the effects of honey on C-peptide levels in type 1 diabetes mellitus. However, several studies were performed in healthy and in type 2 diabetic patients to evaluate the effects of honey on the insulin and C-peptide levels, and the results were controversial. In the study of Al Waili (2003), inhalation of honey solution, when compared with hyperosmolar dextrose and hypoosmolar distilled water, resulted in a significant elevation of plasma insulin and C-peptide in both normal individuals and in patients with type 2 diabetes mellitus. However, in 2004, the same author found that honey ingestion, when compared with sucrose, caused a greater elevation of insulin and C-peptide in type 2 diabetic patients, while in healthy subjects dextrose ingestion caused a significant elevation of plasma insulin and C-peptide when compared with honey. The author hypothesized that honey may have the ability to stimulate insulin production and secretion from the pancreas than do sucrose in type 2 diabetes mellitus. On the other hand, Bornet et al (1985) reported no significant changes in plasma insulin levels after honey ingestion compared to sucrose in type 2 diabetics. Liljeberg et al (1999) found that high-GI foods induced a greater elevation of blood insulin than did low glycemic index meals (like honey). Elliott et al (2002) tried to explore whether fructose consumption might be a contributing factor to the development of obesity and the accompanying metabolic abnormalities observed in the insulin resistance syndrome and they found that honey intake caused a significant lowering of plasma insulin and C-peptide in normal subjects when compared to sucrose and dextrose. They related their findings to the fructose content of honey which does not stimulate insulin secretion from pancreatic beta cells and that consumption of foods and beverages containing fructose produced a smaller postprandial insulin excursions than did consumption of glucose-containing carbohydrates (Glinsmann & Bowman, 1993). Also, Watford et al (2002) stated that very small amounts of fructose, which is the main component of honey, could increase hepatic glucose uptake and glycogen storage, as well as reduce peripheral glycemia and thus insulin levels. Ionescu-Tirgoviste et al (1983) studied the blood glucose and plasma insulin responses to some simple carbohydrates (glucose, fructose, lactose) and some complex ones (apples, potatoes, bread, rice, carrots and honey) in 32 type 2 (non-insulin-dependent) diabetic patients, and they found that increases in plasma insulin were significantly higher after the more refined carbohydrates (glucose, fructose and lactose) than after the more complex ones (apples, potatoes, rice, carrots and honey, P less than 0.01).

We hypothesize that honey might have a direct stimulatory effect on the healthy beta cells of pancreas; an effect which may be related to the non-sugar part of honey. This hypothesis is based on the finding that honey caused significant postprandial increase in the C-peptide level despite its lower glycemic and peak incremental indices when compared to either glucose or sucrose. On the other hand, the lack of significant increase in C-peptide levels among diabetic patients might be due to the minimal residual function of the patient's pancreatic beta cells, which is beyond their capacity of further postprandial response. This proposal is backed up by the findings of Pozzan et al (1997) who investigated the relation between the fasting C-peptide level and the ability to respond to a particular stimulus, and they reported that there is a positive significant correlation between the basal value (BV) and the peak value (PV) of C-peptide in insulin dependent diabetic patients and that positive responses need a minimal basal level of 0.74 ng/ml. In all our studied patients, the basal C-peptide level was less than 0.7 ng/ml. Also other authors found significant correlations between the basal and the maximum C-peptide values after a stimulus. However, they reported different basal values which can respond to stimulation. Such values were 0.09 (Clarson et al., 1987), 0.18 (Eff et al., 1989) and 0.39 ng/ml (Faber & Binder, 1977). The variation in these levels was probably due to the different ages and different diabetes duration of the studied populations (Pozzan et al., 1997).

6. Conclusions and recommendations

1. Honey has a lower glycemic and peak incremental indices compared to glucose and sucrose in both type 1 diabetic patients and non-diabetics. Therefore, we recommend using honey as a sugar substitute in type 1 diabetic patients.

2. In spite of its significantly lower glycemic and peak incremental indices, honey caused significant post- prandial rise of plasma C-peptide levels when compared to glucose and sucrose in non-diabetics; indicating that honey may have a direct stimulatory effect on the healthy beta cells of pancreas. On the other hand, C-peptide levels were not significantly elevated after honey ingestion when compared with either glucose or sucrose in type 1 diabetic patients. Whether or not ingestion of honey in larger doses or/and for an extended period of time would have a significant positive effect on the diseased beta cells, needs further studies.

7. References

Agrawal, O.; Pachauri, A.; Yadav, H.; Urmila, J.; Goswamy, H.; Chapperwal, A.; Bisen, P. & Prasad, G. (2007). Subjects with impaired glucose tolerance exhibit a high degree of tolerance to honey. J Med Food 10(3):473–478

Al Waili, N. (2004). Natural honey lowers plasma glucose, C-reactive protein, homocysteine, and blood lipids in healthy, diabetic, and hyperlipidemic subjects: comparison with dextrose and sucrose. J Med Food 7(1):100-107

Al Waili, N. & Boni, N. (2003). Natural honey lowers plasma prostaglandin concentrations in normal individuals. J Med Food 6(2):129-133

Al-Waili, N. (2003). Intrapulmonary administrations of natural honey solution, hyperosmolar dextrose or hyperosmolar distill water to normal individuals and to patients with type 2 diabetes mellitus or hypertension: their effects on blood glucose level, plasma insulin and C-peptide, blood pressure and peak expiratory flow rate. Eur J Med Res 8(7):295-303

American Diabetes Association. (2001). Report of the expert committee on the diagnosis and classification of diabetes mellitus (committee report).Diabetes care 24, (Suppl.1)

American Diabetes Association (2002). Evidence-based nutrition principles and recommendations for the treatment and prevention of diabetes and related complications. Diabetes Care 25:202-212

Arai, H.; Mizuno, A.; Matsuo, K.; Fukaya, M.; Sasaki, H.; Arima, H.; Matsuura, M.; Taketani, Y.; Doi, T. & Takeda, E. (2004). Effect of a novel palatinose-based liquid balanced formula (MHN-01) on glucose and lipid metabolism in male Sprague-Dawley rats after short- and long-term ingestion. Metabolism 53:977-983

Bogdanov, S. (December 2010). Book of Honey, Chapter 5, Honey Composition, Bee Product Science, available from www.bee-hexagon.net

Bornet, F.; Haardt, M.; Costagliola, D.; Blayo, A. & Slama, G. (1985). Sucrose or honey at breakfast has no additional acute hyper-glycemic effect over an isoglucidic amount of bread in type 2 diabetic patients. Diabetologia 28(4):213-217

Brand, J.; Nicholson, P.; Thorburn, A. & Truswell, A. (1985). Food processing and the glycemic index. Am J Clin Nutr. Dec; 42(6):1192-6

Bretzel, R.; Voigt, K. & Schatz, H. (1998). The United Kingdom Prospective Diabetes Study (UKPDS) implications for the pharmacotherapy of type 2 diabetes mellitus. Exp Clin Endocrinol diabetes 106: 369-372

Chiasson, J.; Josse, R.; Gomis, R.; Hanefeld, M.; Karasik, A. & Laakso, M. (2002). STOP-NIDDM Trial Research Group. Acarbose for prevention of type 2 diabetes mellitus: the STOP- NIDDM trial. Lancet 259: 2072-2077

Clarson, C.; Daneman, D.; Drash, A.; Beckert, D. & Ehelich, R. (1987). Residual B-cell function in children with IDDM; reproducibility of testing and factors influencing insulin secretory reserve. Diabetes Care 10(1):33-38 515

Connors, T. (September 2000). Interpreting your C-peptide values; diabetes health, available from http://www.diabeteshealth.com.html. Updated 2000/09, accessed Jan 2008

Dahlquist, A.; Auricchio, S.; Semenza, G. & Prader, A. (1963). Human intestinal disaccharidases and hereditary disaccharide intolerance: the hydrolysis of sucrose, isomaltose, palatinose (isomaltulose), and 1, 6-a-oligosaccharide (isomalto-oligosaccharide) preparation. J Clin Invest 42:556-562

Daniel, W. (1995). Biostatistics: a foundation for analysis in the health sciences, 6th edn. Wiley, New York

Eff, C.; Fabet, O. & Deckert, T. (1989). Persistent insulin secretion assessed by plasma C-peptide estimation in long-term juvenile diabetes with a low insulin requirement. Diabetologia 32:305- 311

Elliott, S.; Keim, N. & Stern, J. (2002). Fructose, weight gain and the insulin. Am J Clin Nutr 76:911-922

Faber, O. & Binder, C. (1977). B-cell function and blood glucose control in insulin dependent diabetes within the first month of insulin treatment. Diabetologia 13:263–268

FAO/WHO. (1998). Carbohydrates in human nutrition (Paper No. 66). Food and Agricultural Organization and Geneva, World Health Organization, Rome

Frankel, S.; Robinson, G. & Berenbaum, M. (1998). Antioxidant capacity and correlated characteristics of 14 unifloral honeys. J Apic Res 37(1):27–31

Gannon, M.; Nuttall, F.; Westphal, S.; Neil, B. & Seaquist, E. (1989). Effects of dose of ingested glucose on plasma metabolite and hormone responses in type II diabetic subjects. Diabetes Care12:544-552

Gheldof, N. & Engeseth, N. (2002). Antioxidant capacity of honeys from various floral sources based on the determination of oxygen radical absorbance capacity and inhibition of in vitro lipoprotein oxidation in human serum samples. J Agric Food Chem 50(10):3050–3055

Glinsmann, W. & Bowman, B. (1993). The public health significance of crystalline fructose, glucose tolerance. Am J Clin Nutr 77(3):612–621 506

Gross, H.; Polagruto, J.; Zhu, Q.; Kim, S.; Schramm, D. & Keen, C. (2004). Effect of honey consumption on plasma antioxidant status in human subjects. Abstracts of Papers of the American Chemical Society, 227: U29

Hanefeld, M.; Cagatay, M.; Petrowitsch, T.; Neuser, D.; Petzinna, D. & Rupp, M. (2004). Acarbose reduces the risk of myocardial infarction in type 2 diabetic patients: meta-analysis of seven long- term studies. Eur Heart J 25:10-16

Ido, Y.; Vindigni, A. & Chang, K. (1997). Prevention of vascular and neural dysfunction in diabetic rats by C-peptide. Science 277(5325):563–566

Ionescu-Tirgoviste, C.; Popa, E.; Sintu, E.; Mihalache, N.; Cheta, D. & Mincu, I. (1983). Blood glucose and plasma insulin responses to various carbohydrates in type 2 non-insulin-dependent diabetes. Diabetologia 24:80–84

Jenkins, D. (1987). The glycemic index and the dietary treatment of hypertriglyceridemia and diabetes. J Am Coll Nutr 61:11–17

Jenkins, D.; Wolever, T.; Taylor, R.; Barker, H.; Fielden, H.; Baldwin, J.; et al (1981). Glycemic index of foods: a physiological basis for carbohydrate exchange. Am J Clin Nutr 34(3):362– 366

Jennie, B.; Hayne, S.; Petocz, P. & Stephen, C. (2003). Low-glycemic index diets in the management of diabetes. Diabetes Care 26:2261–2267

Kaye, F.; Holt, S. & Janette, C. (2002). International table of glycemic index and glycemic load values. Am J Clin Nutr 76:5n56

Laakso, M. & Lehto, S. (1997). Epidemiology of macrovascular disease in diabetes. J Diabetes Rev 5: 294-315

Liljeberg, H.; Akerberg, A. & Bjorck, I. (1999). Effect of the glycemic index and content of indigestible carbohydrates of cereal-based breakfast meals on glucose tolerance at lunch in healthy subjects. Am J Clin Nutr 69:647–655 503

Lina, B.; Jonker, D. & Kozianowski, G. (2002). Isomaltulose (palatinose): a review of biological and toxicological studies. Food Chem Toxicol 40:1375–1381

Molan, P. (1992). The antibacterial activity of honey. 1. The nature of the antibacterial activity. Bee World 73(1):5-28 (2. Variation in the potency of the antibacterial activity. Bee World 73(2): 59–76)

Molan, P. (1997). Honey as an antimicrobial agent. In: Mizrahi A, Lensky Y (eds) Bee products: properties, applications and api-therapy. Plenum, London, pp 27–37

Nakagami, T. & the DECODA Study Group. (2004). Hyperglycemia and mortality from all causes and from cardiovascular disease in five populations of Asian origin. Diabetologia 47: 385-394

Oizumi, T.; Daimon, M.; Jimbu, Y.; Kameda, W.; Arawaka, N.; Yamaguchi, H.; Ohnuma, H.; Sasaki, H. & Kato, T. (2007). A palatinose- based formula improves glucose tolerance, serum free fatty acid levels and body fat composition. Tohoku J Exp Med 212:91-99

Ostman, E.; Liljeberg, H.; Elmstahl, H. & Bjorck, I. (2001). Inconsistency between glycemic and insulinemic responses to regular and fermented milk products. Am J Clin Nutr 74(1):96-100

Peters, A. & Schriger, D. (1997). Impact of new diagnostic criteria on the diagnosis of diabetes (abstract). Diabetes 46 (Suppl.1):7A

Pozzan, R.; Dimetz, T.; Gazolla, H. & Gomes, M. (1997). Discriminative capacity of fasting C-peptide levels in a functional test according to different criteria of responser to a stimulus; a study of Brazilian insulin-dependent diabetic patients. Braz J Med Biol Res 30(10):1169-1174 511

Risso, A.; Mercuri, F.; Quagliaro, L.; Damante, G. & Ceriello, A. (2001). Intermittent high glucose enhances apoptosis in human umbilical vein endothelial cells in culture. Am J Physiol Endocrinol Metab 281: E924-E930

Samanta, A.; Burden, A. & Jones, G. (1985). Plasma glucose responses to glucose, sucrose, and honey in patients with diabetes mellitus: an analysis of glycemic and peak incremental indices. Diabet Med 2:371-373

Shambaugh, P.; Worthington, V. & Herbert, J. (1990). Differential effects of honey, sucrose, and fructose on blood sugar levels. J Manip Physiol Ther 13:322-325

Steinberg, D.; Kaine, G. & Gedalia, I. (1996). Antibacterial effect of propolis and honey on oral bacteria. Am J Dent 9(6):236-239

Theunissen, F.; Grobler, S. & Gedalia, I. (2001). The antifungal action of three South African honeys on Candida albicans. Apidologie 32(4):371-379

Tominaga, M.; Eguchi, H.; Manaka, H.; Igarashi, K.; Kato, T. & Sekikawa, A. (1999). Impaired glucose tolerance is a risk factor for cardiovascular disease, but not impaired fasting glucose. The Funagata Diabetes Study. Diabetes Care 22: 920-924

Watford, M. (2002). Small amounts of dietary fructose dramatically increase hepatic glucose uptake. Nutr Rev 60(8):253-257

White, JW Jr. (1980). Detection of honey adulteration by carbohydrate analysis. JAOAC 63(1):11-18

White, JW Jr.; et al. (1962). Composition of American honeys. Tech. Bull. 1261. Agricultural Research Service, USDA, Washington DC

White, J. (1975). Composition of honey. In Crane, E (ed.) Honey. A Comprehensive survey, Heinemann Edition; London, pp 157-206

William, C. & Ruchi, M. (2005). Glucose tolerance test, available from http://www.medicinenet.com/glucose_tolerance_test/article.htm. 2005.medicinenet

Wolever, T.; Jenkins, D.; Jenkins, A. & Josse, R. (1991). The glycemic index: methodology and clinical implications. Am J Clin Nutr 54(5):846-854

7

Potentials and Limitations of Bile Acids and Probiotics in Diabetes Mellitus

Momir Mikov[1,2], Hani Al-Salami[3] and Svetlana Golocorbin-Kon[1,2]
*[1]Department of Pharmacology, Toxicology and Clinical
Pharmacology, Medical Faculty, Univeristy of Novi Sad*
[2]Pharmacy Faculty, University of Montenegro, Podgorica
[3]Senior Lecturer, School of Pharmacy, Curtin University, Perth
[1]Serbia
[2]Montenegro
[3]Australia

1. Introduction

Diabetes mellitus is a metabolic disorder classified as Type 1 (T1D) or Type 2 (T2D). T1D is an autoimmune disorder characterized by the destruction of the β-cells of the pancreas resulting in a partial or complete lack of insulin production and the inability of the body to control glucose homeostasis (Akerblom et al. 2002). T1D is also known as juvenile-onset diabetes because it manifests at a young age (Bruno et al. 2005). As it requires the patient to inject insulin to supplement the partial or complete lack of insulin production by the pancreas, it is also called insulin-dependent diabetes mellitus (IDDM). T2D, formerly known as noninsulin-dependent diabetes mellitus (NIDDM) or adult-onset diabetes, is a metabolic disorder with onset most common in middle age and later life (Campbell 1991). T2D may be controlled by diet and exercise and, unlike T1D, does not always require the use of insulin (Campbell 2004). However, the term "noninsulin-dependent" is a misnomer since many patients require insulin therapy at some time in the course of their disease. T2D is often associated with obesity, hypertension and insulin resistance and can result in the complete destruction of beta-cells of the pancreas leading to T1D (Campbell 2004; Weiss & Caprio 2006). The prevalence of T1D and T2D are on the rise worldwide, which has generated a strong drive towards developing preventative measures as well as cure. Recent data published by the International Diabetes Federation highlighted the severity of diabetes epidemic. Data show that the disease is currently affecting 246 million people worldwide, with 46% of all those affected in the 40-59 age group. Previous figures underestimated the scope of the problem, while even the most pessimistic predictions fell short of the current figure. It is predicted that the total number of people living with diabetes will increase to 380 million within twenty years if no new and substantially more effective drugs are produced (Moore et al. 2003a; Rosenbloom et al. 1999). On 2007, the health costs of diabetes have exceeded 200 billion dollars only in the US. This adds to the cost generated from higher rate of hospitalization, higher mortality rate, and impaired performance of workers with diabetes. This has generated a strong drive towards developing preventative measures as well as cure for the disease and its complications. Diabetes is a disease that incorporates various metabolic disturbances such as impaired glucose haemostasis, blood dyscrasias and hyperlipidemia. Major disturbances also include slower gut movement (gastroparesis) and microfloral overgrowth (especially of fermentation bacteria and yeasts due to the slightly more acidic gut contents) (Al-Salami et al. 2007; Husebye 2005). Improving diabetes complications, reducing prevalence and restoring normal physiological patterns should significantly optimise diabetes treatment and the quality of life for diabetic patients.

Side effects associated with diabetes therapy include hypoglycemia, toxin build up in the gut, and lactic acidosis. These remain major issues and cause of death especially in the presence of compromised liver and kidney functions. So despite strict glycemic control, the disease and its complications remain a growing health concern. Diabetic patients suffer complications due to disturbed physiological and biochemical processes associated with the disease including disturbed bile acids production and microfloral composition (Barbeau et al. 2006; Ogura et al. 1986; Peng & Hagopian 2007; Rozanova et al. 2002; Slivka et al. 1979a; Thomson 1983). Thus the use of bile acids and probiotics in diabetes treatment may improve glycemia as well the ameliorate complications. A major improvement would be the discovery of treatments for diabetes that avoid and even replace the absolute requirement for injected insulin. Recent studies in a rat model of Type 1 diabetes show that a multi-therapeutic approach incorporating bile acids and probiotics, as adjunct therapy, exerted better control over glycemia and resulted in ameliorating complications, than when each treatment was administered alone (Al-Salami et al. 2008a; Al-Salami et al. 2008b; Al-Salami et al. 2008e; Al-Salami et al. 2009b). Accordingly, improving diabetes complications, reducing prevalence and restoring normal physiological patterns should significantly optimise diabetes treatment and the quality of life of diabetic patients.

Bile has been used as a therapeutic agent since ancient times. The use of bear gall bladder in treating fever, liver diseases and eye infections has been an ancient phenomenon practiced by many civilizations including the Chinese. Recent studies have showed the therapeutic effects of bear bile in treating gallstones and liver diseases. Bear bile contains substantial amount of ursodeoxycholic acid (UDCA) and chenodeoxycholic acid (CDCA) (Bachrach & Hofmann 1982a; Bachrach & Hofmann 1982b), which recent reports have shown them to also be present in pig bile. Current Chinese medicine uses extracts from pig bile for constipation, jaundice, whooping cough and asthma. Pig bile has also been found to have anti-inflammatory, anticonvulsant and analgesic effects. The applications of bile acids to certain diseases as therapeutic agents have been greatly explored by the ancient Greeks in the sixth century B.C. The ancient Greeks proposed the *Doctrine of Four Humours* or *body fluids* which included yellow bile, black bile, blood and mucus or phlegm. Health is a result of a balanced mixture of the Four Humours (krasis) whereas disease is due to an excess of one of the Four Humours and an imbalance (dyskrasis) of the body fluids (Heaton 1971). Bile therapeutic applications have been explored further by Galen in the second century A.D., and bile was used to facilitate the excretion of stools as a laxative. In 1863 Hoppe-Seyler demonstrated even though bile salts are the major active component in bile, little bile acids is detected in the feces. He proposed bile acids be reabsorbed from the intestine and that bile salts are the major constituents and also proposed continuous recirculation of bile salts, now known as enterohepatic recycling. Heinrich Otto Wieland (1877-1957) won the Nobel Prize in chemistry in 1927 *for his investigations of the constitution of the bile acids and related substances*. In 1940, Roepke and Mason demonstrated that micelle formation was responsible for the solubilisation of non-polar lipids such as cholesterol and fat-soluble vitamins. Twenty years later it was proposed that bile salts were simultaneously absorbed into the ileal mucosa. Heaton and Morris confirmed that active transport of bile salts occurs but only in the ileum (Heaton 1971; Lowbeer et al. 1970).

Primary bile acids are synthesized in hepatocytes from endogenous or dietary cholesterol. They are then conjugated to glycine or taurine to form primary conjugated bile acids. In the small intestine, the conjugated bile acids are metabolised by the gut microflora into secondary bile acids before being reabsorbed in the process of enterohepatic recirculation (Ridlon et al. 2006). Approximately 90-95 % of bile acids secreted into the gut is reabsorbed from the intestine back into the circulation via bile acid transporters, while about 400-800 mg/day is excreted from the body in the faeces (Roberts et al. 2002). The bile acid transporters are mainly the sodium-dependent taurocholate cotransporting polypeptide (NTCP), sodium-independent organic anion transporting protein (OATP), the bile salt export pump (BSEP) (Ballatori et al. 2005a; Higgins & Gottesman 1992; Mao & Unadkat 2005), the organic cation transporter polypeptide (OCTP) and the apical sodium-dependent bile salt transporter (ASBT) (Bodo et al. 2003; Zelcer et al. 2003a; Zelcer et al. 2003b; Zollner et al. 2003). Conjugated bile acids are transported by ASBT, whereas unconjugated bile acids are transported by OATP and by passive diffusion. Conjugated bile acids are transported by intracellular transport mechanisms within hepatocytes to the canalicular poles and secreted into the canalicular lumen by BSEP (Asamoto et al. 2001; Mita et al. 2006).

Cholic acid is an important precursor for the synthesis of steroids and chenodeoxycholic acid, and of recently has been investigated and applied in biliary calculus (cholelith) therapy. To optimise the stability and minimise toxicity of cholic acid, a more stable semisynthetic analogue MKC has been designed and synthesized. This is done on cholic acid through replacing the hydroxyl group on carbon atom 12 with a ketone group. Generally, the hydroxyl groups on the carbon atoms, C7 and C12 are replaced by hydrogen to enhance stability and reduce side effects. However, despite bile acids being endogenous compounds, manufacturing stable analogues can be challenging. The challenges include:
1.   The need for selective protection of 2 hydroxyl groups which is done by acylation.
2.   The choice of a suitable reagent to transform the remaining hydroxyl groups as appropriate.

Although enzymatic dehydroxylation of cholic acid may easily overcome these challenges, chemical reactions involving suitable reagents is still favoured especially for industrial production (Mikov & Fawcett 2006a). 3 hydroxyl groups (C3, C7 and C12) are targeted for acylation. The type of reaction will depend on the type of the bond and its configurational arrangement in the molecule. C3-OH is equatorial thus can be removed through estrification while with C7 and C12 axial groups, oxidation is sufficient. In addition to exploring the potential effect of bile acids, they can also be used as absorption enhancers.

Today it is well known that bile is a complex fluid containing water, electrolytes and other organic molecules including bile salts, cholesterol, phospholipids and bilirubin that flows from the bile duct into the small intestine (Al-Salami et al. 2007). The main endogenous bile acids are primary (cholic and chenodeoxycholic acids) and secondary (deoxycholic and lithocholic acids). Approximately 1 L of bile is secreted by the liver daily. Bile has a pH of 7.8-8.6 and is nearly isotonic with blood. It is secreted from the liver into small ducts that join to form the common hepatic duct. Bile salts are anionic water-soluble products of cholesterol metabolism. Bile salts can form micelles 4-7 nm in diameters which contain fatty acids, monoglycerides and phospholipids. These micelles solubilise lipids and transport them across biological membranes (Hamada et al. 2006; Leng et al. 2003).

In the past, bile acids were considered to have three basic physiological functions (Kuhajda et al. 2006a; Kuhajda et al. 2006b; Mikov & Fawcett 2006b):

1. Elimination of excess cholesterol;
2. Facilitation of the digestion of dietary fats (emulsifying agents);
3. Facilitation of the absorption of fat soluble vitamins such as A, D and K.

However, recent studies have expanded the role of bile acids to include endocrine signalling to regulate glucose, lipid and their own homeostasis and influence energy expenditure and gut microfloral composition (48, 53, 88).

This chapter aims to explore the changes in gut physiology and metabolic pathways which are associated with diabetes. It also aims to identify current and potential applications of bile acids and probiotics in the prevention and treatment of the disease.

2. Glucose regulation and insulin secretion

Glucose is a major source of energy with the normal range (normoglycemia) being 3.5-7.8 mmol/l (Cubeddu & Hoffmann 2002). When the body is at absolute rest (the basal state), glucose consumption is equal to its production (Overkamp et al. 1997; Zisser et al. 2007). When glucose is absorbed into the circulation and the body has no immediate need for energy, glucose is stored in the liver and muscles as glycogen (Overkamp et al. 1997). In healthy individuals, glycogen synthesis (glyconeogenesis) in tissues is stimulated by insulin. When the amount of glucose in the blood gets low, glycogen breaks down in the liver to glucose (glycogenolysis). In healthy individuals, feedback processes ensure that glucose levels are under homeostatic control by balancing glyconeogenesis and glycogenolysis. The liver can also convert lactate to glucose via a process known as gluconeogenesis to further supply the required glucose to the blood when levels are low. Glyconeogenesis, glycogenolysis and gluconeogenesis are controlled by anabolic hormones released from the Islets of Langerhans in the pancreas such as glucagon (released from the α-cells) and insulin (released from the β-cells). These hormones bind to specific receptors to trigger a chain of reactions that control glucose homeostasis. GLUT-2 (mainly in beta-cells) and GLUT-4 (mainly in skeletal muscles) are the dominant glucose transporters. In general, insulin activates to become fully functional pores that are able to transport glucose molecules into tissues (Rosa et al. 2011; Stuart et al. 2009).

The pancreas produces large quantities of insulin which it stores in intracellular secretary granules (Al-Salami et al. 2007). Upon stimulation from rising levels of glucose, these granules release their insulin into the mesenteric veins (Juhl et al. 2002; Just et al. 2008). Insulin secretion is different in healthy and diabetic individuals. In healthy individuals, there are two phases of insulin secretion; first phase insulin secretion (FPIS) which starts immediately after the initial stimulus of raised glucose levels and second phase insulin secretion (SPIS) which starts shortly after FPIS, and has a shorter duration but greater magnitude. FPIS occurs from β-cells of the pancreas as a direct response to high influx of extracellular glucose. In T1D patients, FPIS and SPIS do not exist since there is a complete lack of insulin production while, in T2D patients, FPIS is impaired and further exposure to glucose results in a reduction in insulin secretion in SPIS due to the desensitization of β-cells to glucose.

3. Pathogenesis and risk factors of Type 1 diabetes

Recent studies have shown that the inflammation which leads to the destruction of β-cells is initiated in the gut (Devendra et al. 2004). It is likely to occur within the first three months of life (Notkins & Lernmark 2001) due to different diabetic-causing xenobiotics (diabetogenics) that include gluten (Akerblom et al. 2002), cow milk protein (Barbeau et al. 2007), viruses such as rubella (Vaarala 2006), and food-toxins such as alloxan, streptozotocin and N-nitroso compounds (Vaarala 2006; Ziegler et al. 2003). Although the pathogenesis of T1D remains unclear, the generally accepted explanation is that T1D is a chronic autoimmune disease triggered in genetically susceptible individuals by a primary insult initiated in the gut (Ghosh et al. 2004). T2D develops in adult life probably due to environmental factors (Moore et al. 2003b) that lead to tissue desensitization to insulin. Continuous stimulation of beta-cells through hyperglycemia or certain types of antidiabetic drugs such as sulphonylureas can lead to tissue exhaustion and eventual cessation of insulin production due to tissue damage which results in the development of T1D (Fajans 1987).

The associated-disturbances in the compositions of bile and gut microflora are reported in the literature. However whether the changes in bile and microfloral compositions are caused by diabetes, or diabetes develops as a result of disturbed bile and gut microflora, remains to be determined.

4. Diabetes-associated disturbances in bile acids and gut microflora

Disturbances in bile acids composition may result in tissue necrosis due to higher than normal concentrations of potent bile acids such as lithocholic acid compared with less potent bile acids such as chenodeoxycholic acid. Secondary bile acids are solely produced by the action of gut microflora on primary bile acids, and thus, microfloral composition is directly linked to secondary bile acid production and bile acid composition. This interaction between bile acid composition and the composition of gut microflora represents the base of the hypothesized link between bile acid, gut microflora and energy balance. However, even though the compositions of bile acids and gut microflora are reported to be different in diabetic patients (Duan et al. 2008; Gebel 2011; Morris 1989; Ogura et al. 1986; Slivka et al. 1979a; Thomson 1983), it is still not clear how these changes directly affect the development and progression of diabetes or its complications. These complications include cardiovascular, tissue necrosis and ulcerations, and metabolic disturbances.

The amino acid taurine, which is used by hepatocytes in bile acid conjugation and bile salts formation, has many other physiological functions including the regulation of intracellular osmolarity, cardiomyocytes functions, and as an antioxidant. Accordingly, a clear link between bile compositions, taurine concentrations and diabetes complications can be discussed. A hypoglycemic effect of taurine, directly or through synergizing the effect of insulin, has also been reported (Kulakowski & Maturo 1984). Conjugated bile acids includes glycine and taurine conjugates, both existing in constant ratio. Glycine conjugated bile acids are less soluble and are harder to excrete compared with taurine conjugated bile acids. This result in bile accumulation noticed in T1D subjects (Bennion & Grundy 1977). In T1D patients, who have increased lipid metabolism, the percentage of taurocholic acid in bile is decreased indicating an altered biosynthesis of taurine (Meinders et al. 1981c). In one study, diabetic patients showed altered taurine metabolism causing consequent cellular dysfunctions that resulted in worsening diabetic neuropathy, cardiomyopathy, platelet aggregation and endothelial dysfunction (Hansen 2001). In T1D rats, taurine concentrations were found different in various organs (Goodman & Shihabi 1990; Hansen 2001; Reibel et al. 1979). Taurine concentrations in kidney and liver were low, while they were higher in heart and skeletal muscle. One important diabetic complication, platelet hyperaggregation, has been normalized by the alteration of bile acids composition through the addition of taurine (Franconi et al. 1995). Another complication is T1D retinopathy which have shown significantly less taurine levels in the retina, compared with that in healthy rats (Vilchis & Salceda 1996). Diabetic nephropathy are other major complication of T1D. Taurine consumption has shown to reduce chronic diabetic nephropathy in T1D rats (Trachtman & Sturman 1996). Other diabetic complications can also be reduced or even prevented by the addition of taurine. These include high glucose induced apoptosis in human vascular endothelial cells (Di Wu et al. 1999) and impaired endothelium-dependent vasodilatation in diabetic mice.

Even though the composition of gut microflora has been reported to be different in T1D patients, it may be difficult to quantify or qualify such a difference. Gut microflora interacts closely with the body immune system and has shown to control the immune response to various inflammatory stimuli. The mechanism of action of probiotics could be one or more of the following. Firstly, by competitive exclusion, where gut microfloral bacteria resist colonization of other 'foreign' bacteria. Secondly, by barrier formation where the microflora forms a physical barrier reducing bacterial translocation by forming a wall surrounding the outside part of the gut enterocytes. Thirdly, gut bacteria can produce bacteriocins and change the pH to create a harsher environment for other invading bacteria to settle in the gut. Fourthly, gut microflora can influence the immune system through its effect on gut enterocytes (quorum sensing) and the innate and adaptive immune system (Gareau et al. 2010; Walker 2008a).

It is a common conception that the efficiency of the immune system is compromised in diabetic patients resulting in prolonged healing of infections and diabetic ulcers (Steed et al. 1996). This is also brought about by the higher rates of bacterial infections reported in diabetes and higher rate of antibiotic use (Goldberg & Krause 2009; Paccagnini et al. 2009). In one study, the effect of the probiotic bacteria, Lactobacillus plantarum (Lp) on infected diabetic ulcers, was examined. Topical application of Lp on diabetic ulcers for 30 days induced healing. This effect was observed in almost half of the treated diabetic patients. However, this was not significantly different from healthy treated control suggesting that probiotic treatment is effective in treating diabetic ulcers, but its effect does not vary between diabetic and non-diabetic individuals. It is therefore tempting to speculate that gut microfloral bacteria controls the innate immune responses towards normalizing harmful bacteria in an effort to protect its own environment and keep its own existence.

5. Animal models suitable for investigating bile acids and probiotics effects on Type 1 diabetes

During the process of drug development, various *in vivo*, *ex vivo*, *in situ* and *in silico* methods can be used. Each method has advantages and disadvantages, and so using more than one method can provide better confirmation of findings. *In silico* methods can provide an initial insight into a potential drug candidate with predicted high pharmacological activity and good stability, while *ex vivo* methods can provide more information about a drug's interaction with living tissue, and are more cost-effective compared with *in vivo* animal models (Qin et al. 2010). *In situ* methods can better predict drug absorption compared with *ex vivo* models but *in vivo* models can provide more comprehensive pharmacokinetic profiles and give a better understanding of drug-tissue interactions (Zanchi et al. 1998). *In vivo* studies are usually carried out where drug therapeutic formulations are administered to animals in order to investigate short and long term safety, to explore various clinical effects and to study different physicochemical parameters before confirming suitability of the formulation to a disease condition(s). Various animal models are used to represent various diseases.

Although there is a surplus of animal models (spontaneous and induced) to study T1D, there is no ideal or standard model for studying the effect of bile acids and probiotics on T1D. Rats lack gall bladder which means bile is not stored before secretion but rather is secreted immediately after food intake. However, this does not seem to stop researches from using rats as an animal model of T1D (Al-Salami et al. 2008e). Rats, mice and hamsters have been used to study bile acids and probiotics applications in T1D, however, future research is needed, to compare the effect of bile acids and probiotics on T1D, using different animal models.

An ideal animal model should represent a specific medical condition in terms of disease development, pathophysiology, biological disturbances and short & long term complications.

If we are to create a better model of human T1D, we should carefully consider the disease effect on the following:

1. Relevant end points including primary, secondary and tertiary.
2. The relevant speed and stages of disease development and progression.
3. Disease complications, their progression and the relevant clinical end point(s).
4. Symptomatic/nonsymptomatic signs of the disease.
5. Feasibility of sample collections in terms of tissue site and sample volume.
6. The incidence in males vs. females.

The current therapeutics for T1D are inadequate, which necessitate further drug development and *in vivo* studies. Clinical translation of T1D pathophysiology and clinical manifestations, from animal to human, has been limited and rather difficult. This is because very little is known about T1D; the extent of heterogeneity, polymorphism, genetic distance, the exact site of initial immune response (gut or pancreas), and diabetogenic antigens. Creating a suitable animal model for T1D requires the ability to accurately translate the findings to human. These findings include therapeutic efficacy (prevention/treatment), safety and PK/PD profiles. There are various animal models for T1D, with the nonobese diabetic (NOD) mouse being the 'standard' one. Other models are induction models of rats, mice and hamsters using alloxan or streptozotocin to destroy pancreatic beta cells and induce T1D. The NOD mouse represents the best spontaneous model for a human autoimmune disease, in particular, T1D. NOD mouse model allows the investigation of various immunointerventions that can be used in human T1D. Similar to T1D in human, NOD mice have higher levels of macrophages, dendritic cells, CD4+ and B cells.

The induction of T1D in NOD mouse can be achieved through environmental conditions, mimicking the development of T1D in human. However, the development of T1D in NOD mouse takes place quickly and can produce a significant inflammatory condition that may over-respond to immunomanipulation and exaggerate the effect of a treatment. Also, the incidence of T1D is different between males and females in this model while the incidence is the same in males and females in human. This can further limit the applications and the findings of this animal model (Dieleman et al. 1997). Many therapeutics that showed good efficacy in this model failed to achieve similar results in T1D human subjects (Srinivasan & Ramarao 2007). Having said that and regardless of how different this model is, from the 'true' human TID, NOD mouse remains the most representative of human T1D. Interestingly, in a recently published study, the incidence of T1D was much higher, when the mice were maintained in a germ-free environment suggesting direct connection between gut microflora and the development of T1D (Li-Wen et al. 2007).

The suitable animal model for human T1D should ideally be easy to breed and handle, and can accommodate various medical conditions that may come about or be associated with T1D. Thus, extrapolation of its findings to human should be easily done, and with great accuracy and precision.

6. The therapeutic applications of bile acids and probiotics in Type 1 diabetes

In pathophysiology such as gall stone formations, inflammatory bowel disease and allergic reactions, the administration of probiotics significantly improves body physiology and reduces complications (Cary & Boullata 2010; Gourbeyre et al. 2011; Martin & Walker 2008; Morris et al. 2009; Stephani et al. 2011). In one study, the administration of bile acids and gliclazide to probiotic pre-treated diabetic animals showed efficacy and a significant reduction of diabetic complications (Al-Salami et al. 2008e; Al-Salami et al. 2008g).

The synthesis of bile acids is highly regulated by nuclear hormone receptors and other transcription factors, which ensure a constant supply of bile acids in a very changing metabolic environment. In healthy individuals, bile acids control their own haemostasis through feedback mechanisms involving phosphoenolpyruvate carboxykinase (PEPCK) and farnesoid X receptor alpha (FXR-alpha) nuclear receptors. Their direct effect on diabetes development remains debatable, but through the inhibition of PEPCK and FXR-alpha (via TGR5-D2 signalling pathways), bile acids also inhibits gluconeogenesis. Such mechanisms may seem to oppose that of insulin, which suggests direct effect on glucose haemostasis in healthy individuals. Inherited mutations that impair bile acid synthesis cause many human disorders including early childhood liver inflammation and failure. During the development of diabetes, bile acid synthesis is increased, the bile acid pool is expanded, and bile acid excretion is increased suggesting lack of adequate control over the feedback regulating bile acid haemostasis. Accordingly, several recent studies have investigated the role of and applications of bile acids in glucose haemostasis. Interestingly, where both factors, PEPCK and FXR-alpha fit remains under investigation. During the fasting state, hepatocytes produce more FXR-alpha suggesting that FXR-alpha production takes place in the absent of insulin (Zhang et al, 2004). In another study, when FXR-alpha was tested in diabetic animals, it was noticed to be lower than these in healthy, but when insulin was administered; it normalized such an effect (Duran-Sandoval et al, 2004). Overall, BAs have been reported to inhibit gluconeogenesis via downregulation of phosphoenolpyruvate carboxykinase (PEPCK) mRNA levels in a FXR-alpha-dependent and –independent manner (De Fabiani et al, 2003; Yamagata et al, 2004).

Apart from basic physiological functions like the elimination of cholesterol and the intestinal solubilisation (emulsification) of triacylglycerol, cholesterol and lipid, soluble vitamins, bile acids and their analogues are now recognized as having major therapeutic applications in the treatment of cholelithiasis, as transport promoters for other substances, in potentiating the action of other substances (analgesic, antiviral, hypoglycaemic) and as hypoglycaemic and hypolipidemic agents. In one study, lithocholic acid concentration was higher after diabetes development which resulted in gallstone formation (Chijiiwa 1990). This indicates that diabetes directly altered bile composition. However, the exact mechanism by which diabetes can alter bile acid composition remains unclear.

One hypothesis linking bile acid disturbance with the initiation of diabetes development, is through the over-production of lithocholic acid, brought about by disturbances in the gut microflora (De Leon et al. 1978; Kokk et al. 2005; Meinders et al. 1981a; Meinders et al. 1981b). Diabetes mellitus has been associated with unbalanced secretion of bile (cholelithiasis). In addition, many studies have linked changes in bile composition to the changes in the composition of the gut microflora (Kokk et al. 2005; Mikov et al. 2004; Mikov et al. 2005; Mikov et al. 2006; Mikov & Fawcett 2006b).

Potential therapeutic use of bile acids in T1D can be achieved through two main applications; as hypoglycaemic agents and as absorption-enhancing agent to insulin delivery.

Monoketocholic acid (MKC) (Figure 1) is a stable semisynthetic primary bile acid (cholic acid analogue) with low toxicity that has been shown to enhance the nasal absorption of insulin in rats (89). In addition, MKC has been shown to exert a effect in its own right when administered by the oral route in alloxan-induced T1D rats (Mikov et al. 2007).

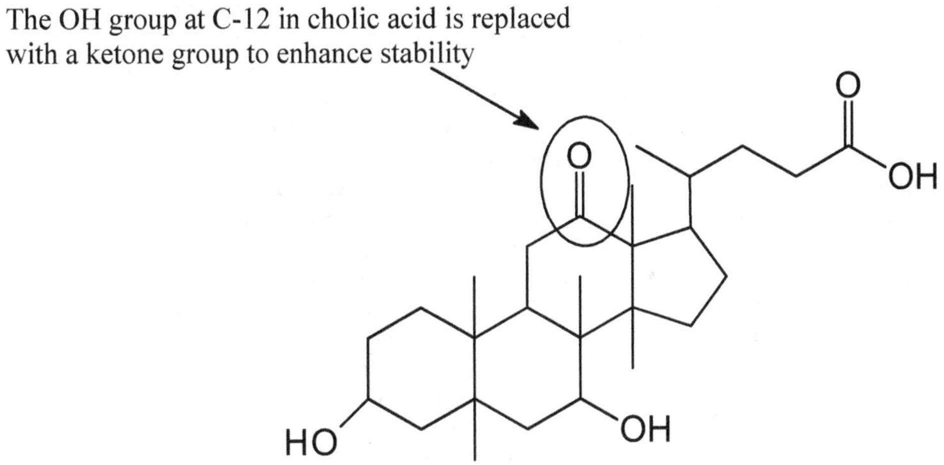

The OH group at C-12 in cholic acid is replaced with a ketone group to enhance stability

Fig. 1. The chemical structure of 12-monoketocholic acid (MKC).

Permeation enhancement through the tissue-solubilising effect of bile salts was found to be one of several mechanisms by which bile salts can facilitate drug absorption. Other mechanisms involve bile salts' effect on efflux and afflux protein transporters on the cell wall of various tissues including gut enterocytes, hepatocytes, nasal mucosa and others (Al-Salami et al. 2008c; Al-Salami et al. 2008d; Al-Salami et al. 2009a).

7. The interaction between protein transportors, bile acid composition and diabetes developement

Bile acids effect on T1D development and progression may also be through their effect on protein transporters, since many transporters have their expression and functionality altered in T1D (Al-Salami et al. 2008c). The exact mechanism associating the change in transporters, bile acids composition and diabetes development, is still unknown but there are few assumptions to explain such an interaction. The first assumption is that T1D starts on the first few months of life with a direct insult in the gut, initiating a disturbance in the gut microflora and a consequent disturbed bile flow. This results in an altered bile feedback mechanisms and a change in the expression of protein transporters responsible for bile enterohepatic recirculation. This results in an inflammatory condition that brings about T1D and beta cells destruction. The second assumption is that disturbance in protein transporters expression and functionality, caused by a genetic mutation, produces a disturbance in bile flow. This leads to disturbances in gut microflora initiating inflammation in the gut affecting beta cells and resulting in T1D. The third assumption is that the functionality of the immune system is altered (due to either an insult in the gut or genetic mutation). This alters the composition of gut microflora resulting in initiating of inflammation reaching the beta cells, as a case of mistaken identity. As a consequence of beta cell inflammation, bile acids synthesis and flow are disturbed resulting in exacerbation of the inflammation and worsening of symptoms. In all these assumptions, genetic susceptibility is expected, and contributes further to T1D development and progression. The above assumptions were based on the work of the authors as well as careful evaluation of the literature.

In recent publications, alterations in the functionality of some transporters have been linked to the development of diabetes; however, the exact mechanism remains not fully understood. Bile salts output in diabetic animals was extremely high compared with healthy, and the expression of Mdr2 was also high after STZ treatment (van Waarde et al. 2002). In another study, a mutation in Zinc transporter 8 (ZT8) located in beta cells, is implicated in the dysregulation of insulin transport and release, and an exacerbation of the inflammatory response leading to T1D. In this study, ZT8 was considered as an autoantigen resulting in the stimulation and production of beta cells autoantibodies and T1D development (Rungby 2010). Moreover, streptozotocin (STZ) had different but significant effect on the expression of Na/Cl/glucose cotransporters, and the administration of insulin reduced such an effect (Vidotti et al. 2008). Hyperglyemia itself directly reduced the activity of Mdr1 suggesting a clear association between pre-T1D hyperglycemia and disturbances in protein transporters (Tramonti et al. 2006). In another recent study, the effect of STZ on cation protein transporters was reported, interestingly, at different levels of protein synthesis; transcriptional and posttranscriptional depending on the type of the transporters affected (Grover et al. 2004). However, some studies suggest a diabetic influence is stronger on enzymatic activities than on protein transporters with the enzymatic influence being the cause of exacerbation of inflammation and development of the disease (Py et al. 2002). The impairment of protein transporters functionality, reported in the diabetic animals can take place either by reduced protein expression or reduced action. When glucose protein transporters in the blood brain barrier were studied under chronic hyperglycemia, their concentrations remain constant but functionality and glucose intake were impaired (Mooradian & Morin 1991). However, under acute hyperglycemia induced by STZ, their concentration decreased suggesting different response at different stages of the disease

(Matthaei et al. 1986). Accordingly, protein transporters have shown strong association with diabetes development and progression as well as diabetic complications.

8. The effect of co-administration of gliclazide on bile acids & probiotics

Gliclazide is used in Type 2 diabetes (T2D) to stimulate insulin production but it also has beneficial extrapancreatic effects which makes it potentially useful in T1D. In fact, some T2D patients continue to use gliclazide even after their diabetes progresses to T1D since it provides better glycemic control than insulin alone. Gliclazide has three main structural features, an aromatic ring, a sulphonylurea group and an azabicyclic ring (Figure 2).

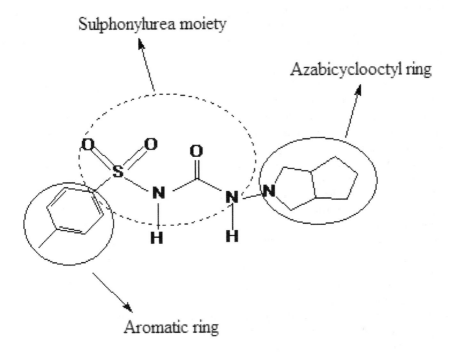

Fig. 2. The chemical structure of gliclazide with three main groups: aromatic ring, sulphonylurea moiety and azabicyclooctyle ring.

In a recent study investigating the applications of bile acids and probiotics in T1D, the bile acid analogue, MKC, was administered i.v. (four groups) and orally (four groups) to healthy, diabetic, probiotic pretreated healthy and probiotic pretreated diabetic rats. The pharmacokinetic parameters of MKC after i.v. administration were found to be similar in all four groups suggesting no significant differences in pharmacokinetic parameters between healthy and diabetic rats irrespective of probiotic pretreatment. C_{max} (maximum concentration), AUC (area under the curve) and F (bioavailability) values after oral administration to untreated healthy rats were also found similar to corresponding values in untreated diabetic rats suggesting similar mechanisms of absorption and systemic distribution of MKC. MKC also showed clear evidence of enterohepatic recycling with probiotic pretreatment delaying its absorption. This suggests different pharmacokinetic properties of the stable bile acid, MKC, in healthy rats compared with diabetic rats. This further supports the authors' previous findings showing that bile acid recirculation in diabetic animals is disturbed compared with healthy ones. When MKC was administered i.v. (to four groups) or orally (to four groups), there was no significant changes in blood glucose in any group of rats after the i.v. dose but, after oral administration to untreated diabetic rats, the elevated blood glucose level was significantly reduced from 23.6 ± 3.1 to 14.1 ± 2.4 mmol/l. Interestingly, diabetic rats pretreated with probiotics showed less weight loss, urine production and water consumption, and improvement in behaviour (curious, active) and survival rate than untreated diabetic rats. In a more recent study, the authors combined bile acid with an antidiabetic drug, gliclazide, and administered that to a rat model of T1D. Interestingly, and through unknown mechanism, the combination of MKC and gliclazide exerted a better hypoglycaemic effect to probiotic pretreated diabetic rats than MKC alone. In this study, pharmacokinetic parameters of i.v. MKC were not affected by the concomitant i.v. administration of gliclazide in either healthy or diabetic rats with and without probiotic pretreatment. Accordingly, even though exact mechanism of interaction, at the molecular level, between MKC and gliclazide is unknown, there is a clear synergistic effect between MKC, gliclazide and probiotic pretreatment in T1D resulting in a profound hypoglycaemic effect and sound reduction in the diabetic complications in those treated diabetic animals.

Overall, the authors confirmed that at the start of experiments, baseline blood glucose levels in each of the four groups (untreated and probiotic treated healthy and diabetic rats) were comparable. the authors also presented initial data supporting the effect of probiotics on the development of T1D. The administration of probiotics to healthy rats had no effect on blood glucose levels but the same treatment of diabetic rats reduced the elevated blood glucose levels by nearly 30% and improved clinical signs and symptoms. These findings present a clear synergistic effect between bile acids, probiotics and gliclazide. More importantly, it shows clearly that intervention by bile acids and probiotics exert a direct and significantly positive effect on glycemic control and the progression of diabetic complications. Even though the details of such effect remains unclear, multitherapeutic approach in treating diabetes showed better efficacy and continue to gain interest worldwide.

Having said that a likely explanation for the effect of probiotics is that they stimulate the GI mucosa to produce insulinotropic polypeptides (Cornell 1985) and glucagon-like peptide-1 (Raymond et al. 1981) and/or induce the gut microflora to release endotoxins which cause an increase in skeletal muscle glucose uptake (Raymond et al. 1980). Probiotic treatment alone was found to influence gliclazide permeation differently in health and diabetic animals (Al-Salami et al. 2008f) while the fact that administration of gliclazide following probiotic pretreatment did not further reduce glucose levels indicates the effect of probiotics is not due to stimulation of insulin release by residual pancreatic cells or to regeneration of functional pancreatic cells. Furthermore, i.v. administration of MKC to healthy and diabetic rats with and without probiotic pretreatment produced little effect. However, oral administration of MKC to diabetic rats produced a significant effect 3 hours after administration suggesting it arises from metabolic activation of MKC in the gut. The effect of oral MKC was not significant in probiotic pretreated diabetic rats that had lower blood glucose levels at the time of MKC administration possibly due to an interaction in the gut. The combination of gliclazide and MKC produced a greater effect in diabetic rats than MKC alone. This synergistic effect could be due to gliclazide enhancing the production and/or absorption of MKC active metabolites in the gut. The administration of gliclazide+MKC also produced the most significant reduction in blood glucose levels in probiotic pretreated diabetic rats (from 12.6 ± 2.0 to 10 ± 2.0 mmol/l, p<0.01). Overall, pretreatment with probiotics and subsequent oral administration of gliclazide+MKC resulted in the greatest effect in this model of T1D as well as in improved signs and symptoms in the animals. In healthy rats, neither probiotic treatment, nor oral administration of gliclazide, MKC or gliclazide+MKC had any effect on blood glucose levels. More interestingly, the authors hypothesized that the chronic treatment of diabetic rats with probiotics may have stimulated the metabolism of the stable bile acid, MKC, in a similar way as reported between cholic acid and *Lactobacilli* (Pigeon et al. 2002). The hypothesis of direct induction of probiotic treatment to bile acid metabolism may explain the therapeutic efficacy of probiotics in treating various disorders implementing a better role of bile acids in such therapeutic effects. Holding true, this should take us a step closer to understand better how probiotic administration exerted a hypoglycaemic effect, when administered alone, to T1D rats. This should also create a new approach to enhancing probiotic efficacy, through the concurrent administration with stable bile acids.

This multidrug therapy shows potential in T1D. This is illustrated by the reduction of blood glucose levels, improvement of diabetic symptoms, and the lower rate of diabetes development by alloxan when injected to rats pretreated with probiotics. Furthermore, the change in PK of gliclazide and MKC after probiotic pretreatment emphasizes the importance of not only investigating the use of probiotics in a disease state, but also investigating the influence of probiotics on drugs that could be used for such a disease. In addition, T1D clearly illustrates different gut biomorphology and response compared with healthy control which should be taken into account when discussing multidrug approach to the disease.

Gliclazide has been used for decades to treat T2D and thus future work should include applying the combination of probiotics, gliclazide and MKC on T2D rats then implications of the findings may be extrapolated to human subjects as appropriate. However, these findings should not be overplayed since variation in gliclazide pharmacokinetics is higher in human than rats (Palmer & Brogden 1993) which may limit further the applications of these findings in human.

One of the applications of the findings is the use of gliclazide, MKC and probiotics in T2D. T2D is characterized by hyperglycemia and hypercholesterolemia and thus bile acids have been used to lower cholesterol levels in diabetic patients (Goldfine 2008). Accordingly, the use of gliclazide, MKC and probiotics may improve glucose and cholesterol unbalance in T2D.

9. The effect of gut microflora and diet on inflammation

There is a great conclusion regarding the importance of gut microflora, made by Sir Henry Shaw (1818–1885): 'I have finally come to the conclusion that a good reliable set of bowels is worth more to a man than any quantity of brains'.

Many autoimmune and inflammatory diseases have shown positive response to probiotic and prebiotic treatments (Sherman et al. 2009; Tlaskalova-Hogenova et al. 2011). These diseases include acute gastroenteritis, antibiotic-associated diarrhoea and colitis, inflammatory bowel disease, type 1 diabetes, irritable bowel syndrome and necrotizing enterocolitis. The composition of the intestinal microflora may also affect mammalian physiology outside the gastrointestinal tract. Recent studies have shown significant changes in gut microfloral and bile acid compositions in T1D (Jaakkola et al. 2003; Siow et al. 1991; Slivka et al. 1979b; Uchida et al. 1979; Uchida et al. 1985). Thus, it is clear that our symbiotic microflora award many metabolic capabilities that our mammalian genomes lack (Zaneveld et al. 2008), and so therapeutics that target microfloral modulation may prove rewarding. When the newborn baby leaves the germ free uterus, she/he enters a highly contaminated extra-uterus environment. This requires the activation of her/his immune system to prevent infection. Over the period of the first year, the newborn's intestinal microflora develops and its composition becomes her/his gut microfloral fingerprint! Gut microflora has been shown to play a major rule in controlling the inflammatory response of the host immune system through direct and indirect bacteria-bacteria and bacteria-host interactions. These interactions include physical and metabolic functions of the gut microfloral bacteria, which protect the intestinal tract from foreign pathogenic bacteria, eliminate the presence of unwanted bacteria through producing bacteriocins and other chemicals, and inform the gut epithelium and the host immune system about whether a local inflammatory response is needed (Shi & Walker 2004; Walker 2008b). Gut microflora can control the host immune system through four main actions. The induction of IgA secretion to protect against infection, triggers localized inflammatory responses, neutralizing T-helper (Th) cell response and also contributing to the induction or inhibition of generalized mucosal immune responses. Recent studies have shown that in autoimmune diseases and gut inflammation disorders, there is a significant disturbances in the ratios of Th cells such as the increase in the Th-2/Th-1 ratio associated with inflammatory bowel diseases, which has been linked to exacerbation of the gut inflammation and the development of the disease. In recent studies, gut-associated dendritic cells in the lamina propria can extend their appendices reaching the gut mucosa and using their Toll-like receptors (TLR) 2 and 4, to sample bacterial metabolites (Rescigno et al. 2001; von & Nepom 2009a). This may result in dendritic cells releasing certain cytokines that stimulate the activation of naive Th-0 into active Th- cells such as 1, 2 and 3/1 (von & Nepom 2009b; Walker 2008b). Interestingly, some microfloral bacteria can actually cross enterocytic microfolds and interact with antigen presenting immune cells in mesenteric lymph nodes to activate naive plasma cells into IgA-producing B cells (Macpherson & Uhr 2004). IgA coats the intestinal mucosa and control further bacterial penetration thus protecting the host from potential pathogenic bacteria. Even more interestingly, gut microflora bacteria have shown ability to not only initiate an inflammatory response but also to control and inhibit such a response. Some microfloral bacteria or their metabolites can interact with the intracellular receptor TLR-9, to which the bacteria activates T cells through the production of potent anti-inflammatory cytokines such as IL-10 (Rachmilewitz et al. 2004). Microfloral bacteria can also produce small molecules that can enter intestinal epithelial cells to inhibit activation of nuclear factor kappa-light-chain-enhancer of activated beta-cells (NFkB) (Neish et al. 2000). Moreover, prolonged exposure to bacterial endotoxins, in particular, LPS (which interacts with TLR 2 and 4) can activate intracellular anti-inflammatory associated proteins that result in an overall anti-inflammatory effect (Otte & Podolsky 2004). Such gut bacterial-host interactions are critical in maintaining a balanced and effective immune response to various infections while maintaining control over prolonged or chronic inflammation and reducing the overstimulation of the host immune system.

Recent evidence suggests that a particular gut microfloral community may favour occurrence of the metabolic diseases. It is well know that the composition of gut microflora changes with diet and also as we age (Rebole et al. 2010; Respondek et al. 2008; Yen et al. 2011). In one study, a high fat diet was associated with higher endotoxaemia and a lowering of bifidobacterium species in mice cecum (Cani et al. 2008). In a follow up study, the administration of prebiotics, in particular, oligofructose, to mice given high fat diet, restored the reduced quantity of bifidobacterium. This also resulted in reducing metabolic endotoxaemia, the inflammatory tone and slowing the development of diabetes. In this study and compared with control mice on chow diet, high fat diet significantly reduced intestinal Gram negative and Gram positive gut bacteria, increased endotoxaemia and diabetes-associated inflammation. However, when diabetic mice on high fat diet were given oligofructose, metabolic normalization took place including the quantity of gut bifidobacteria. In these mice, multiple correlation analyses showed that endotoxaemia negatively correlated with bifidobacteria quantity. By the same token, bifidobacterium quantity significantly and positively correlated with improved glucose tolerance, glucose-induced insulin secretion and normalised inflammatory tone (decreased endotoxaemia and plasma and adipose tissue proinflammatory cytokines) (Cani et al. 2007). In general, the level of microfloral diversity and gut bifidobacteria in human, relate to health status and both decrease with age (Hopkins & Macfarlane 2002).

Compromised gut movement associated with diabetes can result in substantial bacterial and yeast overgrowth which is postulated to disturb bile acids composition and exacerbate the diabetes-associated inflammation (Cani et al. 2009; Fox et al. 2010). Diabetes inflammation and bile acids disturbances can cause chemical unbalance that has been linked to poor tissue sensitivity to insulin (Maki et al. 1995), rise in the levels of reactive radicals in the blood (Jain et al. 2002), poor enterohepatic recirculation and negatively affecting liver detoxification and performance (Oktar et al. 2001; Quraishy et al. 1996). Accordingly, future diabetes therapy should not only focus on rectifying glucose imbalance but also in targeting the disturbances in bile acids composition and the inflammation cascade initiated in the gut. This can be achieved through normalizing the composition of bile acids and microflora, gut immune-response and microflora-epithelial interactions towards maintaining normal biochemical reactions and healthy body physiology. Physiological features of human development including the innate and adaptive immunity, immune tolerance, bioavailability of nutrients, and intestinal barrier functions, are directly related to the composition and functionality of the human microflora. This includes the percentages of what is currently known as good and bad gut microflora. Good microflora includes two main species, Lactobacillius and Bifidobacteria. Microflora modifications may take place due to antibiotics consumption, prebiotic and probiotics administration and the use of drugs which affect gastric motility resulting in changes in gastric pH and gut-emptying rate. These modifications have been shown to be significantly profound in diabetic subjects resulting in the reduction of the percentage of good bacteria, the increase of the percentage of bad bacteria and yeasts and the consequent increase in the percentage of toxic bile salts such as lithocholic acid. This can also contribute to the higher incidence of gall stones and liver necrosis reported in diabetic patients. Accordingly, probiotics can introduce missing microbial components with known beneficial functions for the human host, while prebiotics can enhance the proliferation of beneficial microbes or probiotics, resulting in sustainable changes in the human microflora. Symbiotic relationship between probiotics and prebiotic administration is expected to exert a synergistic effect and in the right dose, may normalize and even reverse dysbiosis-associated complications.

10. The applications of probiotics in diabetes

Probiotics are dietary supplements containing bacteria which, when administered in adequate amounts, confer a health benefit on the host (FAO/WHO 2002). Combinations of different bacterial strains can be used (Bezkorovainy 2001) but a mixture of *Lactobacilli* and *Bifidobacteria* is a common choice (Karimi & Pena 2003). Probiotics have been shown to be beneficial in wide range of conditions including infections, allergies, metabolic disorders such as diabetes mellitus, ulcerative colitis and Crohn's disease (Altenhoefer et al. 2004; Rozanova et al. 2002; Ziegler et al. 2003).

There are reports in the literature that probiotic treatment can be useful in diabetes (Al-Salami et al. 2008b) but there is little explanation of the mechanisms involved. The initial site of diabetogenic cells has been hypothesized to be in the gut whereas pancreatic lymph nodes serve as the site of amplification of the autoimmune response (Jacobs et al. 1989). This autoimmune response may disturb the composition of the normal gut flora. Treatment with *Bifidobacteria* and *Lactobacilli* has been shown to normalize the composition of the gut flora in children with T1D (Rozanova et al. 2002). In addition, the administration of *Lactobacilli* to alloxan-induced diabetic mice prolonged their survival (Matsuzaki et al. 1997a) and administration to non-obese diabetic (NOD, a rodent model of T1D) mice inhibited diabetes development possibly by the regulation of the host immune response and reduction of nitric oxide production (Matsuzaki et al. 1997b). Furthermore, the administration of a mixture of *Bifidobacteria*, *Lactobacilli* and *Streptococci* to NOD mice was protective against T1D development postulated to be through induction of interleukins IL4 and IL10 (Calcinaro et al. 2005).

Slowing of peristalsis (gastroparesis) has been reported in T1D patients. This can result in a bigger population of bacteria in the gut and a subsequent rise in the concentration of secondary bile acids (Meinders et al. 1981a) such as lithocholic acid which is toxic at high concentrations and can induce gut inflammation and blood dyscrasias (Malavolti et al. 1989; Miyai et al. 1982). In addition, the disturbed bile acid composition in T1D (Meinders et al. 1981a) is strongly linked with autoimmune and liver diseases. The administration of *Lactobacilli* and *Bifidobacteria* may restore the bile acid composition (Kurdi et al. 2000; Kurdi et al. 2006). It is important to select the right probiotic species based on efficacy, stability in

Probiotic strain	pH tolerability	Bile tolerability
Lactobacillus rhamnosus	At pH < 2 (after 2 hours) reduction by 2 – 3 log CFU/ml At pH < 1 (after 2 hours), reduction by 6 – 8 log CFU/ml (Succi et al. 2005).	Good survival rate in 3% bile salts for up to 24 hours (Succi et al. 2005).
Lactobacillus acidophilus	At pH < 1 (after 1 hour), reduction by 1 log CFU/ml (Favaro-Trindade & Grosso 2002).	Good survival rate in 4% bile for up to 12 hours (Favaro-Trindade & Grosso 2002).
Bifidobacterium lactis	At pH < 1 (after 1 hour), reduction by 1 log CFU/ml (Favaro-Trindade & Grosso 2002).	Good survival rate in 4% bile for up to 12 hours (Favaro-Trindade & Grosso 2002).

Table 1. pH and bile tolerability of Lactobacillus rhamnosus, Lactobacillus acidophilus and Bifidobacterium lactis.

the gut (bile and pH tolerability) and long term safety. Lactobacillus rhamnosus, Lactobacillus acidophilus and Bifidobacterium lactis show good bile and pH tolerability under normal conditions of pH (1.5-8) and bile acid concentration (0.8 - 3 %) (Table 1), in addition to long term safety (Franz & Bode 1973; Hedenborg & Norman 1984; Hedenborg & Norman 1985).

11. Bile acids as absorption enhancers in Type 1 diabetes therapy

Bile acids and their derivatives can act as absorption enhancers where they are capable of promoting mucosal and systemic drug absorption. Bile acids and their derivatives can increase drug bioavailability, allowing therapeutic doses to be administered by several routes. Bile acids as therapeutic agents have the potential to produce beneficial effects in improving primary biliary cirrhosis and primary sclerosing cholangitis. Bile acids can also control endocrine signalling and enzymatic activities in various disorders. This includes inflammatory diseases (such as diabetes) and cholestatic liver disease in cystic fibrosis.

Permeation of a drug through a biological membranes by passive diffusion is influenced by the drug's solubility and molecular weight, the thickness of both, the mucous and the cytoplasmic membrane, while drug diffusibility is influenced by permeability, surface area and the concentration gradient (Higgins & Gottesman 1992; Maki et al. 2003; Mao & Unadkat 2005; Neubert et al. 1987).

Bile salts (conjugated bile acids) are known to increase the permeation of many drugs. They increase the permeability of the mucosal membrane by breaking down mucous and disrupting cells, thus widening the tight junctions between these cells. This enhances penetration of drugs via the paracellular route. Bile salts can also improve transcellular absorption by increasing drug solubility and dissolution rate. Bile salts can form micelles which increase the permeability of the mucosal membrane by overcoming resistance at the aqueous diffusion layer. They also enhance drug delivery by interacting with membrane lipids and proteins that affect membrane fluidity and the rate of drug trafficking.

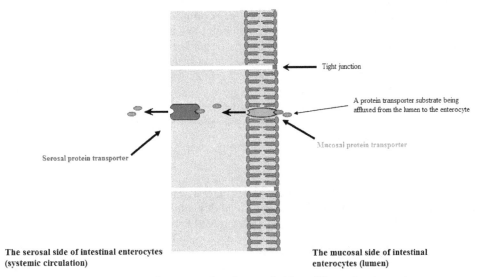

Tight junction

A protein transporter substrate being affluxed from the lumen to the enterocyte

Mucosal protein transporter

Serosal protein transporter

The serosal side of intestinal enterocytes (systemic circulation)

The mucosal side of intestinal enterocytes (lumen)

Fig. 3. Protein transporters in the mucosal and serosal sides of the gut enterocytes.

Recent studies suggest a bigger role for Mdr and Mrp transporters in the enterohepatic recirculation of bile acids (Asamoto et al. 2001). Mrp2 and Mrp3 recognize monovalent (those with a single charge) and divalent (those with a double charge) bile acids as their substrates (St-Pierre et al. 2000; St-Pierre et al. 2001; Zollner et al. 2003) while Mdr1 and Mdr3 recognise bile acid taurocholate, glutathione, bile salt glucuronide and sulfate conjugates (Ballatori et al. 2005a; Ballatori et al. 2005b). Mrp2 is located in the apical membrane of the bile canaliculus where it removes newly formed divalent bile acids into the bile duct. Mrp3 is located in the basolateral membrane of the ileal enterocytes where it removes monovalent bile acids from the gut lumen into the portal vein (Houten et al. 2006a). Figure 3 shows the locations of a mucosal and a serosal protein transporters (mucosal transporter is in green & serosal transporter is in red) expressed in enterocytes.

12. Oral absorption

Drug oral administration is the most convenient and popular route of drug delivery. However, some drugs have low bioavailability and slow absorption rate, thus limited efficacy. Bile salts have been shown to increase the absorption of intestinal insulin by masking its hydrophilic surface resulting in higher permeation through the ileal mucosa and into the systemic circulation, thus enhancing insulin bioavailability. In one study, insulin was formulated with different bile salts and administered orally to rabbits. Bile salts enhanced insulin permeation through the ileal mucosa and resulted in a significant effect which varied based on the type of bile salt used (Mesiha et al. 2002a). When insulin was administered with palmitic acid combined with bile salts, in the form of aqueous fatty acid solution, significant hypoglycaemic effects was observed in the treated diabetic animals. In an aqueous environment, insulin's hypoglycaemic effect was improved by the addition of glycocholate and, to a lesser extent, cholate. Accordingly, bile salts improved insulin's hypoglycaemic effect in the following descending order; sodium deoxycholate > sodium cholate > sodium glycocholate > sodium glycodeoxycholate > sodium taurodeoxycholate (Mesiha et al. 2002b). In general, there are few examples of known bile salt derivatives which are known absorption enhancers. Cholylsarcosine (CS) is an absorption enhancer as well as a non-toxic bile salt derivative. It has good stability and safety profile and is resistant to bacterial degradation in the gastrointestinal tract (Mesiha et al. 2002c; Mikov & Fawcett 2006b). Due to its stability, it does not form deoxycholic acid which can cause hepatotoxicity. Chenodeoxycholic acid and cholyltaurine were more effective than CS, but due to their susceptibility to bacterial degradation, they have poor safety profile. The applications of bile salts as absorption enhances is gaining more interest, especially with the ocular, transermal, nasal, buccal and rectal mucosal routes.

13. Occular absorption

Due to the normally high rates of lacrimation and tear wash-out, occular drug delivery has low efficiency and requires the drug to have high diffusibility through the anterior region of the eye Figure 4. However, when a drug is formulated with a suitable abortion enhancer, its permeation can be doubled or even tripled. A good example of bile salts occular applications is the administration of insulin. In one study that investigated the occular permeation of insulin, less than 1% of insulin reached the systemic circulation via the ocular route. The addition of some absorption enhancers may improve the permeation to around

4%. This still remains a limiting factor in insulin clinical applications (25). An estimated 80% of administered drug is eliminated through the nasal cavity after occular application (26). Another study (Yamamoto et al. 1989) determined the extent to which absorption promoters could enhance the absorption of insulin via the ocular route. When administered alone, occular insulin serum levels reached Cmax within 15 minutes of occular administration while when formulated with sodium glycocholate, sodium taurocholate and sodium deoxycholate (as absorption enhancers), insulin Cmax was reached within 5 minutes. When insulin was co-administered with sodium glycocholate, the amount of insulin permeating the eyes and reaching the systemic circulation increased from 1% to 5.5%. Sodium deoxycholate was found to be more effective and sodium taurocholate least effective at enhancing the occular absorption of insulin. This implies a good potential of bile acid applications in insulin occular delivery in T1D, when other routes as less desirable.

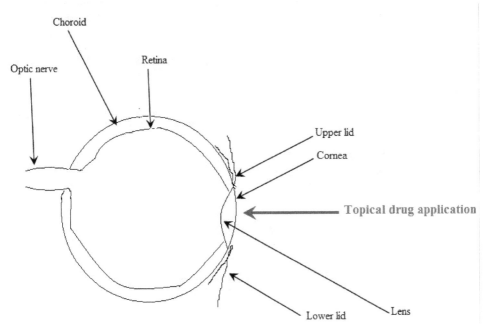

Fig. 4. The general structure of the eye.

14. Nasal absorption

The Nasal route is a convenient and popular method of drug administration as it is feasible and it has fast absorption rate. It also provides reasonable bioavailability as it bypasses first pass hepatic metabolism. However, pharmacologically active peptides such as hormones and proteins with molecular weights > 10 kDa do not have the ability to permeate the nasal mucosal layer without being significantly trapped, washed out (through the nasopharyngeal cavity), or degraded before reaching the systemic circulation. In order to optimise nasal drug delivery to drugs such as insulin, suitable permeation enhancers such as bile salts may be appropriate. For insulin to be delivered nasally, it has to permeate the nasal mucosa and into the systemic circulation (nasal vasculature). Large peptides such as insulin are not easily absorbed through the nasal mucosa when administered via a nasal spray (Hirai et al. 1978). Insulin must be transported between or through the apical and basal membranes of columnar cells, basal cells and capillary endothelial cells of blood vessels (Figure 5) (Gordon et al. 1985a; Li et al. 1992). However, it must first cross the mucous layer which varies in thickness averaging between 5 and 20 mm in depth. Mucociliary clearance washes out mucous and entrapped particles from the anterior to the posterior nasal cavity and down the oesophagus. Drugs administered through the nasal route must dissolve rapidly in the mucous before reaching the epithelium. The drug must then move between tight junctions, survive the intercellular matrix and diffuse between the basolateral cells to reach the subepithelial space through which it can enter the nasal vasculature (Junginger 1992). Bile salts exert their permeation enhancing effect through solubilising cellular proteins, membrane phospholipids and through limiting the effect of metabolizing enzymes. Although the exact mechanism by which bile salts solubilise cellular components without necessarily damaging tissues is unknown, bile salts enhance absorption of drugs across membranes. The solubilisation of membrane components may be related to the ability of bile acids to overcome nasal membrane barrier resistance (Shao et al. 1992a). In one study (Shao et al. 1992b), the effect of bile salts on the structure, integrity, configuration and strength of the nasal mucosa, was study. The effect was investigated through administering bile salts to animal's nasal cavity then measuring the levels of cellular proteins (in the cell membrane and the cytoplasm), DNA-metabolizing enzymes and other biomarkers. The study concluded that deoxycholate caused the greatest solubilising effect on the nasal mucosa while taurocholate caused the least effect. Another study (Gordon et al. 1985a) was carried out in human, to investigate the physicochemical properties of bile salts and their relations to the permeation effect in nasal drug delivery. As expected, the rate of absorption of drug molecules was directly correlated to the bile salt's lipophilicity and their permeation effect. The most effective permeation enhancer, through the nasal mucosa, was deoxycholate, followed by, chenodeoxycholate, cholate then finally ursodeoxycholate.

However, large or too frequent doses of bile salts have been found to cause significant damage to the nasal mucosa and subsequent nasal bleeding (Hersey & Jackson 1987a). Moreover, enhancing further the nasal absorption of an insulin-bile salt formulation, through the use of starch microspheres, has been investigated (Illum et al. 2001). Microspheres are non-toxic and biocompatible with rabbit nasal mucosa (Bjork et al. 1991). Illum et al. examined the effect of starch microspheres on the absorption enhancing efficiency of bile salts in formulations with insulin, after application in the nasal cavity of sheep. The enhancers were selected on the basis of their perceived or proven mechanism of action and worked predominantly by interacting with the lipid membrane. The microsphere formulation was placed in the anterior part of the nasal cavity where few cilia are present. The bioadhesive properties provide a high drug concentration in close contact with the epithelial surface for an extended time period. Generally, microspheres can assist the passage of small drug molecules but an absorption enhancer is necessary for polypeptides with molecular weights above 6000 Da. Bioadhesive starch microspheres synergistically increase the effect of absorption enhancers on the absorption of insulin across the nasal membrane in sheep. The bioadhesive starch microspheres were shown to increase synergistically the effect of the bile salts on the transport of the insulin across the nasal mucosa. So when bile salts were used in conjunction with bioadhesive starch microspheres, they increased the amount of absorption by a factor ranging from 1 to 5, compared to bile salts alone (Illum et al. 2001). Such maximization of insulin-bile salt mucosal permeation was successful to enhance insulin absorption through the nasal mucosa, and thus shows great potential in insulin nasal delivery.

The ability of a bile acid to enhance permeation is heavily dependent on its hydroxyl groups and the concentration of bile acid present in solution. Insulin absorption increases when the concentration of bile salt exceeds its aqueous critical mice concentration (CMC). The amount of insulin absorbed also increases with increasing hydrophobicity of the bile salt. The order of bile salts' ability to increase insulin absorption is DCA>CDCA>CA>UDCA (Gordon et al. 1985b). When sodium deoxycholate, the most hydrophobic bile salt, is co-administered with insulin, the absorbed insulin causes more than 30% reduction in blood glucose levels in diabetic subjects (Moses et al. 1983). When a bile salt possess poor hydrophobicity, its efficacy is significantly reduced. When the highly hydrophilic sodium ursodeoxycholate is formulated with insulin then administered to diabetic subjects, the bile salt showed no significant permeation enhancing effect on insulin, and almost no decrease in blood sugar was reported in the treated diabetic subjects. Bile salts may increase the absorption of insulin by forming micelles in which the insulin resides in high concentrations. Another proposed mechanism is that bile acids form reverse micelles which form channels across the nasal membrane through which insulin can move to reach the bloodstream (Gordon et al. 1985b). Bile salts may also bind and trap Ca^{2+} causing tight junctions to loosen and allowing insulin to pass. In addition, sodium lauryl sulphate (SLS) may enhance drug absorption via the nasal route by lyzing biological membranes. This involves lipid solubilisation and subsequent protein denaturation and dissolution (Donovan et al. 1990). Accordingly, SLS has a unique ability to enhance absorption efficiently and at low concentration.

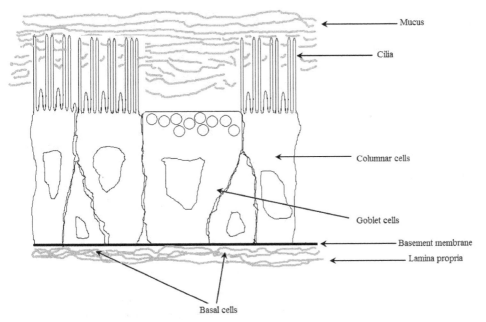

Fig. 5. The mucosal layer of the nasal cavity.

15. Rectal absorption

The rectum is the final part of the intestinal tract and about 4-5 inches long. It is the part of the gastrointestinal tract that extends from the colon in the lower left part of the abdomen to the anus. Its temperature is the same as the body temperature, constant at 37 °C. For insulin to be administered rectally, it needs to pass through the rectal epithelia, lamina propria and muscularis mucosa. The rectum has a rich vasculature making it a good site for drug administration.

For maximum absorption, insulin suppositories should not be inserted too high into the rectum since the superior rectal vein takes blood straight to the liver, where first pass effect is taking place. Inserting insulin to the lower part of the rectum will result in insulin permeation to the inferior or middle rectal veins which drain into the inferior vena cava bypassing the liver and avoiding first pass metabolism. However, reaching the higher part of the colon is not feasible thus rendering insulin rectal delivery ineffective. Enhancing insulin rectal absorption can be achieved using bile salts (Sayani & Chien 1996).

Bile acids have shown good efficacy in enhancing rectal absorption when complexed with or added to drug formulations. In human, INF-α, an antiviral, antineoplastic and immunoregulatory molecule, was not absorbed when administered rectally in a hydrophilic suppository, but when sodium ursodeoxycholate was incorporated into the suppository base, detectable levels were obtained (Lee et al. 1991; Lee 1991). By the same token, the effect of bile salts in insulin rectal absorption was investigated. Rectal administration with 5% sodium glycocholate produced a large increase in the effect of a 10 U/kg dose. Rectal and nasal administration reduced plasma glucose approximately half as effectively as intramuscular insulin in the presence of this bile salt (Aungst & Rogers 1988). This method of administration may be beneficial to those requiring only small doses of insulin or those uncomfortable with injection. Thus, it is clear that bile salts are effective promoters for rectal administration of insulin. The proposed mechanism of action involves enhanced membrane permeability, lipid solubilizing and the inhibition of proteolytic enzymes at the absorption site. However, rectal drug administration remains unfavorable and invasive and thus remains a major limitation for such a drug delivery system.

16. Pulmonary absorption

Pulmonary drug delivery is effective due to fast and convenient drug absorption. Lungs have rich vasculature and their blood output bypasses the liver metabolism, resulting in high drug bioavailability. It is commonly used to deliver anti-inflammatory therapeutics such as in asthma treatment. To maximize drug permeation through the lungs, reducing particle size may be appropriate. Particle size less than 5 μm ensures high absorbability but very low particle size (1 μm or less) makes particle-expulsion most likely and thus renders drug ineffective (Agu et al. 2001a; Agu et al. 2001b). Administration of insulin through inhalation may be effective but faces many challenges including mucous, mucociliary clearance, lung surfactants and proteases and peptidases at the alveolar surface (Heinemann et al. 2000). The addition of bile acids to insulin should minimise such challenges through enhancing mucus permeation and reducing enzymatic degradation. This is particularly interesting since current subcutaneous insulin injection causes wide range of side effects such as irritation and scarring as well as being highly unfavourable by patients due to its invasiveness and discomfort. In one study (45), the bioavailability of inhaled insulin was measured with and without the addition of bile acids. The bioavailability of inhaled insulin was 7.8% but, with the addition of a bile acid, absolute bioavailability reached 10.2% (p < 0.05). This was a small but significant increase which presents bile acids as permeation enhancers in pulmonary drug applications. Bile acids could have enhanced insulin effect through exerting their own hypoglycemic effect causing a further reduction in glucose levels after administration with insulin. The study also reported that the onset of the hypoglycemic effect after insulin inhalation with bile acids was more than ten times faster, then when insulin was injected SC alone. However, interpatient variation was large in terms of hypoglycemia, which was a disadvantage for such a method of insulin delivery. In other studies (Agu et al. 2001a; Agu et al. 2001b), insulin was administered via the lung with and without sodium glycocholate. The addition of 1% sodium glycocholate inhibited insulin degradation within the lung. Although neither the types of proteolytic enzymes involved in insulin hydrolysis nor the specific mode of stabilization by bile acids were investigated, sodium glycocholate was suggested to be an aminopeptidase inhibitor. Bile acids wide use in pulmonary drug formulation is limited by their safety profile. at the dose required to increase absorption, bile acids are non-toxic and relatively safe. However, when aspirated in large amounts, bile acids have been shown to cause pulmonary oedema and haemorrhage due to dissolution of pulmonary membranes (Kaneko et al. 1990).

17. Bile acids as hypoglycemic agents

Recent studies have shown that the semisynthetic bile acid analogue, 12-monoketocholic acid (MKC) exerted a significant hypoglycemic effect when administered alone to a rat model of T1D. When administered with insulin, MKC exerted a synergistic effect potentiating the hypoglycemic effect of insulin (Kuhajda et al. 2000; Mikov et al. 2008). MKC hypoglycemic effect was studied using various formulations including the oral, nasal, ocular and rectal applications. Then, the hypoglycemic effect was compared with that of insulin injected subcutaneously. The mixture of MKC and insulin also tested for hypoglycemic activity. Nasal administration of the insulin-MKC mixture resulted in a decrease of blood glucose concentration that reached 54% of that obtained after subcutaneous application of insulin. However, following nasal administration of the MKC, the decrease in blood glucose reached 36% of that obtained after subcutaneous application of insulin. The discovery of a link between bile acids and glucose regulation offers a new perspective in the design of hypoglycaemic drugs in treating diabetes (Miljkovic et al. 2000). The mechanisms by which, bile acids such as MKC exerts its hypoglycemic effect in T1D, was explored further. The hypoglycemic effect of bile acids on T1D rats could be explained through their effect on FXR and PPARs metabolic pathways (Houten et al. 2006b; Trauner et al. 2010). However such mechanisms remain to be fully characterized.

18. Safety of bile acids and probiotics

Many studies have been conducted to test the toxicity and safety of primary and secondary bile salts and their derivatives. Some bile salts have excellent safety profiles while others are not safe. Bile salts can be used as therapeutic agents, as absorption enhancers and as formulation excipients. Deoxycholic acid is used in manufacturing steroids and in vaccine production (e.g. influenza vaccine). However, its use is severely limited by its narrow safety profile. In relatively high doses, deoxycholic acid can cause hepatotoxicity and can damage the gastric mucosa. Cholylsarcosine (CS) is a stable bile salt derivative of deoxycholic acid. It resists bacterial activation to the more toxic bile acid, deoxycholic acid, and thus has a good safety profile. It is commonly used as an absorption enhancer in the treatment of primary biliary cirrhosis (Ricci et al. 1998). Deoxycholic acid salt is also used in the formulation of Amphotericin B, which is commonly used for treating fungal infections of the eyes (Samiy et al. 1996). However, due to its limited safety profile, Amphotericin B in doses as low as 1 μg has been shown to cause retinal damage despite the fact that the recommended dose is 5-10 μg (Souri & Green 1974). The administration of Amphotericin B deoxycholate may also result in cataract formation, opacity, retinal necrosis and retinal ganglion cell loss (Cannon et al. 2003).

When it comes to predicting the toxicity of bile salts, it seems that toxicity increases with their permeation ability. The more capable bile salts are to solubilizing membrane proteins, the more toxic they are (Shao et al. 1992a). In one study (Hersey & Jackson 1987b), bile acids damaged nasal epithelium causing nasal irritation, congestion and bleeding. The authors concluded that nasal applications of bile salts should be limited with infrequent dosing regimen.

Formulation of bile salts in inhalations can cause pulmonary oedema, when inhaled in large quantities. This is due to the solubilization and dissolution of the pulmonary membranes and pulmonary hemorrhage (Kaneko et al. 1990). However, such side effects are only caused by largely inhaled doses.

Probiotic administration has shown good safety profile in individuals with overall good health status, and may be suffering from mild infections or GI disorders (Luoto et al. 2010). Probiotic safety stems from the fact that many strains are of human origin and present in large numbers in human GIT (Rozanova & Voevodin 2008). Accordingly, the reported incidences of probiotics inducing bacterial infection and bacteremia are very low (Snydman 2008). The only major concern with probiotic administration is the potential of bacterial translocation resulting in the induction of antibiotic-resistance strains that may lead to pathogenesis and haemodyscrasia (Liong 2008; Snydman 2008). Having said that risks of infections caused by probiotic treatment is expected to be significant in immunocompromised patients (Marteau & Shanahan 2003; Rayes et al. 2005).

If the use of probiotics and bile acids is to become part of T1D therapy, their safety concerns may be overcome by thoroughly studying appropriate dosing and frequency, their short and long term effect on mucosal membranes and the variation of their effect in different populations.

19. Conclusion

Conjugated bile acids (bile salts) can form micelles that solubilise and transport lipids across biological membranes. Bile acids as absorption promoters have the potential to aid intestinal, ocular, nasal, pulmonary and rectal absorption of insulin. Bile acids are hypoglycemic agents on their own and thus can be used as adjunct therapy in treating T1D. However, in high concentrations, bile acids may damage tissue, so it is important to examine their safety profile thoroughly before application e.g. in buccal formulations as there is conflicting evidence on the morphological changes that occur in the buccal epithelium upon contact with bile acids. However, such an improvement in insulin absorption is still insufficient and subcutaneous injection remains the commonly used method. Nasal administration has certain advantages such as ease of use and high bioavailability. However, it does not allow transport of high molecular weight proteins and peptides. Bile acids have demonstrated the ability to enhance the nasal absorption of insulin and other drugs. One of the main disadvantages of the applications of bile acids as permeation enhancers is that the greater the bile acid is at promoting permeation of through mucosa, the more toxic it becomes. Accordingly, it is important to determine the mechanism of action by which bile acids enhance absorption in order to design absorption promoting agents that are not toxic or irritant. In addition, knowledge of the mechanism of action may allow prediction of the exact amount of a therapeutic substance that will reach the systemic circulation. The metabolism and deconjugation of bile acids are brought about by the gut microflora. Interestingly, gut microflora plays a major rule in energy balance and gut inflammation. Probiotics have shown hypoglycemic effect, when administered alone, thus, their use in T1D should be studied further.

Type 1 diabetes and its complications cannot be cured by the best most intensive insulin therapy (Shamoon et al. 1993). This clearly emphasizes the fact that the disease is more complex, interdependent, and challenging to treat than being a simple hyperglycemia. That is why, in our opinion, multidrug approach which integrates a comprehensive, targeted, and tailored treatment should guarantee the best outcome for diabetic patients.

20. Acknowledgement

This work has been supported by Ministry of Science and Technology of Serbia Research grant No 41012.

21. References

Agu, R.U., Jorissen, M., Willems, T., Augustijns, P., Kinget, R. & Verbeke, N. (2001a) In-vitro nasal drug delivery studies: comparison of derivatised, fibrillar and polymerised collagen matrix-based human nasal primary culture systems for nasal drug delivery studies. *Journal of Pharmacy and Pharmacology*, 53, 1447-1456.

Agu, R.U., Ugwoke, M.I., Armand, M., Kinget, R. & Verbeke, N. (2001b) The lung as a route for systemic delivery of therapeutic proteins and peptides. *Respiratory Research*, 2, 198-209.

Akerblom, H.K., Vaarala, O., Hyoty, H., Ilonen, J. & Knip, M. (2002) Environmental factors in the etiology of type 1 diabetes. 115, 18-29.

Al-Salami, H., Butt, G., Fawcett, J.P., Tucker, I.G., Golocorbin-Kon, S. & Mikov, M. (2008a) Probiotic treatment reduces blood glucose levels and increases systemic absorption of gliclazide in diabetic rats. *Eur.J.Drug Metab Pharmacokinet.*, 33, 101-106.

Al-Salami, H., Butt, G., Fawcett, J.P., Tucker, I.G., Golocorbin-Kon, S. & Mikov, M. (2008b) Probiotic treatment reduces blood glucose levels and increases systemic absorption of gliclazide in diabetic rats. *European Journal of Drug Metabolism and Pharmacokinetics*, 33, 101-106.

Al-Salami, H., Butt, G., Tucker, I., Fawcett, P.J., Golocorbin-Kon, S., Mikov, I. & Mikov, M. (2009a) Gliclazide reduces MKC intestinal transport in healthy but not diabetic rats. *European Journal of Drug Metabolism and Pharmacokinetics*, 34, 43-50.

Al-Salami, H., Butt, G., Tucker, I. & Mikov, M. (2008c) Influence of the semisynthetic bile acid (MKC) on the ileal permeation of gliclazide in healthy and diabetic rats. *Pharmacol.Rep.*, 60, 532-541.

Al-Salami, H., Butt, G., Tucker, I. & Mikov, M. (2008d) Influence of the semisynthetic bile acid MKC on the ileal permeation of gliclazide ex vivo in healthy and diabetic rats treated with probiotics. *Methods and Findings in Experimental and Clinical Pharmacology*, 30, 107-113.

Al-Salami, H., Butt, G., Tucker, I. & Mikov, M. (2008e) Probiotic treatment proceeded by a single dose of bile acid and gliclazide exert the most hypoglycemic effect in Type 1 diabetic rats. *Medical Hypothesis Research*, 4, 93-101.

Al-Salami, H., Butt, G., Tucker, I., Skrbic, R., Golocorbin-Kon, S. & Mikov, M. (2008f) Probiotic Pre-treatment Reduces Gliclazide Permeation (ex vivo) in Healthy Rats but Increases It in Diabetic Rats to the Level Seen in Untreated Healthy Rats. *Arch.Drug Inf.*, 1, 35-41.

Al-Salami, H., Butt, G., Tucker, I.G., Fawcett, J.P. & Mikov, M. (2009b) Probiotic treatment decreases the oral absorption of the semisynthetic bile acid, MKC, in healthy and diabetic rats. *The European journal of drug metabolism and pharmacokinetics*.

Al-Salami, H., Grant, B., Ian, T. & Mikov, M. (2008g) The influence of probiotics pre-treatment, on the ileal permeation of gliclazide, in healthy and diabetic rats. *The archives of drug information*, 1, 35-41.

Al-Salami, H., Kansara, H., King, J., Morar, B., Jayathilaka, B., Fawcett, P.J. & Mikov, M. (2007) Bile acids: a bitter sweet remedy for diabetes. *The New Zealand Pharmacy Journal*, 27, 17-20.

Altenhoefer, A., Oswald, S., Sonnenborn, U., Enders, C., Schulze, J., Hacker, J. & Oelschlaeger, T.A. (2004) The probiotic Escherichia coli strain Nissle 1917 interferes with invasion of human intestinal epithelial cells by different enteroinvasive bacterial pathogens. 40, 223-229.

Asamoto, Y., Tazuma, S., Ochi, H., Chayama, K. & Suzuki, H. (2001) Bile-salt hydrophobicity is a key factor regulating rat liver plasma-membrane communication: relation to bilayer structure, fluidity and transporter expression and function. 359, 605-610.

Aungst, B.J. & Rogers, N.J. (1988) Site Dependence of Absorption-Promoting Actions of Laureth-9, Na Salicylate, Na2Edta, and Aprotinin on Rectal, Nasal, and Buccal Insulin Delivery. *Pharmaceutical Research*, 5, 305-308.

Bachrach, W.H. & Hofmann, A.F. (1982a) Ursodeoxycholic Acid in the Treatment of Cholesterol Cholelithiasis .1. *Digestive Diseases and Sciences*, 27, 737-761.

Bachrach, W.H. & Hofmann, A.F. (1982b) Ursodeoxycholic Acid in the Treatment of Cholesterol Cholelithiasis .2. *Digestive Diseases and Sciences*, 27, 833-856.

Ballatori, N., Christian, W.V., Lee, J.Y., Dawson, P.A., Soroka, C.J., Boyer, J.L., Madejczyk, M.S. & Li, N. (2005a) OSTalpha-OSTbeta: a major basolateral bile acid and steroid transporter in human intestinal, renal, and biliary epithelia. 42, 1270-1279.

Ballatori, N., Hammond, C.L., Cunningham, J.B., Krance, S.M. & Marchan, R. (2005b) Molecular mechanisms of reduced glutathione transport: role of the MRP/CFTR/ABCC and OATP/SLC21A families of membrane proteins. 204, 238-255.

Barbeau, W.E., Bassaganya-Riera, J. & Hontecillas, R. (2006) Putting the pieces of the puzzle together - a series of hypotheses on the etiology and pathogenesis of type 1 diabetes. 68, 607-609.

Barbeau, W.E., Bassaganya-Riera, J. & Hontecillas, R. (2007) Putting the pieces of the puzzle together - a series of hypotheses on the etiology and pathogenesis of type 1 diabetes. 68, 607-619.

Bennion, L.J. & Grundy, S.M. (1977) Effects of diabetes mellitus on cholesterol metabolism in man. 296, 1365-1371.

Bezkorovainy, A. (2001) Probiotics: determinants of survival and growth in the gut. 73, 399S-405S.

Bjork, E., Bjurstrom, S. & Edman, P. (1991) Morphological Examination of Rabbit Nasal-Mucosa After Nasal Administration of Degradable Starch Microspheres. *International Journal of Pharmaceutics*, 75, 73-80.

Bodo, A., Bakos, E., Szeri, F., Varadi, A. & Sarkadi, B. (2003) Differential modulation of the human liver conjugate transporters MRP2 and MRP3 by bile acids and organic anions. 278, 23529-23537.

Bruno, G., Runzo, C., Cavallo-Perin, P., Merletti, F., Rivetti, M., Pinach, S., Novelli, G., Trovati, M., Cerutti, F. & Pagano, G. (2005) Incidence of type 1 and type 2 diabetes in adults aged 30-49 years: the population-based registry in the province of Turin, Italy. 28, 2613-2619.

Calcinaro, F., Dionisi, S., Marinaro, M., Candeloro, P., Bonato, V., Marzotti, S., Corneli, R.B., Ferretti, E., Gulino, A., Grasso, F., De Simone, C., Di Mario, U., Falorni, A., Boirivant, M. & Dotta, F. (2005) Oral probiotic administration induces interleukin-10 production and prevents spontaneous autoimmune diabetes in the non-obese diabetic mouse. *Diabetologia*, 48, 1565-1575.

Campbell, I.W. (1991) Management of type 2 diabetes mellitus with special reference to metformin therapy. 17, 191-196.

Campbell, I.W. (2004) Long-term glycaemic control with pioglitazone in patients with type 2 diabetes. 58, 192-200.

Cani, P.D., Bibiloni, R., Knauf, C., Neyrinck, A.M., Neyrinck, A.M., Delzenne, N.M. & Burcelin, R. (2008) Changes in gut microbiota control metabolic endotoxemia-induced inflammation in high-fat diet-induced obesity and diabetes in mice. *Diabetes*, 57, 1470-1481.

Cani, P.D., Neyrinck, A.M., Fava, F., Knauf, C., Burcelin, R.G., Tuohy, K.M., Gibson, G.R. & Delzenne, N.M. (2007) Selective increases of bifidobacteria in gut microflora improve high-fat-diet-induced diabetes in mice through a mechanism associated with endotoxaemia. *Diabetologia*, 50, 2374-2383.

Cani, P.D., Possemiers, S., Van de Wiele, T., Guiot, Y., Everard, A., Rottier, O., Geurts, L., Naslain, D., Neyrinck, A., Lambert, D.M., Muccioli, G.G. & Delzenne, N.M. (2009) Changes in gut microbiota control inflammation in obese mice through a mechanism involving GLP-2-driven improvement of gut permeability. *Gut*, 58, 1091-1103.

Cannon, J.P., Fiscella, R., Pattharachayakul, S., Garey, K.W., De Alba, F., Piscitelli, S., Edward, D.P. & Danziger, L.H. (2003) Comparative toxicity and concentrations of intravitreal amphotericin B formulations in a rabbit model. *Investigative Ophthalmology & Visual Science*, 44, 2112-2117.

Cary, V.A. & Boullata, J. (2010) What is the evidence for the use of probiotics in the treatment of inflammatory bowel disease? *J.Clin.Nurs.*, 19, 904-916.

Chijiiwa, K. (1990) The effects of ethinylestradiol, a glucose diet and streptozotocin induced diabetes mellitus on gallstone formation and biliary lipid composition in the hamster. *Jpn.J.Surg.*, 20, 567-576.

Cornell, R.P. (1985) Endogenous Gut-Derived Bacterial-Endotoxin Tonically Primes Pancreatic-Secretion of Insulin in Normal Rats. *Diabetes*, 34, 1253-1259.

Cubeddu, L.X. & Hoffmann, I.S. (2002) Insulin resistance and upper-normal glucose levels in hypertension: a review. *J.Hum.Hypertens.*, 16 Suppl 1, S52-S55.

De Leon, M., Ferenderes, R. & Carulli, N. (1978) Bile lipid composition and bile acid pool size in diabetes. 23, 710-716.

Devendra, D., Liu, E. & Eisenbarth, G.S. (2004) Type 1 diabetes: recent developments. 328, 750-754.

Di Wu, Q., Wang, J.H., Fennessy, F., Redmond, H.P. & Bouchier-Hayes, D. (1999) Taurine prevents high-glucose-induced human vascular endothelial cell apoptosis. *American Journal of Physiology-Cell Physiology*, 277, C1229-C1238.

Dieleman, L.A., Pena, A.S., Meuwissen, S.G. & van Rees, E.P. (1997) Role of animal models for the pathogenesis and treatment of inflammatory bowel disease. 223, 99-104.

Donovan, M.D., Flynn, G.L. & Amidon, G.L. (1990) The Molecular-Weight Dependence of Nasal Absorption - the Effect of Absorption Enhancers. *Pharmaceutical Research*, 7, 808-815.

Duan, F., Curtis, K.L. & March, J.C. (2008) Secretion of insulinotropic proteins by commensal bacteria: rewiring the gut to treat diabetes. *Appl.Environ.Microbiol.*, 74, 7437-7438.

Fajans, S. (1987) [Classification, pathogenesis and course of various types of diabetes mellitus]. 93, 139-144.

FAO/WHO. (2002) guidelines for the evaluation of probiotics in food.

Favaro-Trindade, C.S. & Grosso, C.R. (2002) Microencapsulation of L. acidophilus (La-05) and B. lactis (Bb-12) and evaluation of their survival at the pH values of the stomach and in bile. 19, 485-494.

Fox, J.G., Feng, Y., Theve, E.J., Raczynski, A.R., Fiala, J.L.A., Doernte, A.L., Williams, M., McFaline, J.L., Essigmann, J.M., Schauer, D.B., Tannenbaum, S.R., Dedon, P.C., Weinman, S.A., Lemon, S.M., Fry, R.C. & Rogers, A.B. (2010) Gut microbes define liver cancer risk in mice exposed to chemical and viral transgenic hepatocarcinogens. *Gut*, 59, 88-97.

Franconi, F., Bennardini, F., Mattana, A., Miceli, M., Ciuti, M., Mian, M., Gironi, A., Anichini, R. & Seghieri, G. (1995) Plasma and Platelet Taurine Are Reduced in Subjects with Insulin-Dependent Diabetes-Mellitus - Effects of Taurine Supplementation. *American Journal of Clinical Nutrition*, 61, 1115-1119.

Franz, B. & Bode, J.C. (1973) [Plasma bile acid concentration (PGK): fasting values, daily fluctuations and effect of intraduodenal bile acid administration in healthy subjects and patients with chronic liver diseases]. *Z Gastroenterol*, 11, 131-134.

Gareau, M.G., Sherman, P.M. & Walker, W.A. (2010) Probiotics and the gut microbiota in intestinal health and disease. *Nature Reviews Gastroenterology & Hepatology*, 7, 503-514.

Gebel, E. (2011) The host with the most. A human body's bacteria may offer clues to why diabetes develops. *Diabetes Forecast.*, 64, 36-39.

Ghosh, S., van Heel, D. & Playford, R.J. (2004) Probiotics in inflammatory bowel disease: is it all gut flora modulation? 53, 620-622.

Goldberg, E. & Krause, I. (2009) Infection and type 1 diabetes mellitus - a two edged sword? *Autoimmun.Rev.*, 8, 682-686.

Goldfine, A.B. (2008) Modulating LDL cholesterol and glucose in patients with type 2 diabetes mellitus: targeting the bile acid pathway. 23, 502-511.

Goodman, H.O. & Shihabi, Z.K. (1990) Supplemental Taurine in Diabetic Rats - Effects on Plasma-Glucose and Triglycerides. *Biochemical Medicine and Metabolic Biology*, 43, 1-9.

Gordon, G.S., Moses, A.C., Silver, R.D., Flier, J.S. & Carey, M.C. (1985a) Nasal Absorption of Insulin - Enhancement by Hydrophobic Bile-Salts. *Proceedings of the National Academy of Sciences of the United States of America*, 82, 7419-7423.

Gordon, G.S., Moses, A.C., Silver, R.D., Flier, J.S. & Carey, M.C. (1985b) Nasal absorption of insulin: enhancement by hydrophobic bile salts. 82, 7419-7423.

Gourbeyre, P., Denery, S. & Bodinier, M. (2011) Probiotics, prebiotics, and synbiotics: impact on the gut immune system and allergic reactions. *J.Leukoc.Biol.*, 89, 685-695.

Grover, B., Buckley, D., Buckley, A.R. & Cacini, W. (2004) Reduced expression of organic cation transporters rOCT1 and rOCT2 in experimental diabetes. *J.Pharmacol.Exp Ther.*, 308, 949-956.

Hamada, T., Goto, H., Yamahira, T., Sugawara, T., Imaizumi, K. & Ikeda, I. (2006) Solubility in and affinity for the bile salt micelle of plant sterols are important determinants of their intestinal absorption in rats. *Lipids*, 41, 551-556.

Hansen, S.H. (2001) The role of taurine in diabetes and the development of diabetic complications. *Diabetes Metab Res.Rev.*, 17, 330-346.

Heaton, K.W. (1971) Abnormal Bile Or Faulty Gall Bladder. *British Medical Journal*, 1, 289-&.

Hedenborg, G. & Norman, A. (1984) The nature of urinary bile acid conjugates in patients with extrahepatic cholestasis. 44, 725-733.

Hedenborg, G. & Norman, A. (1985) Fasting and postprandial serum bile acid concentration with special reference to variations in the conjugate profile. 45, 151-156.

Heinemann, L., Klappoth, W., Rave, K., Hompesch, B., Linkeschowa, R. & Heise, T. (2000) Intra-individual variability of the metabolic effect of inhaled insulin together with an absorption enhancer. *Diabetes Care*, 23, 1343-1347.

Hersey, S.J. & Jackson, R.T. (1987a) Effect of bile salts on nasal permeability in vitro. *J.Pharm.Sci.*, 76, 876-879.

Hersey, S.J. & Jackson, R.T. (1987b) Effect of bile salts on nasal permeability in vitro. *J.Pharm.Sci.*, 76, 876-879.

Higgins, C.F. & Gottesman, M.M. (1992) Is the multidrug transporter a flippase? 17, 18-21.

Hirai, S., Ikenaga, T. & Matsuzawa, T. (1978) Nasal Absorption of Insulin in Dogs. *Diabetes*, 27, 296-299.

Hopkins, M.J. & Macfarlane, G.T. (2002) Changes in predominant bacterial populations in human faeces with age and with Clostridium difficile infection. *Journal of Medical Microbiology*, 51, 448-454.

Houten, S., Watanabe, M. & Auwerx, J. (2006a) Endocrine functions of bile acids. 25, 1419-1425.

Houten, S.M., Watanabe, M. & Auwerx, J. (2006b) Endocrine functions of bile acids. *Embo Journal*, 25, 1419-1425.

Husebye, E. (2005) The pathogenesis of gastrointestinal bacterial overgrowth. *Chemotherapy*, 51 Suppl 1, 1-22.

Illum, L., Fisher, A.N., Jabbal-Gill, I. & Davis, S.S. (2001) Bioadhesive starch microspheres and absorption enhancing agents act synergistically to enhance the nasal absorption of polypeptides. *International Journal of Pharmaceutics*, 222, 109-119.

Jaakkola, I., Jalkanen, S. & Hanninen, A. (2003) Diabetogenic T cells are primed both in pancreatic and gut-associated lymph nodes in NOD mice. *Eur J Immunol*, 33, 3255-3264.

Jacobs, D.B., Hayes, G.R. & Lockwood, D.H. (1989) In vitro effects of sulfonylurea on glucose transport and translocation of glucose transporters in adipocytes from streptozocin-induced diabetic rats. 38, 205-211.

Jain, S.K., Kannan, K., Lim, G., Mcvie, R. & Bocchini, J.A. (2002) Hyperketonemia increases tumor necrosis factor-alpha secretion in cultured U937 monocytes and type 1 diabetic patients and is apparently mediated by oxidative stress and cAMP deficiency. *Diabetes*, 51, 2287-2293.

Juhl, C., Grofte, T., Butler, P.C., Veldhuis, J.D., Schmitz, O. & Porksen, N. (2002) Effects of fasting on physiologically pulsatile insulin release in healthy humans. *Diabetes*, 51 Suppl 1, S255-S257.

Junginger, H.E. (1992) Formulation Aspects on Dermatological Preparations and Transdermal Drug Delivery Systems. *Acta Pharmaceutica Nordica*, 4, 117.

Just, T., Pau, H.W., Engel, U. & Hummel, T. (2008) Cephalic phase insulin release in healthy humans after taste stimulation? *Appetite*, 51, 622-627.

Kaneko, T., Sato, T., Katsuya, H. & Miyauchi, Y. (1990) Surfactant Therapy for Pulmonary-Edema Due to Intratracheally Injected Bile-Acid. *Critical Care Medicine*, 18, 77-83.

Karimi, O. & Pena, A.S. (2003) Probiotics: Isolated bacteria strain or mixtures of different strains? Two different approaches in the use of probiotics as therapeutics. 39, 565-597.

Kokk, K., Verajankorva, E., Laato, M., Wu, X.K., Tapfer, H. & Pollanen, P. (2005) Expression of insulin receptor substrates 1-3, glucose transporters GLUT-1-4, signal regulatory protein 1alpha, phosphatidylinositol 3-kinase and protein kinase B at the protein level in the human testis. 80, 91-96.

Kuhajda, K., Kandrac, J., Kevresan, S., Mikov, M. & Fawcett, J.P. (2006a) Structure and origin of bile acids: an overview. 31, 135-143.

Kuhajda, K., Kevresan, S., Kandrac, J., Fawcett, J.P. & Mikov, M. (2006b) Chemical and metabolic transformations of selected bile acids. 31, 179-235.

Kuhajda, K., Kevresan, S., Mikov, M., Sabo, A. & D., M. (2000) Influence of 3a,7a-dihydroxy-12-keto-5ß-cholanate on blood glucose level in rats. 8, 304-308.

Kulakowski, E.C. & Maturo, J. (1984) Hypoglycemic Properties of Taurine - Not Mediated by Enhanced Insulin Release. *Biochemical Pharmacology*, 33, 2835-2838.

Kurdi, P., Kawanishi, K., Mizutani, K. & Yokota, A. (2006) Mechanism of growth inhibition by free bile acids in lactobacilli and bifidobacteria. 188, 1979-1986.

Kurdi, P., van Veen, H.W., Tanaka, H., Mierau, I., Konings, W.N., Tannock, G.W., Tomita, F. & Yokota, A. (2000) Cholic acid is accumulated spontaneously, driven by membrane deltapH, in many lactobacilli. 182, 6525-6528.

Lee, V.H.L. (1991) Trends in Peptide and Protein Drug Delivery. *Biopharm-the Technology & Business of Biopharmaceuticals*, 4, 22-25.

Lee, V.H.L., Yamamoto, A. & Kompella, U.B. (1991) Mucosal Penetration Enhancers for Facilitation of Peptide and Protein Drug Absorption. *Critical Reviews in Therapeutic Drug Carrier Systems*, 8, 91-192.

Leng, J., Egelhaaf, S.U. & Cates, M.E. (2003) Kinetics of the micelle-to-vesicle transition: aqueous lecithin-bile salt mixtures. *Biophys.J.*, 85, 1624-1646.

Li, Y.P., Shao, Z.Z. & Mitra, A.K. (1992) Dissociation of Insulin Oligomers by Bile-Salt Micelles and Its Effect on Alpha-Chymotrypsin-Mediated Proteolytic Degradation. *Pharmaceutical Research*, 9, 864-869.

Li-Wen, H., Bi-Zhou, L., Xue-Zhong, L., Xiu-Feng, H. & Ling, B. (2007) Synthesis, structure and characterization of [Cu(2,2 '-bpy)(2)][{Cu(2,2 '-bpy)(2)}(2)W12O40(H-2)]center dot 4H(2)O. *Chinese Journal of Structural Chemistry*, 26, 1435-1440.

Liong, M.T. (2008) Safety of probiotics: translocation and infection. *Nutr.Rev.*, 66, 192-202.

Lowbeer, T.S., Heaton, K.W. & Read, A.E. (1970) Gallbladder Inertia in Adult Coeliac Disease. *Gut*, 11, 1057-&.

Luoto, R., Laitinen, K., Nermes, M. & Isolauri, E. (2010) Impact of maternal probiotic-supplemented dietary counselling on pregnancy outcome and prenatal and postnatal growth: a double-blind, placebo-controlled study. *Br J Nutr*, 103, 1792-1799.

Macpherson, A.J. & Uhr, T. (2004) Induction of protective IgA by intestinal dendritic cells carrying commensal bacteria. *Science*, 303, 1662-1665.

Maki, M., Huupponen, T., Holm, K. & Hallstrom, O. (1995) Seroconversion of Reticulin Autoantibodies Predicts Celiac-Disease in Insulin-Dependent Diabetes-Mellitus. *Gut*, 36, 239-242.

Maki, N., Hafkemeyer, P. & Dey, S. (2003) Allosteric modulation of human P-glycoprotein. Inhibition of transport by preventing substrate translocation and dissociation. 278, 18132-18139.

Malavolti, M., Fromm, H., Ceryak, S. & Shehan, K.L. (1989) Interaction of Potentially Toxic Bile-Acids with Human-Plasma Proteins - Binding of Lithocholic (3-Alpha-Hydroxy-5-Beta-Cholan-24-Oic) Acid to Lipoproteins and Albumin. *Lipids*, 24, 673-676.

Mao, Q. & Unadkat, J.D. (2005) Role of the breast cancer resistance protein (ABCG2) in drug transport. 2005/09/09, E118-E133.

Marteau, P. & Shanahan, F. (2003) Basic aspects and pharmacology of probiotics: an overview of pharmacokinetics, mechanisms of action and side-effects. *Best.Pract.Res.Clin.Gastroenterol.*, 17, 725-740.

Martin, C.R. & Walker, W.A. (2008) Probiotics: role in pathophysiology and prevention in necrotizing enterocolitis. *Semin.Perinatol.*, 32, 127-137.

Matsuzaki, T., Nagata, Y., Kado, S., Uchida, K., Hashimoto, S. & Yokokura, T. (1997a) Effect of oral administration of Lactobacillus casei on alloxan-induced diabetes in mice. 105, 637-642.

Matsuzaki, T., Nagata, Y., Kado, S., Uchida, K., Kato, I., Hashimoto, S. & Yokokura, T. (1997b) Prevention of onset in an insulin-dependent diabetes mellitus model, NOD mice, by oral feeding of Lactobacillus casei. 105, 643-649.

Matthaei, S., Horuk, R. & Olefsky, J.M. (1986) Blood-brain glucose transfer in diabetes mellitus. Decreased number of glucose transporters at blood-brain barrier. *Diabetes*, 35, 1181-1184.

Meinders, A.E., Henegouwen, V.B., Willekens, F.L.A., Schwerzel, A.L., Ruben, B.A. & Huybregts, A.W.M. (1981a) Biliary lipid and bile acid composition in insulin-dependent diabetes mellitus. 26, 402-408.

Meinders, A.E., Van Berge Henegouwen, G.P., Willekens, F.L., Schwerzel, A.L., Ruben, A. & Huybregts, A.W. (1981b) Biliary lipid and bile acid composition in insulin-dependent diabetes mellitus. Arguments for increased intestinal bacterial bile acid degradation. 26, 402-408.

Meinders, A.E., Vanbergehenegouwen, G.P., Willekens, F.L.A., Schwerzel, A.L., Ruben, A. & Huybregts, A.W.M. (1981c) Biliary Lipid and Bile-Acid Composition in Insulin-Dependent Diabetes-Mellitus - Arguments for Increased Intestinal Bacterial Bile-Acid Degradation. *Digestive Diseases and Sciences*, 26, 402-408.

Mesiha, M.S., Ponnapula, S. & Plakogiannis, F. (2002a) Oral absorption of insulin encapsulated in artificial chyles of bile salts, palmitic acid and alpha-tocopherol dispersions. 249, 1-5.

Mesiha, M.S., Ponnapula, S. & Plakogiannis, F. (2002b) Oral absorption of insulin encapsulated in artificial chyles of bile salts, palmitic acid and alpha-tocopherol dispersions. *International Journal of Pharmaceutics*, 249, 1-5.

Mesiha, M.S., Ponnapula, S. & Plakogiannis, F. (2002c) Oral absorption of insulin encapsulated in artificial chyles of bile salts, palmitic acid and alpha-tocopherol dispersions. *International Journal of Pharmaceutics*, 249, 1-5.

Mikov, M., Al-Salami, H., Golocorbin-Kon, S., Skrbic, R., Raskovic, A. & Fawcett, J.P. (2008) The influence of 3 alpha,7 alpha-dihydroxy-12-keto-5 beta-cholanate on gliclazide pharmacokinetics and glucose levels in a rat model of diabetes. *European Journal of Drug Metabolism and Pharmacokinetics*, 33, 137-142.

Mikov, M., Boni, N.S., Al-Salami, H., Kuhajda, K., Kevresan, S., Golocorbin-Kon, S. & Fawcett, J.P. (2007) Bioavailability and hypoglycemic activity of the semisynthetic bile acid salt, sodium 3alpha,7alpha-dihydroxy-12-oxo-5beta-cholanate, in healthy and diabetic rats. *Eur.J.Drug Metab Pharmacokinet.*, 32, 7-12.

Mikov, M. & Fawcett, J.P. (2006a) Bile acids - Chemistry, biosynthesis, analysis, chemical & metabolic transformations and pharmacology. *European Journal of Drug Metabolism and Pharmacokinetics*, 31, 133-134.

Mikov, M. & Fawcett, J.P. (2006b) Chemistry, biosynthesis, analysis, chemical & metabolic transformations and pharmacology. 31, 133-134.

Mikov, M., Fawcett, J.P., Kuhajda, K. & Kevresan, S. (2006) Pharmacology of bile acids and their derivatives: absorption promoters and therapeutic agents. 31, 237-251.

Mikov, M., Raskovic, A., Jakovljevic, E., Dudvarski, D. & Fawcett, J.P. (2005) Influence of the bile salt sodium 3alfa,7alfa-dihydroxy-12-oxo-5beta-cholanate on ampicillin pharmacokinetics in rats. 5, 197-200.

Mikov, M., Raskovic, A., Kuhajda, K., Kevresan, S. & Potsides, C.Y. (2004) Therapeutic perspective of bile acids-Toxicity and interaction. 1, S-1.

Miljkovic, D., Kuhajda, K., Mikov, M., Kevresan, S. & A., S. (2000) US patent No. 6060465 on bile acids and their derivatives as glycoregulatory agents. *US*.

Mita, S., Suzuki, H., Akita, H., Hayashi, H., Onuki, R., Hofmann, A.F. & Sugiyama, Y. (2006) Inhibition of bile acid transport across Na+/taurocholate cotransporting polypeptide (SLC10A1) and bile salt export pump (ABCB 11)-coexpressing LLC-PK1 cells by cholestasis-inducing drugs. 34, 1575-1581.

Miyai, K., Javitt, N.B., Gochman, N., Jones, H.M. & Baker, D. (1982) Hepatotoxicity of Bile-Acids in Rabbits - Ursodeoxycholic Acid Is Less Toxic Than Chenodeoxycholic Acid. *Laboratory Investigation*, 46, 428-437.

Mooradian, A.D. & Morin, A.M. (1991) Brain uptake of glucose in diabetes mellitus: the role of glucose transporters. *Am.J.Med.Sci.*, 301, 173-177.

Moore, P.A., Zgibor, J.C. & Dasanayake, A.P. (2003a) Diabetes: a growing epidemic of all ages. *J Am Dent Assoc*, 134 Spec No, 11S-15S.

Moore, P.A., Zgibor, J.C. & Dasanayake, A.P. (2003b) Diabetes: a growing epidemic of all ages. *J Am Dent Assoc*, 134 Spec No, 11S-15S.

Morris, J.A. (1989) A possible role for bacteria in the pathogenesis of insulin dependent diabetes mellitus. *Med.Hypotheses*, 29, 231-235.

Morris, J.D., Diamond, K.A. & Balart, L.A. (2009) Do probiotics have a role in the management of inflammatory bowel disease? *J.La State Med.Soc.*, 161, 155-159.

Moses, A.C., Gordon, G.S., Carey, M.C. & Flier, J.S. (1983) Insulin Administered Intranasally As An Insulin-Bile Salt Aerosol - Effectiveness and Reproducibility in Normal and Diabetic Subjects. *Diabetes*, 32, 1040-1047.

Neish, A.S., Gewirtz, A.T., Zeng, H., Young, A.N., Hobert, M.E., Karmali, V., Rao, A.S. & Madara, J.L. (2000) Prokaryotic regulation of epithelial responses by inhibition of IkappaB-alpha ubiquitination. *Science*, 289, 1560-1563.

Neubert, R., Furst, W. & Wurschi, B. (1987) [Drug permeation through artificial lipoid membranes. 20. The effectiveness of multiple-lamellar liposomes for evaluating drug transport]. *Pharmazie*, 42, 102-103.

Notkins, A.L. & Lernmark, A. (2001) Autoimmune type 1 diabetes: resolved and unresolved issues. 108, 1247-1252.

Ogura, Y., Ito, T. & Ogura, M. (1986) Effect of diabetes and of 7 alpha-hydroxycholesterol infusion on the profile of bile acids secreted by the isolated rat livers. *Biol.Chem.Hoppe Seyler*, 367, 1095-1099.

Oktar, B.K., Gulpinar, M.A., Ercan, F., Cingi, A., Alican, I. & Yegen, B.C. (2001) Beneficial effects of glycocholic acid (GCA) on gut mucosal damage in bile duct ligated rats. *Inflammation*, 25, 311-318.

Otte, J.M. & Podolsky, D.K. (2004) Functional modulation of enterocytes by gram-positive and gram-negative microorganisms. *Am.J.Physiol Gastrointest.Liver Physiol*, 286, G613-G626.

Overkamp, D., Gautier, J.F., Renn, W., Pickert, A., Scheen, A.J., Schmulling, R.M., Eggstein, M. & Lefebvre, P.J. (1997) Glucose turnover in humans in the basal state and after intravenous glucose: a comparison of two models. *Am.J.Physiol*, 273, E284-E296.

Paccagnini, D., Sieswerda, L., Rosu, V., Masala, S., Pacifico, A., Gazouli, M., Ikonomopoulos, J., Ahmed, N., Zanetti, S. & Sechi, L.A. (2009) Linking chronic infection and autoimmune diseases: Mycobacterium avium subspecies paratuberculosis, SLC11A1 polymorphisms and type-1 diabetes mellitus. *PLoS One*, 4, e7109.

Palmer, K.J. & Brogden, R.N. (1993) Gliclazide. An update of its pharmacological properties and therapeutic efficacy in non-insulin-dependent diabetes mellitus. 46, 92-125.

Peng, H. & Hagopian, W. (2007) Environmental factors in the development of Type 1 diabetes.

Pigeon, R.M., Cuesta, E.P. & Gililliand, S.E. (2002) Binding of free bile acids by cells of yogurt starter culture bacteria. 85, 2705-2710.

Py, G., Lambert, K., Milhavet, O., Eydoux, N., Prefaut, C. & Mercier, J. (2002) Effects of streptozotocin-induced diabetes on markers of skeletal muscle metabolism and monocarboxylate transporter 1 to monocarboxylate transporter 4 transporters. *Metabolism*, 51, 807-813.

Qin, X., Yuan, F., Zhou, D. & Huang, Y. (2010) Oral characteristics of bergenin and the effect of absorption enhancers in situ, in vitro and in vivo. *Arzneimittelforschung.*, 60, 198-204.

Quraishy, M.S., Chescoe, D., Mullervy, J., Coates, M., Hinton, R.H. & Bailey, M.E. (1996) Influence of the gut microflora and of biliary constituents on morphological changes in the small intestine in obstructive jaundice. *HPB Surg*, 10, 11-20.

Rachmilewitz, D., Katakura, K., Karmeli, F., Hayashi, T., Reinus, C., Rudensky, B., Akira, S., Takeda, K., Lee, J., Takabayashi, K. & Raz, E. (2004) Toll-like receptor 9 signaling mediates the anti-inflammatory effects of probiotics in murine experimental colitis. *Gastroenterology*, 126, 520-528.

Rayes, N., Seehofer, D., Theruvath, T., Schiller, R.A., Langrehr, J.M., Jonas, S., Bengmark, S. & Neuhaus, P. (2005) Supply of pre- and probiotics reduces bacterial infection rates after liver transplantation--a randomized, double-blind trial. *Am.J.Transplant.*, 5, 125-130.

Raymond, R.M., Harkema, J.M. & Emerson, T.E. (1980) Direct Effects of Escherichia-Coli Endotoxin in Promoting Skeletal-Muscle Glucose-Uptake in the Dog. *Circulatory Shock*, 7, 218-219.

Raymond, R.M., Harkema, J.M. & Emerson, T.E. (1981) Direct Effects of Gram-Negative Endotoxin on Skeletal-Muscle Glucose-Uptake. *American Journal of Physiology*, 240, H342-H347.

Rebole, A., Ortiz, L.T., Rodriguez, M.L., Alzueta, C., Trevino, J. & Velasco, S. (2010) Effects of inulin and enzyme complex, individually or in combination, on growth performance, intestinal microflora, cecal fermentation characteristics, and jejunal histomorphology in broiler chickens fed a wheat- and barley-based diet. *Poult.Sci.*, 89, 276-286.

Reibel, D.K., Shaffer, J.E., Kocsis, J.J. & Neely, J.R. (1979) Changes in Taurine Content in Heart and Other Organs of Diabetic Rats. *Journal of Molecular and Cellular Cardiology*, 11, 827-830.

Rescigno, M., Urbano, M., Valzasina, B., Francolini, M., Rotta, G., Bonasio, R., Granucci, F., Kraehenbuhl, J.P. & Ricciardi-Castagnoli, P. (2001) Dendritic cells express tight junction proteins and penetrate gut epithelial monolayers to sample bacteria. *Nat.Immunol.*, 2, 361-367.

Respondek, F., Goachet, A.G. & Julliand, V. (2008) Effects of dietary short-chain fructooligosaccharides on the intestinal microflora of horses subjected to a sudden change in diet. *J.Anim Sci.*, 86, 316-323.

Ricci, P., Hofmann, A.F., Hagey, L.R., Jorgensen, R.A., Dickson, E.R. & Lindor, K.D. (1998) Adjuvant cholylsarcosine during ursodeoxycholic acid treatment of primary biliary cirrhosis. *Digestive Diseases and Sciences*, 43, 1292-1295.

Ridlon, J.M., Kang, D.J. & Hylemon, P.B. (2006) Bile salt biotransformations by human intestinal bacteria. 47, 241-259.

Roberts, M.S., Magnusson, B.M., Burczynski, F.J. & Weiss, M. (2002) Enterohepatic circulation: physiological, pharmacokinetic and clinical implications. 41, 751-790.

Rosa, S.C., Rufino, A.T., Judas, F., Tenreiro, C., Lopes, M.C. & Mendes, A.F. (2011) Expression and function of the insulin receptor in normal and osteoarthritic human chondrocytes: modulation of anabolic gene expression, glucose transport and GLUT-1 content by insulin. *Osteoarthritis.Cartilage.*

Rosenbloom, A.L., Joe, J.R., Young, R.S. & Winter, W.E. (1999) Emerging epidemic of type 2 diabetes in youth. *Diabetes Care*, 22, 345-354.

Rozanova, G.N. & Voevodin, D.A. (2008) [A case of an effective application of probiotics in the complex therapy of severe type 1 diabetes mellitus and intestinal disbacteriosis]. *Klin.Med (Mosk)*, 86, 67-68.

Rozanova, G.N., Voevodin, D.A., Stenina, M.A. & Kushnareva, M.V. (2002) Pathogenetic role of dysbacteriosis in the development of complications of type 1 diabetes mellitus in children. 133, 164-166.

Rungby, J. (2010) Zinc, zinc transporters and diabetes. *Diabetologia*, 53, 1549-1551.

Samiy, N., Ng, E.W.M., Ruoff, K., Baker, A.S. & Damico, D.J. (1996) Pneumococcal endophthalmitis in the rat: Clinical and histological characterization. *Investigative Ophthalmology & Visual Science*, 37, 3556.

Sayani, A.P. & Chien, Y.W. (1996) Systemic delivery of peptides and proteins across absorptive mucosae. *Critical Reviews in Therapeutic Drug Carrier Systems*, 13, 85-184.

Shamoon, H., Duffy, H., Fleischer, N., Engel, S., Saenger, P., Strelzyn, M., Litwak, M., Wylierosett, J., Farkash, A., Geiger, D., Engel, H., Fleischman, J., Pompi, D., Ginsberg, N., Glover, M., Brisman, M., Walker, E., Thomashunis, A., Gonzalez, J., Genuth, S., Brown, E., Dahms, W., Pugsley, P., Mayer, L., Kerr, D., Landau, B., Singerman, L., Rice, T., Novak, M., Smithbrewer, S., Mcconnell, J., Drotar, D., Woods, D., Katirgi, B., Litvene, M., Brown, C., Lusk, M., Campbell, R., Lackaye, M., Richardson, M., Levy, B., Chang, S., Heinheinemann, M., Barron, S., Astor, L., Lebeck, D., Brillon, D., Diamond, B., Vasilasdwoskin, A., Laurenzi, B., Foldi, N., Rubin, M., Flynn, T., Reppucci, V., Heise, C., Sanchez, A., Whitehouse, F., Kruger, D., Kahkonen, D., Fachnie, J., Fisk, J., Carey, J., Cox, M., Ahmad, B., Angus, E., Campbell, H., Fields, D., Croswell, M., Basha, K., Chung, P., Schoenherr, A., Mobley, M., Marchiori, K., Francis, J., Kelly, J., Etzwiler, D., Callahan, P., Hollander, P., Castle, G., Bergenstal, R., Spencer, M., Nelson, J., Bezecny, L., Roethke, C., Orban, M., Ulrich, C., Gill, L., Morgan, K., Laechelt, J., Taylor, F., Freking, D., Towey, A., Lieppman, M., Rakes, S., Mangum, J., Cooper, N., Upham, P., Jacobson, A., Crowell, S., Wolfsdorf, J., Beaser, R., Ganda, O., Rosenzweig, J., Stewart, C., Halford, B., Friedlander, E., Tarsy, D., Arrigg, P., Sharuk, G., Shah, S., Wu, G., Cavallerano, J., Poole, R., Silver, P., Cavicchi, R., Fleming, D., Marcus, J., Griffiths, C., Cappella, N., Nathan, D., Larkin, M., Godine, J., Lynch, J., Norman, D., Mckitrick, C., Haggen, C., Delahanty, L., Anderson, E., Lou, P., Taylor, C., Cros, D., Folino, K., Brink, S., Abbott, K., Sicotte, K., Service, F.J., Schmidt, A., Rizza, R., Zimmerman, B., Schwenk, W., Mortenson, J., Ziegler, G., Lucas, A., Hanson, N., Sellnow, S., Pach, J., Stein, D., Eickhoff, B., Woodwick, R., Tackmann, R., Trautmann, J., Rostvold, J., Link, T., Dyck, P., Daube, J., Colligan, R., Windebank, A., King, J., Colwell, J., Wood, D., Mayfield, R., Picket, J., Chitwood, M., Billings, D., Dabney, Y., Buse, J., King, L., Vale, S., Thompson, T., Bohm, B., Lyons, T., Hermayer, K., Rice, A., Molitch, M., Schaefer, B., Johnson, C., Lyons, J., Metzger, B., Cohen, B., Nishida, T., Parque, K., Yusim, V., Moore, M., Jampol, L., Dineen, K.,

Stahl, J., Richine, L., Weinberg, D., Loose, I., Kushner, M., Morrison, A., Jalbert, A., Tildesley, H., Leung, S., Begg, I., Johnson, D., Lalani, S., Kennedy, T., Meadows, G., Kolterman, O., Lorenzi, G., Jones, K., Goldbaum, M., Swenson, M., Lyon, R., Giotta, M., Kadlec, K., Reed, R., Kirsch, L., Goodman, J., Cahill, S., Clark, T., Abram, R., Sayner, L., Ochabski, R., Gloria, R., Birchler, G., Grant, J., Grasse, B., Christle, L., Abreu, B., Grant, I., Heaton, R., Zeitler, R., Sivitz, W., Bayless, M., Schrott, H., Olson, N., Tindal, B., Snetselaar, L., Mueller, D., Dudler, A., Swartzendruber, J., Hoffman, R., Macindoe, J., Kramer, J., Weingeist, T., Kimura, A., Stone, E., Grout, T., Fountain, C., Karakas, S., Vogel, C., Montague, P., Keyser, D., Mennen, S., Doggett, C., Rose, G., Devet, K., Muhle, P., Kowarski, A., Ostrowski, D., Levin, P., Chalew, S. & Hylton, J. (1993) The Effect of Intensive Treatment of Diabetes on the Development and Progression of Long-Term Complications in Insulin-Dependent Diabetes-Mellitus. *New England Journal of Medicine*, 329, 977-986.

Shao, Z., Krishnamoorthy, R. & Mitra, A.K. (1992a) Cyclodextrins As Nasal Absorption Promoters of Insulin - Mechanistic Evaluations. *Pharmaceutical Research*, 9, 1157-1163.

Shao, Z., Krishnamoorthy, R. & Mitra, A.K. (1992b) Cyclodextrins As Nasal Absorption Promoters of Insulin - Mechanistic Evaluations. *Pharmaceutical Research*, 9, 1157-1163.

Sherman, P.M., Cabana, M., Gibson, G.R., Koletzko, B.V., Neu, J., Veereman-Wauters, G., Ziegler, E.E. & Walker, W.A. (2009) Potential roles and clinical utility of prebiotics in newborns, infants, and children: proceedings from a global prebiotic summit meeting, New York City, June 27-28, 2008. *J.Pediatr.*, 155, S61-S70.

Shi, H.N. & Walker, A. (2004) Bacterial colonization and the development of intestinal defences. *Can.J.Gastroenterol.*, 18, 493-500.

Siow, Y., Schurr, A. & Vitale, G.C. (1991) Diabetes-induced bile acid composition changes in rat bile determined by high performance liquid chromatography. *Life Sci.*, 49, 1301-1308.

Slivka, O.I., Zelinskii, B.A. & Zelinskii, S.T. (1979a) [Bile acids in the bile in diabetes mellitus]. *Probl.Endokrinol.(Mosk)*, 25, 16-19.

Slivka, O.I., Zelinskii, B.A. & Zelinskii, S.T. (1979b) [Bile acids in the bile in diabetes mellitus]. 25, 16-19.

Snydman, D.R. (2008) The safety of probiotics. *Clin.Infect.Dis.*, 46 Suppl 2, S104-S111.

Souri, E.N. & Green, W.R. (1974) Intravitreal Amphotericin-B Toxicity. *American Journal of Ophthalmology*, 78, 77-81.

Srinivasan, K. & Ramarao, P. (2007) Animal models in type 2 diabetes research: an overview. 125, 451-472.

St-Pierre, M.V., Kullak-Ublick, G.A., Hagenbuch, B. & Meier, P.J. (2001) Transport of bile acids in hepatic and non-hepatic tissues. 204, 1673-1686.

St-Pierre, M.V., Serrano, M.A., Macias, R.I., Dubs, U., Hoechli, M., Lauper, U., Meier, P.J. & Marin, J.J. (2000) Expression of members of the multidrug resistance protein family in human term placenta. 279, R1495-R1503.

Steed, D.L., Donohoe, D., Webster, M.W. & Lindsley, L. (1996) Effect of extensive debridement and treatment on the healing of diabetic foot ulcers. Diabetic Ulcer Study Group. *J.Am.Coll.Surg.*, 183, 61-64.

Stephani, J., Radulovic, K. & Niess, J.H. (2011) Gut microbiota, probiotics and inflammatory bowel disease. *Arch.Immunol.Ther.Exp (Warsz.)*, 59, 161-177.

Stuart, C.A., Howell, M.E., Zhang, Y. & Yin, D. (2009) Insulin-stimulated translocation of glucose transporter (GLUT) 12 parallels that of GLUT4 in normal muscle. *J.Clin.Endocrinol Metab*, 94, 3535-3542.

Succi, M., Tremonte, P., Reale, A., Sorrentino, E., Grazia, L., Pacifico, S. & Coppola, R. (2005) Bile salt and acid tolerance of Lactobacillus rhamnosus strains isolated from Parmigiano Reggiano cheese. 244, 129-137.

Thomson, A.B. (1983) Uptake of bile acids into rat intestine. Effect of diabetes mellitus. *Diabetes*, 32, 900-907.

Tlaskalova-Hogenova, H., Stepankova, R., Kozakova, H., Hudcovic, T., Vannucci, L., Tuckova, L., Rossmann, P., Hrncir, T., Kverka, M., Zakostelska, Z., Klimesova, K., Pribylova, J., Bartova, J., Sanchez, D., Fundova, P., Borovska, D., Srutkova, D., Zidek, Z., Schwarzer, M., Drastich, P. & Funda, D.P. (2011) The role of gut microbiota (commensal bacteria) and the mucosal barrier in the pathogenesis of inflammatory and autoimmune diseases and cancer: contribution of germ-free and gnotobiotic animal models of human diseases. *Cell Mol.Immunol.*, 8, 110-120.

Trachtman, H. & Sturman, J.A. (1996) Taurine: A therapeutic agent in experimental kidney disease. *Amino Acids*, 11, 1-13.

Tramonti, G., Xie, P., Wallner, E.I., Danesh, F.R. & Kanwar, Y.S. (2006) Expression and functional characteristics of tubular transporters: P-glycoprotein, PEPT1, and PEPT2 in renal mass reduction and diabetes. *Am.J.Physiol Renal Physiol*, 291, F972-F980.

Trauner, M., Claudel, T., Fickert, P., Moustafa, T. & Wagner, M. (2010) Bile Acids as Regulators of Hepatic Lipid and Glucose Metabolism. *Digestive Diseases*, 28, 220-224.

Uchida, K., Makino, S. & Akiyoshi, T. (1985) Altered bile acid metabolism in nonobese, spontaneously diabetic (NOD) mice. 34, 79-83.

Uchida, K., Takase, H., Kadowaki, M., Nomura, Y., Matsubara, T. & Takeuchi, N. (1979) Altered bile acid metabolism in alloxan diabetic rats. 29, 553-562.

Vaarala, O. (2006) Is it dietary insulin? 1079, 350-359.

van Waarde, W.M., Verkade, H.J., Wolters, H., Havinga, R., Baller, J., Bloks, V., Muller, M., Sauer, P.J. & Kuipers, F. (2002) Differential effects of streptozotocin-induced diabetes on expression of hepatic ABC-transporters in rats. *Gastroenterology*, 122, 1842-1852.

Vidotti, D.B., Arnoni, C.P., Maquigussa, E. & Boim, M.A. (2008) Effect of long-term type 1 diabetes on renal sodium and water transporters in rats. *Am.J.Nephrol.*, 28, 107-114.

Vilchis, C. & Salceda, R. (1996) Effect of diabetes on levels and uptake of putative amino acid neurotransmitters in rat retina and retinal pigment epithelium. *Neurochemical Research*, 21, 1167-1171.

von, H.M. & Nepom, G.T. (2009a) Animal models of human type 1 diabetes. *Nat.Immunol.*, 10, 129-132.

von, H.M. & Nepom, G.T. (2009b) Animal models of human type 1 diabetes. *Nat.Immunol.*, 10, 129-132.

Walker, W.A. (2008a) Mechanisms of action of probiotics. *Clinical Infectious Diseases*, 46, S87-S91.

Walker, W.A. (2008b) Mechanisms of action of probiotics. *Clinical Infectious Diseases*, 46, S87-S91.

Weiss, R. & Caprio, S. (2006) Development of type 2 diabetes in children and adolescents. 97, 263-269.

Yamamoto, A., Luo, A.M., Doddakashi, S. & Lee, V.H.L. (1989) The Ocular Route for Systemic Insulin Delivery in the Albino Rabbit. *Journal of Pharmacology and Experimental Therapeutics*, 249, 249-255.

Yen, C.H., Tseng, Y.H., Kuo, Y.W., Lee, M.C. & Chen, H.L. (2011) Long-term supplementation of isomalto-oligosaccharides improved colonic microflora profile, bowel function, and blood cholesterol levels in constipated elderly people--a placebo-controlled, diet-controlled trial. *Nutrition*, 27, 445-450.

Zanchi, A., Stergiopulos, N., Brunner, H.R. & Hayoz, D. (1998) Differences in the mechanical properties of the rat carotid artery in vivo, in situ, and in vitro. *Hypertension*, 32, 180-185.

Zaneveld, J., Turnbaugh, P.J., Lozupone, C., Ley, R.E., Hamady, M., Gordon, J.I. & Knight, R. (2008) Host-bacterial coevolution and the search for new drug targets. *Curr Opin Chem Biol*, 12, 109-114.

Zelcer, N., Reid, G., Wielinga, P., Kuil, A., van der Heijden, I., Schuetz, J.D. & Borst, P. (2003a) Steroid and bile acid conjugates are substrates of human multidrug-resistance protein (MRP) 4 (ATP-binding cassette C4). 371, 361-367.

Zelcer, N., Saeki, T., Bot, I., Kuil, A. & Borst, P. (2003b) Transport of bile acids in multidrug-resistance-protein 3-overexpressing cells co-transfected with the ileal Na+-dependent bile-acid transporter. 369, 23-30.

Ziegler, A.G., Schmid, S., Huber, D., Hummel, M. & Bonifacio, E. (2003) Early infant feeding and risk of developing type 1 diabetes-associated autoantibodies. 290, 1721-1728.

Zisser, H.C., Bevier, W.C. & Jovanovic, L. (2007) Restoring euglycemia in the basal state using continuous glucose monitoring in subjects with type 1 diabetes mellitus. *Diabetes Technol.Ther.*, 9, 509-515.

Zollner, G., Fickert, P., Fuchsbichler, A., Silbert, D., Wagner, M., Arbeiter, S., Gonzalez, F.J., Marschall, H.U., Zatloukal, K., Denk, H. & Trauner, M. (2003) Role of nuclear bile acid receptor, FXR, in adaptive ABC transporter regulation by cholic and ursodeoxycholic acid in mouse liver, kidney and intestine. 39, 480-488.

8

Role of Vitamin D in the Pathogenesis and Therapy of Type 1 Diabetes Mellitus

Agustin Busta, Bianca Alfonso and Leonid Poretsky
Albert Einstein College of Medicine, Beth Israel
Medical Center New York
U.S.A.

1. Introduction

This chapter will review the role of vitamin D in the pathogenesis and treatment of type 1 diabetes mellitus.
We will discuss the mechanisms through which vitamin D might affect pancreatic function. We will summarize the results of in-vitro and animal studies and will conclude with a review of the relevant clinical trials.

2. Definition

Type 1 diabetes mellitus is an autoimmune disease in which the pancreas is unable to respond to secretagogue stimulation with appropriate insulin secretion. Hyperglycemia develops when more than 70-90% of the insulin-producing beta cells are destroyed. An autoimmune destructive process, which plays a central role in the development of type 1 diabetes mellitus, is facilitated by the subject's own genetic susceptibility and by non-genetic factors. Non-genetic factors include viral infections, toxic chemicals, and others. Vitamin D deficiency is a non-genetic factor that appears to be associated with an increased risk of developing type 1 diabetes mellitus.
Type 1 diabetes mellitus complications are classified into acute and chronic. The acute complications include life-threatening conditions like severe hypoglycemia or diabetic ketoacidosis (DKA). Chronic diabetic complications can be divided into microvascular complications (retinopathy, neuropathy and nephropathy) and macrovascular complications (cardiovascular, cerebrovascular and peripheral vascular disease). Severe microvascular and macrovascular complications can lead to renal failure (the most common cause of hemodialysis in the US), blindness or lower extremity amputations.
Overall, uncontrolled diabetes mellitus in patients over 50 years of age reduces life expectancy in males and females by 7.5 and 8.2 years respectively (Franco et al.,2007).

3. Epidemiology

In 2010, about 215,000 people younger than 20 years of age had diabetes (type 1 or type 2) in the United States._ A 2011 Centers for Disease Control and Prevention (CDC) report estimates that nearly 26 million Americans have diabetes._ Diabetes affects 8.3% of

Americans of all ages and 11.3% of adults aged 20 years and older, according to the National Diabetes Fact Sheet for 2011. About 27% of those with diabetes (approximately 7 million Americans) do not know they have the disease. 1 in every 400 children and adolescents has type 1 diabetes.

Type 1 diabetes mellitus continues to be highly prevalent in many countries, with an overall annual increase estimated at 3% (International Diabetes Federation [IDF] 2010). Worldwide, it is more common in males than in females, with a ratio of 1.5.

The 4th edition of the IDF Diabetes Atlas, released in 2009 at the 20th World Diabetes Congress, estimated that in 2010, 285 million people would have diabetes (6.4% of world's adult population). The same forum predicts that by 2030, 438 million people will have diabetes world-wide. Type 1 diabetes in children is estimated at 480,000 patients worldwide in 2010, and the number of newly diagnosed cases per year is 75,800 (IDF 2010).

3.1 Natural history

The natural history of type 1 diabetes is characterized by an autoimmune destruction of the beta cells in the islands of Langerhans in the pancreas. The autoimmune process has cellular and humoral components, leading to the destruction of the beta cells and a decreased insulin secretion. As beta-cell mass declines, insulin secretion decreases until the available insulin no longer is adequate to maintain normal blood glucose levels. After 70-90% of the beta cells are destroyed, hyperglycemia develops and diabetes may be diagnosed.

The natural history of type 1 diabetes has 4 stages: genetic susceptibility, autoimmune process, pre-diabetes and diabetes.

The rate of beta cell destruction is variable. In some patients years will go by before the onset of diabetes, while other patients may never develop beta cell insufficiency, perhaps due to the regaining of tolerance. Most patients with type 1 diabetes mellitus have one or more susceptible human leukocyte antigen (HLA) class II, and over 90% have beta cell autoantibodies present. The appearance of circulating islet cell autoantibodies is the first detectable sign of this immune process.

4. Pathogenesis of type 1 diabetes mellitus

4.1 Genetic component

Genetics has an important role in the etiology of type 1 diabetes. However, extra-genetic components influence the penetrance of diabetes susceptibility genes. If data are obtained at a single point in time, the risk of type 1 diabetes mellitus between monozygotic twins can be as low as 30%, but if the monozygotic twins are followed long-term, the cumulative incidence of diabetes reaches 65% (Redondo et al., 2008). In the same cohort of monozygotic twins, the rate of persistent autoantibody positivity, type 1 diabetes mellitus, or both, reached 78% (Redondo et al., 2008).

To better understand the genetic susceptibility to diabetes, candidate gene studies were conducted in order to identify genes that are associated with autoimmune type 1 diabetes.

Human leukocyte antigen (HLA) associations have been long recognized in many autoimmune diseases. In type 1 diabetes mellitus, the HLA on chromosome 6p21 is well described and is considered to play an important role in more than 50% of the familial cases in Caucasians (Noble et al., 1996). HLA DR4-DQ8 or DR3-DQ2 haplotypes are detected in up to 90% of patients with type 1 diabetes mellitus (Devendra & Eisenbarth, 2003). The combination of these 2 types, DR4-DQ8/DR3-DQ2, carries the highest risk and type 1 diabetes mellitus occurs at a very early age in this population. First-degree relatives of the patients who carry the highest risk haplotype combination also have a higher risk of developing diabetes mellitus as compared to the relatives of diabetes patients who do not have this haplotype and who develop type 1 diabetes mellitus later in life (Gillespie et al., 2002).

Another HLA haplotype (DR15-DQ6) might have protective properties, and is found in a much larger percentage in the general population (20%) as compared to less than 1% in patients with type 1 diabetes mellitus (Eisenbarth & Gottlieb, 2004).

HLA haplotypes appear to have an association with islet autoantibodies. Glutamic acid decarboxylase (GAD) antibodies are more frequent in patients with HLA DR3-DQ2, whereas insulin auto-antibodies (IAA) and protein tyrosine phosphatase-like protein antibodies (IA-2 antibodies) are more frequent in patients with HLA DR4-DQ8. Patients that do not have these haplotypes are less likely to develop islet autoantibodies (Achenbach et al., 2005).

Another key genetic factor is the insulin gene (INS), with different forms of the promoter region conferring either protection or increased susceptibility to autoimmune diabetes mellitus (Bennett et al., 1995). The insulin gene contributes 10% to the genetic susceptibility in developing autoimmune diabetes (Bell et al., 1984). The risk of developing diabetes depends on the expression of the insulin protein in the thymus which can cause a defective central tolerance to the insulin molecule. The degree of immune tolerance may be reflected by the less common presence of insulin autoantibodies (IAA) in patients or relatives who have the protective INS class I/III or III/III genotypes (Vafiadis et al., 1997).

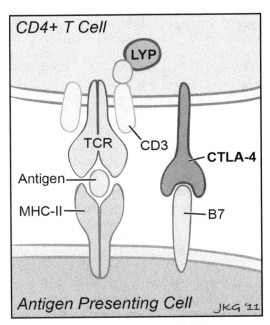

Fig. 1. Antigen Presenting Cell. The activation of the T-cell by various stimuli (antigens), is brought by major histocompatibility complex (MHC-HLA II). This figure shows also, inhibitors of T-cell activation: cytotoxic T lymphocyte antigen 4 (CTLA-4) and lymphoid tyrosine phosphatase (LYP).

T cells are recognized to be a major part of the immune process in diabetes mellitus, and several genes involved in T cell regulation are associated with type 1 diabetes mellitus. Two genes encoding factors that are suppressive to the T cell activation appear to have a close association with autoimmune diabetes: lymphoid tyrosine phosphatase locus (LYP/PTPN22) (Smyth et al., 2004), and cytotoxic T lymphocyte antigen 4 (CTLA-4) (Ueda et al., 2003) (Figure 1), located on chromosome 2q33.

The CTLA-4, which is a T-Lymphocyte receptor, is expressed after T-cell activation (Greenwald et al., 2005). It turns off T-cell responses by inhibiting the production of interleukine-2. CTLA-4 polymorphism in humans has been associated with an increased risk of autoimmune disease, including type 1 diabetes mellitus (Gough et al., 2005).

Another gene linked to an increased risk for type 1 diabetes is the gene for the intercellular adhesion molecule (ICAM-1) (Nejentsev et al., 2003). A recent genome-wide association study described over 40 loci associated with an increased risk for type 1 diabetes (Barrett et al., 2009).

4.2 Autoimmune process

One of the best animal models for type 1 diabetes mellitus is the nonobese diabetic mouse (NOD). NOD mouse develops type 1 diabetes mellitus spontaneously, over the course of a few months, allowing the investigators to study this process stage by stage. Many reports describe in detail the genetics, the immune process, the influence of the environment and most importantly, the potential therapies to prevent, delay or reverse the destructive process that leads to type 1 diabetes mellitus in this model. Delovitch and Singh (Delovitch & Singh, 1997) reviewed the use of NOD mouse in the studies of type 1 diabetes mellitus. In NOD mice, the first step is the infiltration of the peri-islet regions of the pancreatic islets by dendritic cells (DC) and macrophages, followed by T cells (CD4+ and CD8+). This stage is known as peri-insulitis, occurring around 3-4 weeks of age. It is followed by a slower, progressive T cell destruction of the beta cells (insulitis), by 4-6 months of age (Delovitch & Singh, 1997). Thus, the T cells and the dendritic cells are key players in the immune process leading to type 1 diabetes mellitus.

The dendritic cells (DC) are antigen-presenting cells which originate from the bone marrow. They become active once they capture and process the antigens. After infiltrating the pancreas and undergoing antigenic maturation, DC secrete IL-12 and present the processed antigen (on their surface and in association with the major histocompatibility complex [MHC] class II) to other cells of the immune system (i.e. T cells) (see Fig 1).

T cells are categorized mainly based on their immune actions, achieved via the different cytokines they secrete. Cytokines are classified into two types: type 1 cytokines, which activate the cellular immunity and suppress the humoral immune response, and type 2 cytokines, which activate the humoral immunity and inhibit the cellular immune process (Rabinovitch, 1998).

Th1 cells are preferentially formed from their T cell precursors (T helper 0) under the direct influence of mature DC and IL-12 (Banchereau & Steinman, 1998).

T helper 1 cells (Th1) are involved in cell-mediated immune responses (inflammation, cytotoxicity, delayed hypersensitivity) and produce type 1 cytokines: tumor necrosis factor β (TNFβ), interferon γ (IFNγ), and interleukin 2 (IL-2). T helper 2 cells (Th2) are important in humoral immunity (activate B cells and antibody production, down regulating Th 1 cells) and secrete type 2 cytokines: interleukins 4, 5, 6, 9 and 10 (Rabinovitch, 1998) (Fig. 2).

The Th2 cells are protective for the beta cells. They have an inhibitory effect on the Th1 cells, which are destructive to the pancreatic beta cells. In the NOD mouse, it appears that the immunologic self-tolerance to pancreatic beta cells is lost. The disruption of the equilibrium between Th1 and Th2 cells in the thymus and in the periphery is believed to play a crucial role in the pathogenesis of autoimmune diabetes mellitus (Delovitch & Singh, 1997). Once Th1 cells are produced they will secrete interferon γ (IFN γ) and IL-2, leading to the activation of macrophages and cytotoxic T cells, which are destructive to the pancreatic beta cells (Adorini, 2001). The same Th1 cells will stimulate the IgG2a autoantibodies against the islet beta cells autoantigens (Delovitch & Singh, 1997). Autoimmune diabetes can be transferred from a diabetic NOD mouse to an unaffected mouse via T cells (Bendelac et al., 1987). NOD mice develop a spontaneous loss of T-cell tolerance to glutamic acid decarboxylase antibodies (GAD), leading to autoimmune diabetes (Kaufman et al., 1993). In NOD mice, there is an increased resistance to apoptosis in immunocytes (Leijon et al., 1995, Penha-Goncalves et al., 1995).

Immune responses to several beta-cell proteins have been described (auto-antigens). Exposure to glutamic acid decarboxylase (GAD65 and GAD67) led to an increased T cell proliferation as early as 4 weeks of life in NOD mice, coinciding with the onset of insulitis (Tisch 1993). Some of the other beta-cell antigens elicited an increased immune response after a few more weeks, but there were other beta-cell antigens that did not trigger an immune reaction (for example, amylin) (Tisch 1993). The same study showed that intrathymic injections of GAD65 had a protective effect from autoimmune diabetes in NOD mice (delaying the onset of disease and decreasing the frequency) (Tisch etal., 1993)

GAD65- reactive T cells were proven to have the ability to transfer diabetes to NOD/SCID (severe combined immunodeficiency) mice (Zekzer et al., 1998). To further support the central role of GAD antigen in autoimmune diabetes, the beta-cell-specific suppression of GAD expression in antisense GAD transgenic NOD mice was demonstrated to prevent the production of diabetogenic T cells and the onset of diabetes (Yoon et al., 1999)

In humans, the pancreas becomes infiltrated with mononuclear cells. Autoantibodies to insulin (IAA), glutamic acid decarboxylase (GAD) and insulinoma associated-2 antibody (IA-2) are demonstrated years before the clinical symptoms of diabetes. (Kulmala et al., 1998) T cell responses to several islet cells antigens (insulin, GAD, IA-2) have been reported in IDDM (MacCuish et al., 1975). The presence of autoantibodies alone does not explain the development of diabetes, since it is recognized now that children born to type 1 diabetic mother with high antibody titers transferred through the umbilical cord do not develop diabetes more often than expected. An interesting case was published by Martin et al in 2001, describing a case of type 1 diabetes mellitus occurring in a patient that had a hereditary B-cell defect (Martin et al., 2001).

4.3 Environmental component
The environment is implicated in the pathogenesis of type 1 diabetes mellitus by many studies.

Environmental factors have an important role in initiating an immune process that ultimately leads to pancreatic beta cell destruction and clinically apparent diabetes mellitus. Many environmental factors have been proposed, including viruses (rubella, mumps or coxsackievirus B4), toxic substances and cytotoxins. Nutritional status and diet have also been implicated as potential players in type 1 diabetes pathogenesis: vitamin D deficiency, early protein diet exposure or exposure to cow's milk in infancy.

Viruses are among the main culprits studied. Before the eradication of rubella in most countries, congenital rubella was strongly associated with the development of type 1 diabetes mellitus (Menser et al., 1978). A recent meta analysis of observational studies has shown an association between type 1 diabetes and enterovirus infection (Yeung 2011).

While some theories implicate viral infections in the pathogenesis of type 1 diabetes, a recent hypothesis argues that a decreased exposure to microbes may contribute to the current increase in autoimmune disease. This theory is known as "the hygiene hypothesis" (Gale, 2002).

It is a known fact that the incidence of autoimmune diabetes follows a geographical pattern, with many studies reporting an association between type 1 diabetes and vitamin D status. A few large ecological studies describe a pattern of geographical variation, with an increased incidence of type 1 diabetes in the areas located north of the equator. Furthermore, seasons appear to also influence the incidence of type 1 diabetes, with the highest incidence during winter and the lowest during summer. The month of birth during springtime is associated with a higher risk of type 1 diabetes (Kahn et al., 2009), a finding that could be explained by possible low circulating vitamin D levels in both mother and fetus through the winter months of the pregnancy.

In order to develop more information about environmental factors that play a role in the pathogenesis of diabetes, an international initiative (the Environmental Determinants of Diabetes in the Young) will be following thousands of infants with an increased genetic risk from birth until adolescence and will gather data about infectious agents, dietary or other environmental factors.

Typically, the treatment for type 1 diabetes mellitus involves insulin therapy, but in the last few years new therapies have been approved as well (for example, Symlin). For newly diagnosed patients with autoimmune diabetes, combination therapy has been suggested in an attempt to minimize beta cell destruction and prolong pancreatic function. The new therapeutic options include: immunotherapy, vaccines, drugs that influence T cell action, anti-inflammatory drugs (for example, one time use of anti-IL-1R drug), or long-term treatment with B cell components to induce regulatory T cells (oral or nasal insulin, insulin peptide therapy, GAD-Alum or the proinsulin DNA vaccines). Glucagon-like peptide 1-related drugs (GLP-1) could be also considered as a therapeutic option because they promote peritubular pancreatic cell growth (Von Herrath, 2010).

5. Vitamin D

Although initially described as a "vitamin", vitamin D is now recognized to be a hormone, synthesized in the human body and exerting its action on other organs via a nuclear receptor (vitamin D receptor, VDR).

Even though vitamin D can be obtained from the diet in small quantities, the main source of vitamin D is the skin. Under the direct influence of ultra violet B light (UVB light), 7-dehydrocholesterol (DHC) (provitamin D3) is converted into pre-vitamin D3, which is then further converted into cholecalciferol (vitamin D3) via thermal isomerization. Interestingly, if pre-vitamin D3 continues to be exposed to UVB, it will be converted into biologically inactive metabolites (tachysterol and lumisterol), preventing a potential UVB- induced vitamin D intoxication (Holick, 1999) The other source of vitamin D is the diet, which contains cholecalciferol (vitamin D3), originating from animal sources, and ergocalciferol (vitamin D2), deriving from plants (Holick, 1999).

Regardless of their source, once they enter into the circulation, forms of inactive vitamin D3 or D2 bind to the vitamin D-binding protein (DBP) and are transported to the liver. The inactive vitamin D is activated through a 2-step hydroxylation process via two hydroxylases that belong to the cytochrome P450- dependent steroid hydroxylases (CYP450). In the liver, vitamin D undergoes the first hydroxylation at C-25 via some of the CYP 450 vitamin D 25-hydroxylases, forming calcidiol (25-hydroxyvitamin D) (Prosser & Jones, 2004). This is the major circulating form of vitamin D. At the level of the proximal renal tubule, 25-OH vitamin D is further hydroxylated to calcitriol (1,25 dihydroxyvitamin D, the active form of vitamin D) by the 1α-hydroxylase (1α(OH)ase, CYP27B1) (Prosser & Jones, 2004). Both calcidiol and calcitriol are inactivated via the 25-hydroxyvitamin D3-24-hydroxylase (CYP24), forming the inactive metabolite 24,25- dihydroxyvitamin D (Holick, 1999).

1α-hydroxylase has been described in many extrarenal tissues: macrophages, monocytes, and placenta, rendering these cells capable of synthesizing 1α-,25(OH)$_2$D$_3$from 25(OH)vitamin D (Weisman et al., 1979, Bhalla et al., 1983, Stoffels et al., 2007, Adams et al., 1983). The activity of 1α-hydroxylase in the immune cells is not under the regulation of parathyroid hormone and 1α-,25(OH)$_2$D$_3$, but rather under immune cytokine regulation. A defect in the up-regulation of 1α-hydroxylase after immune stimulation is described in NOD mouse (Overbergh et al., 2000). Extrarenal distribution of 1α-hydroxylase becomes important in understanding the extra-skeletal effects of vitamin D.

VDR is part of the nuclear receptor super family of ligand-activated transcription factors, which also includes glucocorticoid, thyroid hormone and estrogen receptors. The gene for VDR is located on chromosome 12q12-14, and shows great polymorphism (Haussler et al., 1998). After 1,25 (OH)$_2$D$_3$ binds to VDR, it induces conformational changes that facilitate heterodimerization with the retinoid X receptor and the recruitment of nuclear receptor coactivator proteins, which then act on the chromatin. The specific DNA sequence that is ultimately affected by the vitamin D is known as the vitamin D responsive element (VDRE) (Carlberg & Polly, 1998).

The discovery of the vitamin D receptor (VDR) on the immune cells (Strugnell & DeLuca, 1997), led to the hypothesis that vitamin D could affect the autoimmune processes. However, in VDR deficient mice models, there is no increase in autoimmune diseases (Mathieu et al., 2001)

The protective effects of vitamin D in several autoimmune diseases have been described in animal models (experimental autoimmune encephalomyelitis (Lemire, 1995), murine models of human multiple sclerosis and murine models of rheumatoid arthritis (Cantorna et al., 1996). In other autoimmune diseases, like psoriasis, vitamin D analogues are the mainstay of treatment today.

The extraskeletal effects of 1α-,25(OH)$_2$D$_3$ can usually be observed only at very high concentrations (10^{-10}mol/l), higher than physiological levels needed for calcium balance (concentrations that could probably be achieved in specific target tissues via the macrophages' 1α-hydroxylase) (Mathieu et al., 2005). Thus a risk of hypercalcemia and other side effects of 1α-25(OH)$_2$D$_3$ could occur if it were used for its anti-autoimmune properties. Numerous vitamin D analogs have been developed to exert extraskeletal effects, with less pronounced action on the calcium metabolism. Most of these analogs are used for laboratory research purposes, but some are part of standard treatment for certain autoimmune diseases (for example, calcipotriol for psoriasis).

There are several theories that attempt to explain the link between Vitamin D and autoimmune diabetes. This relationship appears to be complex, with actions at multiples levels: genetic, autoimmune and also direct action on the pancreatic beta cells.

6. Vitamin D and type 1 diabetes

Animal studies and clinical trials in patients with new onset of type 1 diabetes show that the replacement of vitamin D may arrest the deterioration of pancreatic function and improve C-peptide levels.

There is strong epidemiologic data showing that the population in countries with a high prevalence of type 1 diabetes mellitus is commonly vitamin D deficient. Vitamin D supplementation during pregnancy decreased the risk of the development of type 1 diabetes mellitus for offspring (Fronczak et al., 2003). Supplementation of vitamin D at an early age also decreases the risk for developing type 1 diabetes (Hypponen et al., 2001)

The vitamin D receptor (VDR) has been described on almost every tissue in the human body, including the cells of the immune system, as discussed earlier.

The VDR gene is located on chromosome 12, and has a few allelic variants. It has been reported that some of these allelic variations of the VDR gene are linked to an increased risk of type 1 diabetes mellitus in the German and the Indian Asian population (Pani et al., 2000, Chang et al., 2000). On the other hand, the same association was not found in another population sample (British, Portuguese and Finnish origin) (Guo et al., 2006, Lemos, 2008, Turpeinen, 2002).

An interaction between specific VDR polymorphisms and predisposing HLA DRB1 0301 allele was described in North Indian patients (Israni et al., 2009) and is associated with an increased risk of developing type 1 diabetes mellitus.

As discussed earlier, the last step in the activation of vitamin D is facilitated by the key enzyme 1α-hydroxylase, encoded by the CYP27B1 gene on the chromosome 12q13.1-q13.3. Polymorphism in this gene is described as being associated with an increased risk of type 1 diabetes mellitus (Lopez et al., 2004, Bailey et al., 2007). The polymorphism in the CYP27B1 gene could potentially lead to the reduced expression of 1α-hydroxylase, less production of the active 1α,25 (OH) $_2$ D$_3$, and ultimately, to the increased risk of type 1 diabetes.

6.1 Vitamin D and type 1 diabetes: The effects on the immune processes

Vitamin D interacts with most immune cells and affects their cytokine production. Overall, vitamin D has a protective effect on the pancreatic beta cells (Figure 2).

DCs are affected by 1α,25 (OH)$_2$D$_3$ in many ways. DCs mature after they engulf the antigen, increasing the expression of MHC-II molecules on their surface and secreting IL-12. Studies show that vitamin D analogs suppress the expression of MHC-II molecules (Griffin 2000) The cytokine secretion by DC is affected as well: the IL-12 is inhibited (D'Ambrosio 1998), while IL-10 production is increased (Penna 2000). Furthermore, DC apoptosis is promoted by exposure to vitamin D (Penna 2000).

If DC are exposed to 1α,25 (OH)$_2$ D$_3$, they do not mature at a subsequent exposure to an antigen, becoming tolerogenic (Griffin et al., 2001). After being treated with a vitamin D analog, the DC do not simply remain immature, but instead are transformed into tolerogenic DC with special endocytic properties (Ferreira et al., 2009). Adorini et al published a paper describing how 1α,25(OH)₂ D₃ can change the dendritic cells into a tolerogenic phenotype which is thought to induce T regulatory cells and inhibit autoimmune diseases, like type 1 diabetes (Adorini, 2003) (Fig 2).

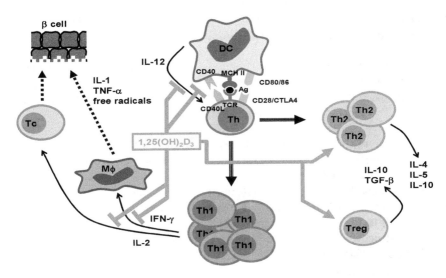

Fig. 2. The immunomodulatory effects of 1α,25(OH)2D3. At the level of the antigen-presenting cell (such as dendritic cells; DCs), 1α,25(OH)2D3 inhibits the surface expression of MHC class II-complexed antigen and of co-stimulatory molecules, in addition to production of the cytokine IL-12, thereby indirectly shifting the polarization of T cells from a Th1 towards a Th2 phenotype. In addition, 1α,25(OH)2D3 has immunomodulatory effects directly at the level of the T cell, by inhibiting the production of the Th1 cytokines IL-2 and IFN-γ and stimulating the production of Th2 cytokines. Moreover, 1α,25(OH)2D3 favors the induction of regulatory T cells. Both Th2 and Tregs can inhibit Th1 cells through the production of counteracting or inhibitory cytokines. Together, these immunomodulatory effects of 1α,25(OH)2D3 can lead to the protection of target tissues, such as β cells, in autoimmune diseases and transplantation. CD40L, CD40 ligand; Mf, macrophage; Tc, cytotoxic T cell; TGF- β, transforming growth factor β; Th1,T helper type 1; TNF-α, tumor necrosis factor α; Treg, regulatory T cell. This figure was published in Trends in Endocrinology and Metabolism Vol.16 No.6 August 2005. Vitamin D and type 1 diabetes mellitus: state of art. Chantal Mathieu and Klaus Badenhoop. Copyright @ Elsevier 2005. Used with permission.

Descriptions of the VDR on T lymphocytes lead to the subsequent investigation of vitamin D actions on these immune cells. Interestingly, 1α-hydroxylase is not expressed in the T cells, and vitamin D activated in the macrophages acts on the T cells, suggesting an autocrine action of 1α,25 dihydroxyvitamin D₃.

Rigby and his team proved that cytokine production by T cells is influenced by vitamin D analogs: IL-2 and IFN γ are inhibited (Rigby et al., 1987), while production of some of the type 2 cytokines (IL-4, 5, and 10) is enhanced (Boonstra et al., 2001)

Inhibition of mitogen-stimulated T-cell cultures by vitamin D has been also reported (Rigby et al., 1984)

On the other hand, suppressor T cells are stimulated by vitamin D, leading to the inhibition of T-cell mediated immunity (Mathieu et al., 1994).

While inhibiting the IL-12 production from the DC, vitamin D is able to shift the differentiation of T naïve cells into Th0 cells and further into Th2 cells (IL-12 is an important cytokine that preferentially promotes the Th1 cell formation from the Th0 cells) (Willheim et al., 1999).

A recent study reported the direct modulation of CD4+ T cell function by active vitamin D, describing the inhibition of IL-17, IL-21, IFNγ, and the induction of T reg cells expressing CTLA-4 and FoxP3. If the T cells are grown in an environment rich in IL-2 and vitamin D, they express the highest levels of CTLA-4 and FoxP3, and are able to suppress the proliferation of the resting CD4+ T cells (Jeffery et al., 2009).

VDR is normally expressed on the B cells only upon their activation. Chen reported that $1\alpha,25$ $(OH)_2D_3$ decreased B cell proliferation and immunoglobulin production and induced cell death (Chen et al., 2007).

Vitamin D inhibits the production of inflammatory interleukins: IL-12, IL-2, interferon γ, tumor necrosis factor (TNF)-α, and TNF-β ,while the production of anti-inflammatory cytokines (IL-4, IL-10, TGF-β) is stimulated. This may disrupt the production of Th1 cells, which are destructive for the pancreatic beta cells, with a resultant beneficial effect on the beta cells (Lemire, 1995, van Etten & Mathieu 2005).

6.2 Vitamin D and type 1 diabetes: Direct effects on pancreatic cells

$1\alpha,25$ $(OH)_2$ D_3 appears to have a direct protective effect against pancreatic beta cell destruction by reducing the expression of MHC class I molecules (Hahn et al, 1997). In addition, vitamin D appears to increase islet cell expression of the A20 protein, which has antiapoptotic function (Riachy et al., 2002) (Fig 2). Vitamin D also decreases the expression of Fas, which is a transmembrane cell surface receptor mediator, involved in pancreatic beta cell apoptosis (Riachy et al., 2006).

7. Animal studies – vitamin D and type 1 diabetes

Insulitis can be inhibited by the administration of high doses of vitamin D in NOD mice (Mathieu et al., 1992), and $1\alpha,25(OH)_2D_3$ can prevent autoimmune diabetes in these animals (Mathieu et al., 1994). In both spontaneously developing and cyclophosphamide induced models of diabetes mellitus, vitamin D protects against autoimmune diabetes in NOD mice through restoration of the deficient suppressor cell function (Mathieu et al., 1995). VDR ligands enhance CD4+CD25+ regulatory T cells; these cells may play a role in protecting against insulitis in NOD mice (Adorini, 2003).

The loss of balance between the Th1 cells and Th2 cells, with the overproduction of the Th1 cells, appears to be central in the autoimmune diabetes pathogenesis. In NOD mice, the exposure to GAD65 leads to T cell proliferation and antibody production (Kaufman et al., 1993), at the same time as insulitis develops. 1,25 dihydroxyvitamin D_3 administration leads to a local immune shift of the balance between the Th1 cells and Th2 cells, favoring the increase in IL-4 production and the decrease in the γ interferon secretion.

Overbergh et al demonstrated that in NOD mice the immune shift between Th1/Th2 cells occurs in the periphery and is not limited to the pancreas (Overbergh et al., 2000). Furthermore, this change in the immune milieu occurs only in the autoantigen–specific immune response (exposure to GAD65, insulin B-chain, heat shock protein 65), and is not observed in the immune response associated with other antigens (ovalbumin, tetanus toxins, etc).

The recurrence of autoimmune diabetes mellitus after islet cell transplant was prevented in NOD mice by treatment with vitamin D analogs in combination with cyclosporine A (Casteels et al., 1998). Further, the administration of a nonhypercalcemic vitamin D analog in combination with an immunosuppressant (cyclosporine A) prevented progression to overt diabetes mellitus, even after the insulitis developed (Casteels et al., 1998). This effect, however, could not be reproduced when the vitamin D analog was administered without the addition of cyclosporine.

The NOD mice have an increased resistance to apoptosis in their immune cells. 1,25-dihydroxyvitamin D3 restores apoptosis in NOD mice in the thymus, leading to the increased destruction of autoimmune effector cells (Casteels et al., 1998).

In the BB rat, another animal model for autoimmune diabetes mellitus, 1,25-dihydroxyvitamin D did not lead to any significant difference in the incidence of diabetes when given from weaning to 120 days (Mathieu et al., 1997). This finding illustrates the issue of potentially different disease mechanisms in various animals and the difficulty of applying research findings from one animal model to another, or to humans.

8. Clinical studies – vitamin D and type 1 diabetes

The data available from human studies is scant and controversial.

A few ecological studies support the theory that vitamin D is a major player in the autoimmune disease pathogenesis, including type 1 diabetes mellitus.

A study in Northern Europe described the seasonal pattern of disease onset for autoimmune diabetes mellitus (Karvonen et al., 1998). The Diabetes Epidemiology Research International Group reported in 1988 an increased incidence of autoimmune diabetes with lower average yearly temperatures, which, in turn, was strongly associated with increasing latitude distances from the equator. This variation is thought to be due to the decreased exposure of the skin to the UV radiation.

In a very large worldwide study, Mohr et al analyzed the data from the Diabetes Mondial Project Group and found that in children younger than 14 years of age, the incidence rates of type 1 diabetes mellitus were significantly increased at higher latitudes and with low UVB exposure. Incidence rates of type 1 diabetes mellitus approached zero in the region with high UVB irradiance (Mohr et al., 2008).

Several European studies reported a decreased risk of diabetes in infants supplemented with high doses of vitamin D. The EURODIAB substudy 2 study group in seven European centers reported that vitamin D supplementation in infancy decreased the risk of autoimmune diabetes in a fairly consistent manner (Dalquist et al., 1999). Hypponen et al published the results of a birth-cohort study in northern Finland that included all pregnant women who were due to give birth in 1966, and recorded the frequency and the dosing of the vitamin D supplementation in the first year of life, as well as the presence of suspected rickets. 30 years later, the authors found that there was a lower incidence of diabetes mellitus in children who took any dose of vitamin D as compared with children that did not take any vitamin D supplementation. Even more so, the risk was lower in children that took the highest dose (2000 IU daily) as compared to the lower dose of vitamin D. Children with suspected rickets had a 3 fold increased risk of developing insulin-dependent diabetes mellitus (Hypponen et al., 2001). The risk of developing islet auto-antibodies in the children of mothers that took vitamin D during pregnancy was decreased in the Diabetes Autoimmunity Study in the Young (DAISY) (Fronczak et al., 2003). It is unclear from these studies if the protective effect is due to the supplementation with extra doses of vitamin D or prevention of vitamin D deficiency.

Two new interventional trials have been published in the last 2 years supporting the beneficial effect of vitamin D on the development of autoimmune diabetes.

A pilot study looking at patients with adult-onset latent autoimmune diabetes (LADA) demonstrated that supplementation with 1,25 dihydroxyvitamin D3 for 1 year resulted in beta cell preservation, as assessed by C-peptide levels (Li et al., 2009).

Aljabri et al conducted a prospective study in which patients with vitamin D deficiency were assigned to receive 4000 IU of vitamin D3 daily and had vitamin D 25 (OH) levels and hemoglobin A1c measured at baseline and at 12 weeks. The results revealed that the patients who achieved higher circulating levels of vitamin D 25 (OH) had a lower hemoglobin A1c (Aljabri et al., 2010).

Other studies, however, did not find similar results. A study which examined the effects of supplementation with cod liver oil during the first year of life, found that the infants who were supplemented had a decreased risk of developing childhood-onset type 1 diabetes. However, this decreased risk of type 1 diabetes mellitus was not observed in the infants if the cod liver oil was supplemented during pregnancy or if the vitamin D preparations were supplemented during the first year of the infant's life. Since cod liver oil has a high content of vitamin D along with the long-chain n-3 fatty acids (eicosapentaenoic and docosahexaenoic), it is not clear if these effects are due to the high vitamin D content of the cod liver oil or due to the fatty acids (Stene et al., 2003).

Pittoco et al reported the results of an interventional trial in children with newly diagnosed type 1 diabetes, in which the patients were administered calcitriol or nicotinamide in order to preserve beta-cell function. Even though there was a decrease in the insulin requirements at 3 and 6 months in the calcitriol treated group, at the end of the first year there was no difference between the C-peptide levels or hemoglobin A1c between the two groups (Pitocco et al., 2006).

Bizzarri et al investigated whether supplementation with calcitriol in recent onset autoimmune diabetes has a protective effect on the pancreatic beta cells and found that, at the doses used in the study, calcitriol did not confer protection against the autoimmune destruction of the beta cells (Bizzarri et al., 2010). In Germany, Walter et al supplemented newly diagnosed adult patients with 1,25(OH)2D3 for 18 months. At the end of the study there was no difference in the areas under the curve (AUC) for C-peptide, peak C-peptide, or fasting C-peptide after a mixed meal tolerance test between the treatment and the placebo groups (Walter et al., 2010).

9. Conclusion

In conclusion, the data on the role of vitamin D in the pathogenesis of autoimmune diabetes mellitus is inconclusive. More studies, particularly, interventional trials, with vitamin D or vitamin D nonhypercalcemic analogs need to be performed before the interaction between autoimmunity, diabetes mellitus and vitamin D is completely understood.

10. Acknowledgements

We would like to thank Barbara Pietrzyk-Busta, RN, MA for her invaluable assistance in the preparation and editing of this manuscript, and to Jill Gregory, CMI, FAMI for designing an illustration of Figure 1.

11. References

Adams JS, Singer FR, Gacad MA, Sharma OP, Hayes MJ, Vouros P & Holick M (1995). Isolation and structural identification of 1,25-dihydroxyvitamin D3 produced by cultured alveolar macrophages in sarcoidosis. J Clin Endocrinol Metab, 60:960-966.

Adams JS, Sharma OP, Gacad MA & Singer FR (1983). Metabolism of 25-hydroxyvitamin D3 by cultured pulmonary alveolar macrophages in sarcoidosis. J Clin Invest, 72:1856–1860.

Adorini L (2003) Tolerogenic dendritic cells induced by vitamin D receptor ligands enhance regulatory T cells inhibiting autoimmune diabetes. Ann N Y Acad Sci, 987:258–261.

Adorini L (2001). Interleukin 12 and autoimmune diabetes. Nat Genet 27(2):131–132.

Aljabri KS, Bokhari SA & Khan MJ. (2010). Glycemic changes after vitamin D supplementation in patients with type 1 diabetes mellitus and vitamin D deficiency. Ann Saudi Med, 30(6):454-458.

Achenbach P, Bonifacio E, Koczwara K & Ziegler AG (2005). Natural history of type 1 diabetes. Diabetes,54(Suppl2):S25-S31.

Banchereau J & Steinman RM. (1998). Dendritic cells and the control of immunity. Nature 392(6673):245–252.

Bailey R , Cooper JD, Zeitels L,Smyth DJ, Yang JH, Walker NM, Hypponen E, Dunger DB, Ramos-Lopez E, Badenhoop K, Nejentsev S & Todd JA (2007). Association of the Vitamin D metabolism gene CYP27B1 with type 1 diabetes. Diabetes,56(10):2616-2621.

Barrett JC, Clayton DG, Concannon P, Akolkar B, Cooper JD, Erlich HA, Julier C, Morahan G, Nerup J, Nierras C, Plagnol V, Pociot F, Schuilenburg H, Smyth DJ, Stevens H, Todd JA, Walker NM & Rich SS (2009). Genome-wide association study and a meta-analysis find that over 40 loci affect risk of type 1 diabetes. Nature Genetics. 41(6):703-707.

Bhalla AK, Amento EP, Clemens TL, Holick MF & Krane SM. (1983). Specific high-affinity receptors for 1,25 dihydroxyvitamin D3 in human peripheral mononuclear cells: Presence in monocytes and induction in T lymphocytes following activation. J Clin Endocrinol Metab 57(6):1308-1310.

Bendelac A, Carnaud C, Boitard C & Bach JF. (1987). Syngeneic transfer of autoimmune diabetes from diabetic NOD mice to healthy neonates. Requirement for both L3T4+ and Lyt-2+ T cells. J Exp Med 166:823-832.

Bennett ST, Lucassen AM, Gough SC, Powell EE, Undlien DE, Pritchard LE, Merriman ME, Kawaguchi Y, Dronsfield MJ & Pociot F (1995). Susceptibility to human type 1 diabetes at IDDM2 is determined by tandem repeat variation at the insulin gene mini satellite locus. Nat Genet, 9:284-292.

Bell GI, Horita S & Kharam JH (1994). A polymorphic locus near the insulin gene is associated with insulin-dependent diabetes mellitus. Diabetes ,33:176-83.

Benoist C & Mathis D. 1997. Cell death mediators in autoimmune diabetes – No shortage of suspects. Cell 89(1):1-3.

Bizzarri C, Pitocco D, Napoli N, Di Stasi E, Maggi D, Manfrini S, Suraci C, Cavallo MG, Cappa M, Ghirlanda G, Pozzilli P & IMDIAB Group. 2010. No protective effect of calcitriol on beta-cell function in recent-onset type 1 diabetes .Diabetes Care 33:1962-1963.

Boonstra A, Barrat FJ, Crain C, Heath VL, Savelkoul HF & O'Garra A. 1alpha,25-Dihydroxyvitamin D3 has a direct effect on naïve CD4+ T cells to enhance the development of Th2 cells. J Immunol 2001;167(9):4974-4980.

Bonifacio E & Ziegler AG (2010). Advances in the prediction and natural history of type 1 diabetes. Endocrinol Metab Clin N Am 39: 513-525.

Cantorna MT, Hayes CE & DeLuca HF (1996). 1,25-dihydroxyvitamin D3 reversibly blocks the progressions of relapsing encephalomyelitis, a model of multiple sclerosis. Proc Natl Acad Sci USA 93(15):7861-7864.

Cantorna MT, Hayes CE & DeLuca HF (1998). 1,25-dihydroxyvitamin D3 prevents and ameliorates symptoms in two experimental models of human arthritis. J Nutr 128(1):68–72.

Carlberg C & Polly P (1998). Gene regulation by vitamin D3. Crit. Rev. Eukaryot. Gene Expr. 8, 19–42.

Casteels K, Waer M, Bouillon R, Depovere J, Bouillon R & Mathieu C (1998). 1,25-dihydroxy-vitamin D3 restores sensitivity to cyclophosphamide-induced apoptosis in non-obese diabetic (NOD) mice and protects against diabetes. Clin Exp Immunol 112:181-187.

Casteels KM, Waer M, Laureys J, Valckx D, Depovere J, Bouillon R & Mathieu C (1998). Prevention of autoimmune destruction of syngeneic islet grafts in spontaneously diabetic nonobese diabetic mice by a combination of a vitamin D3 analog and cyclosporine. Transplantation 65:1225-1232.

Chang TJ, Lei HH, Yeh JI, Chiu KC, Lee KC, Chen MC, Tai TY & Chuang LM (2000). Vitamin D receptor gene polymorphisms influence susceptibility to type 1 diabetes mellitus in the Taiwanese population. Clin Endocrinol (Oxf ,52(5):575-580.

Casteels KM, Mathieu C, Ware M, Valckx D, Overbergh L, Laureys JM & Bouillon R (1998). Prevention of type 1 diabetes in nonobese diabetic mice by late intervention with nonhyperclcemic analogs of 1,25-dihydroxyvitamin D3 in combination with a short induction course of cyclosporine A. Endocrinology. 139:95-102.

Chen S, Sims GP, Chen XX, Gu YY, Chen S & Lipsky PE (2007). Modulatory effects of 1,25-dihydroxyvitamin D3on human B cell differentiation. J Immunol,179(3):1634-1647.

Clemes DL & Mahan KJ (2010). Alcoholic pancreatitis: lessons from the liver. World J Gastroenterol, 16(11):1314-1320.

Dalquist G et al (1999). The EURODIAB Substudy 2 Study Group. Vitamin D supplement in early childhood and risk for type 1 (insulin-dependent) diabetes mellitus. Diabetologia 42:51-54.

Delovitch TL & Singh B (1997). The nonobese diabetic mouse as a model of autoimmune diabetes: Immune dysregulation gets the NOD. Immunity 7(6):727-738.

Devendra D & Eisenbarth GS (2003). Immunologic endocrine disorders. J Allergy Clin Immunol ,111:S624-S636.

D'Ambrosio D, Cippitelli M, Cocciolo MG, Mazzeo D, Lucia PD, Lang R, Sinigaglia F & Panina-Bordignon P (1998). Inhibition of IL12 production by 1,25-dihydroxyvitamin D3: involvement of NF-□B down regulation by 1,25-dihydroxy vitamin D3. J Clin Invest 101:252–262.

Diabetes Epidemiology Research International Group (1988). Geographic patterns of childhood insulin-dependent diabetes mellitus. Diabetes 37(8):1113–1119.

Eisenbarth GS & Gottlieb PA (2004). Autoimmune polyendocrine syndromes. N Engl J Med, 350:2068-2079.

Ferreira GB, van Etten E, Lage K, Hansen DA, Moreau Y, Workman CT, Waer M, Verstuyf A, Waelkens E, Overbergh L & Mathieu C (2009). Proteome analysis demonstrates profound alterations in human dendritici cell nature by TX527, an analogue of vitamin D. Proteomics , 9(14):3752-3764.

Franco OH, Steyerberg EW, Hu FB, Mackenbach J, Nusselder W (2007). Associations of diabetes mellitus with total life expectancy and life expectancy with and without cardiovascular disease. Arch Intern Med.;167:1145-1151.

Fronczak CM, Baron AE, Chase HP Ross C, Brady HL, Hoffman M, Eisenbarth GS, Rewers & Norris JM (2003) In utero dietary exposures and risk of islet autoimmunity in children. Diabetes Care 26:3237–3242.

Gamble DR & Taylor KW (1969). Seasonal incidence of diabetes mellitus. Br Med J 3:631-633.

Gamble DR, Kinsley ML, Fitzgerald MG Bolton R & Taylor KW (1969). Viral antibodies in diabetes mellitus. Br Med J 3:627-630.

Gale EA (2002). A missing link in the hygiene hypothesis? Diabetologia, 45:588-94.

Guo SW, Magnuson VL, Schiller JJ, Wang X, Wu Y & Ghosh S (2006). Meta-analysis of vitamin D receptor polymorphism and type 1 diabetes: a HuGE review of genetic association studies. Am J Epidemiol,164(8):711-724.

Gillespie KM (2006). Type 1 diabetes: pathogenesis and prevention. CMAJ,175(2):165-170.

Gillespie KM, Gale EAM & Bingley PJ (2002). High familial risk and genetic susceptibility in early onset childhood diabetes. Diabetes ,51:210-214.

Giulietti A, Gysemans C, Stoffels K, VAN Etten E, Decallonne B, Overbergh L, Bouillon R & Mathieu C (2004) Vitamin D deficiency in early life accelerates type 1 diabetes in non-obese diabetic mice. Diabetologia 47:451-462.

Gough SC, Walker LS & Sansom DM (2005): CTLA4 gene polymorphism and autoimmunity. Immunol, 204:102-115.

Griffin MD, Lutz WH, Phan VA, Bachman LA, McKean DJ & Kumar R (2000). Potent inhibition of dendritic cell differentiation and maturation by vitamin D analogs. Biochem Biphys Res Commun, 270(3):701-708.

Griffin MD, Lutz W, Phan VA, Bachman LA, McKean DJ & Kumar R (2001). Dendritic cell modulation by 1alpha,25 dihydroxyvitamin D3 and its analogs: A vitamin D receptor-dependent pathway that promotes a persistent state of immaturity in vitro and in vivo. Proc Natl Acad Sci USA 98:6800–6805.

Gregori S, Giarratana N, Smiroldo S, Uskokovic M & Adorini L (2002). A 1alpha,25-dihydroxyvitamin D(3) analog enhances regulatory T-cells and arrests autoimmune diabetes in NOD mice. Diabetes 51:1367–1374.

Greenwald RJ, Freeman GJ & Sharpe AH (2005). The B7 family revisited. Annu Rev Immunol 2005;23:515-548.

Hahn HJ Kuttler B, Mathieu C & Bouillon R (1997). 1,25 dihydroxyvitamin D3 reduces MHC antigen expression on pancreatic beta-cells in vitro. Transplant Proc,29(4):2156-2157.

Haussler MR, Whitfield GK, Haussler CA, Hsieh JC, Thompson PD, Selznick SH, Dominguez CE & Jurutka PW (1998). The nuclear vitamin D receptor: biological and molecular regulatory properties revealed. J Bone Miner Res 13:325-349.

Helfand RF, Gary HE Jr, Freeman CY, Anderson LJ & Pallansch MA (1995). Serologic evidence of an association between enteroviruses and the onset of type 1 diabetes mellitus. Pittsburgh Diabetes Reseacrh Group. J Infect Dis 172:1206-1211.

Hypponen E, Laara E, Reunanen A, Jarvelin MR & Virtanen SM (2001). Intake of vitamin D and risk of type 1 diabetes: a birth-cohort study. Lancet,358: 1500-1503.

Holick MF (1999). Vitamin D: photobiology, metabolism, mechanism of action, and clinical applications. In: Favus M, editor. Primer on the metaboilic bone diseases and disorders of mineral metabolism. Philadelphia: Lippincott Williams and Wilkins, pp92-98.

IDF. International Diabetes Federation World Atlas of Diabetes. 2006.

Israni N, Goswami R, Kumar A & Rani R (2009). Interaction of vitamin D receptor with HLA DRB1 0301 in type 1 diabetes patients from North India. PLoS One , 4(12):e8023.

Jeffery LE, Burke F, Mura M, Zheng Y, Qureshi OS, Hewison , Walker LS, Lammas DA, Raza K & Sansom DM (2009). 1,25-Dihydroxyvitamin D3 and IL-2 combine to inhibit T cell production of inflammatory cytokines and promote development of regulatory T cells expressing CTLA-4 and FoxP3. J Immunol;183(9):5458-5467.

Kahn HS, Morgan TM, Case LD, Dabelea D, Mayer-Davis EJ, Lawrence JM, Marcovina SM & Imperatore G (2009). Association of type 1 diabetes with month of birth among US youth: the SEARCH for diabetes in Youth study. Diabetes Care, 32(11):2010-2015.

Karvonen M, Jantti V, Muntoni S, Stabilini M, Stabilini L, Muntoni S & Tuomilehto J (1998) Comparison of the seasonal pattern in the clinical onset of IDDM in Finland and Sardinia. Diabetes Care 21:1101-1109.

Kaufman DL, Clare-Salzler M, Tian J, Forsthuber T, Ting GST, Robinson P, Atkinson MA, Sercarz EE, Tobin AJ & Lehmann PV (1993). Spontaneous loss of T-cell tolerance to glutamic acid decarboxylase in murine insulin-dependent diabetes. Nature 366:69-72.

Kulmala P, Savola K, Peteren JS, Vähäsalo P, Karjalainen J, Löppönen T, Dyrberg T, Akerblom HK & Knip M. The Childhood Diabetes in Finland Study Group (1998). Prediction of insulin-dependent diabetes mellitus in siblings of children with diabetes. A population-based study. J Clin Invest 101:327-336.

Lampeter E, Signore A, Gale E & Pozzilli P (1989). Lessons from the NOD mouse for the pathogenesis and immunotherapy of human type I (insulin-dependent) dia- betes mellitus. Diabetologia 32:703-708, 1989.

Lemire JM (1995). Immunomodulatory actions of 1,25 dihydroxyvitamin D3. J Steroid Biochem Mol Biol, 53(1-6): 599-602.

Lemire JM (1995). 1, 25 dihydroxylase vitamin D3 prevents the in vivo induction of murine experimental autoimmune encephalomyelitis. J Clin Invest 87(3): 1103-1107.

Lemos MC (2008). Lack of association of vitamin D receptor gene polymorphism with susceptibility to type 1 diabtes mellitus in the Portughese population Hum Immunol, 69(2):134-138.

Leijon K, Hammarström B & Holmberg D (1994). NOD mice display enhanced immune responses and prolonged survival of lymphoid cells. Int Immunol 6:339-345.

Li X, Liao L, Yan X, Huang G, Lin J, Lei M, Wang X & Zhou Z (2009). Protective effects of 1-α-hydroxyvitamin D3 on residual β-cell function in patients with adult-onset latent autoimmune diabetes (LADA). Diabetes Metab Res Rev. 25(5): 411-416.

Lopez, ER, O Zwermann, M Segni, G Meyer, M Reincke, J Seissler, J Herwig, KH Usadel, & K Badenhoop (2004). A promoter polymorphism of the CYP27B1 gene is associated with Addison's disease, Hashimoto's thyroiditis, Graves' disease and type 1 diabetes mellitus in Germans. Eur. J. Endocrinol. 151, 193-197.

Lopez ER, Regulla K, Pani MA, Krause M, Usadel KH & Badenhoop K (2004). CYP27B1 polymorphism variants are associated with type 1 diabetes mellitus in Germans. J. Steroid Biochem. Mol. Biol. 89-90, 155-157.

Mathieu C, Laureys J, Sobis H, Vandeputte M, Waer M & Bouillon R (1992). 1,25-Dihydroxyvitamin D3 prevents insulitis in NOD mice. Diabetes 41:1491-1495.

Mathieu C, Waer M, Laureys J, Rutgeerts O & Bouillon R (1994). Prevention of autoimmune diabetes in NOD mice by 1, 25 dihydroxyvitamin D3. Diabetologia, 37:552-558.

Mathieu C, Waer M, Casteels K, Laureys J & Bouillon R (1995). Prevention of type I diabetes in NOD mice by nonhypercalcemic doses of a new structural analog of 1,25-dihydroxyvitamin D3, KH1060. Endocrinology 136:866-872.

Mathieu C, Casteels K & Bouillon R (1997). Vitamin D and diabetes. In: Feldman D, Glorieux F, Pike J (eds) Vitamin D. Academic, San Diego, pp 1183-1196.

Mathieu C, Van Etten E, Gysemans C, Decallonne B, Kato S, Laureys J, Depovere J, Valckx D, Verstuyf A & Bouillon R (2001). In vitro and in vivo analysis of the immune system of vitamin D receptor-knock out mice. J. Bone Miner. Res. 16, 2057-2065.

Mathieu C, Gysemans C, Giulietti A & Bouillon R (2005). Vitamin D and diabetes. Diabetologia. 48:1247-1257.

MacCuish AC, Jordan J, Campbell CJ, Duncan LJ & Irvine WJ (1975). Cell-mediated immunity in diabetes mellitus: lymphocyte transformation by insulin and insulin fragments by insulin and insulin fragments in insulin-treated and newly-diagnosed diabetics. Diabetes 24:36-43.

Makino S, Kunimoto K, Muraoka Y, Katakiri K & Tochino Y (1980). Breeding of a non-obese, diabetic starin of mice. Exp Anim, 29:1-8.

Martin S, Wolf-Eichbaum D, Duinkerken G, Scherbaum WA, Kolb H, Noordzij JG, & Roep OP (2001). Development of type 1 diabetes despite severe hereditary B-lymphocyte deficiency. N Engl J Med 345:1036-1040.

Mohr SB, Garland CF, Gorham ED & Garland FC (2008). The association between ultraviolet B irradiance, vitamin D status and incidence rates of type 1 diabetes in 51 regions worldwide. Diabetologia, 51(8);1391-1398.

Menser MA, Forrest JM & Bransby RD (1978). Rubella infection and diabetes melliyus. Lancet i:57-60.

Nakayama M, Abiru N,Moriyama H, Babaya N, Liu E, Miao L, Yu L, Wegmann DR, Hutton JC, Elliott JF & Eisenbarth GS (2005). Prime role for an insulin epitope in the development of type 1 diabetes in NOD mice. Nature, 435:220.

Nejentsev S, Guja C, McCormack R, , Cooper J, Howson S, Nutland S, Rance H,Neil Walker N, Undlien D, Ronningen KS, Tuomilehto-Wolf E, Tuomilehto J, Ionescu-Tirgoviste C, Gale EAM, Bingley PJ , Gillespie KM, Savage DA , Carson JD, Patterson CC, Maxwell AP & Todd JA (2003). Association of intercellular adhesion molecule-1 gene with type 1 diabetes. Lancet, 362:1723-4.

Noble JA, Valdes AM, Cook M, Klitz W, Thomson G & Erlich HA (1996). The role of HLA class II genes in insulin-dependent diabetes mellitus: molecular analysis of 180 Caucasian, multiplex families. Am J Hum Genet 59:1134-1148.

Overbergh L, Decallonne B, Valckx D, Verstuyf A, Depovere J, Laureys J, Rutgeerts O, Saint-Arnaud R, Bouillon R & C Mathieu (2000). Identification and immune regulation of 25-hydroxyvitamin D-1-alpha-hydroxylase in murine macrophages. Clin Exp Immunol 120: 139-146.

Overbergh L, Decallonne B, Waer M, Rutgeerts O, Valkx D, Casteels KM, Laureys J, Bouillon R & Mathieu C (2000). 1alpha,25- dihydroxyvitamin D3 induces an autoantigen-specific T-helper 1/T-helper 2 immune shift in NOD mice immunized with GAD65 (p524-543). Diabetes 49:1301-1307.

Pani MA, Knapp M, Donner H, Braun J, Baur M & Usadel K (2000). Vitamin D receptor allele combinations influence genetic susceptibility to type 1 diabetes in Germans. Diabetes,49(3):504-507.

Penna G & Adorini L (2000). 1 Alpha,25-dihydroxyvitamin D3 inhibits differentiation, maturation, activation, and survival of dendritic cells leading to impaired alloreactive T cell activation. J Immunol, 164(5):2405-2411.

Penha-Goncalves C, Leijon K, Persson L & Holmberg D (1995). Type I diabetes and the control of dexamethasone-induced apoptosis in mice maps to the same region on chromosome 6. Genomics 28:398-404.

Prosser DE & Jones G (2004). Enzymes involved in the activation and inactivation of vitamin D. Trends Biochem Sci,29:664-673.

Pitocco D, Crinò A, Di Stasio E, Manfrini S, Guglielmi C, Spera S, Anguissola GB, Visalli N, Suraci C, Matteoli MC, Patera I P, Cavallo MG, Bizzarri C & Pozzilli P on behalf of the IMDIAB Group (2006). The effects of calcitriol and nicotinamide on residual pancreatic beta-cell function in patients with recent-onset type 1 diabetes (IMDIAB XI). Diabet Med, 23(8):920-923.

Rabinovitch A (1998). An update on cytokines in the pathogenesis of insulin-dependent diabetes mellitus. Diabetes Metab Rev 14(2):129-151.

Redondo MJ, Jeffrey J, Fain PR, Eisenbarth GS & Orban T (2008). Concordance for islet autoimmunity among monozygotic twins. NEJM, 359;26:2849-2850.

Riachy R, Vandewalle B, Kerr Conte, Riachy J, Moerman E, Sacchetti P, Lukowiak B, Gmyr V, Bouckenooghe T, Dubois M, Pattou F (2002). 1,25 dihydroxy vitamin D protects RINm5F and human islet cells against cytokine-induced apoptosis: implications of the antiapoptoctic protein A20. Endocrinology 2002;143(12):4809-4819.

Riachy R, Vandewalle B, Moerman E, Belaich S, Lukowiak B, Gmyr V, Muharram G, Kerr Conte J & Pattou F (2006). 1,25 dihydroxy vitamin D protects human pancreatic islets against cytokine-induced apoptosis via down-regulation of the Fas receptor . Apoptosis, 11(2):151-159.

Rigby WF, Denome S & Fanger MW (1987). Regulation of lymphokine production and human T lymphocyte activation by 1,25-dihydroxyvitamin D3. Specific inhibition at the level of messenger RNA. J Clin Invest, 79(6):1659-1664.

Rigby WF, Stacy T & Fanger MW (1984). Inhibition of T lymphocyte mitogenesis by 1,25-dihydroxyvitamin D3 (calcitriol). J Clin Invest, 74(4):1451-1455.

Stene LC, Joner G & Norwegian Childhood Diabetes Study Group (2003). Norwegian Childhood Diabetes Study Group.Use of cod liver oil during the first year of life is associated with lower risk of childhood-onset type 1 diabetes: a large, population-based, case-control study. Am J Clin Nutr, 78: 1128–1134.

Smyth D, Cooper JD, Collins JE, Heward JM, Franklyn JA, Howson JMM, Vella A, Nutland S, Rance HE, Maier L, Barratt BJ, Guja C, Ionescu-Tîrgoviste C, Savage DA, Dunger DB, Widmer B, Strachan DP, Ring SM, Walker N, Clayton DG, Twells RCJ, Gough SCL & Todd JA (2004). Replication of an association between the lymphoid tyrosine phosphatase locus (LYP/PTPN22) with type 1 diabetes, and evidence for its role as a general autoimmunity locus. Diabetes, 53:3020-2023.

Stoffels K, Overbergh L, Bouillon R & Mathieu C (2007). Immune regulation of 1 alpha-hydroxylase in murine peritoneal macrophages: unraveling the IFNgamma pathway. J Steroid biochem Mol Biol, 103:567-571.

Strandell E, Eizirik DL & Sandler S (1994). Reversal of beta-cell suppression in vitro in pancreatic islets isolated from nonobese diabetic mice during the phase preceding insulin-dependent diabtes mellitus. J Clin Invest, 85:1944-1950.

Strugnell SA & DeLuca HF (1997). The vitamin D receptor - structure and transcriptional activation. Proc Soc Exp Biol Med 215:223-228.

Tisch R, Yang XD, Singer SM, Liblau RS, Fugger L & McDevitt HO (1993). Immune response to glutamic acid decarboxylase correlates with insulitis in nonobese diabetic mice. Nature 366:72–75.

Turpeinen H (2003).Vitamin D receptor polymorphism: no association with type 1 diabtes in the Finnish population. Eur J Endocrinol, 149(6):591-596.

Ueda H, Howson JM, Esposito L, Heward J, Snook H, Chamberlain G, Rainbow DB, Hunter KM, Smith AN, Di Genova G, Herr MH, Dahlman I, Payne F, Smyth D, Lowe C, Twells RC, Howlett S, Healy B, Nutland S, Rance HE, Everett V, Smink LJ, Lam AC, Cordell HJ, Walker NM, Bordin C, Hulme J, Motzo C, Cucca F, Hess JF, Metzker ML, Rogers J, Gregory S, Allahabadia A, Nithiyananthan R, Tuomilehto-Wolf E, Tuomilehto J, Bingley P, Gillespie KM, Undlien DE, Rønningen KS, Guja C, Ionescu-Tîrgovişte C, Savage DA, Maxwell AP, Carson DJ, Patterson CC, Franklyn JA, Clayton DG, Peterson LB, Wicker LS, Todd JA & Gough SC (2003) Association of the T-cell regulatory gene CTLA4 with susceptibility to autoimmune disease. Nature , 423:506-511.

Van Etten E & Mathieu C (2005). Immunoregulation by 1,25-dihydroxyvitamin D3: basic concepts J Steroid Biochem Mol Biol , 97(1-2):93-101.

Vafiadis P, Bennett ST, Todd JA, Nadeau J, Grabs R, Goodyer CG, Wickramasinghe S, Colle E & Polychronakos C (1997). Insulin expression in human thymus is modulated by INS VNTR alleles at the IDDM2 locus. Nat Genet 15:289-292.

Walter M Kaupper T, Adler K, Foersch J, Bonifacio E & Ziegler AG (2010). No effect of the 1alpha,25-dihydroxyvitamin D3 on beta-cell residual function and insulin requirement in adults with new onset type 1 diabetes. Diabetes Care 33:1443-1448.

Weisman Y, Harell A, Edelstein S, et al. (1979) 1 alpha, 25-hydroxyvitamin D3 and 24,25-dihydroxyvitamin D3 in vitro synthesis by human decidua and placenta. Nature 281:317-319.

Yeung WG , Rawlinson WD, Craig ME (2011). Enterovirus infecction and type 1 diabetes mellitus:systemic review and meta-analysis of observational molecular studies BMJ, 342:d35.

Willheim M, Thien R, Schrattbauer K, Bajna E, Holub M, Gruber R, Baier K, Pietschmann P, Reinisch W, scheiner O, Peterlik M (1999). Regulatory effects of 1alpha,25-dihydroxyvitamin D3 on the cytokine production of human peripheral blood lymphocytes. J Clin Endocrinol Metab, 84(10):3739-3744.

Von Herrath M (2010). Combination therapies for type 1 diabetes: why not now? Immunotherapy, 2(3):289–291.

Yoon J-W, Yoon C-S, Lim H-W, Huang Q, Kang Y, Pyun K, Hirasawa K, Sherwin R &

Jun H-S (1999). Control of autoimmune diabetes in NOD mice by GAD expression or suppression in β cells. Science 284:1183–1187.

Zekzer D, Wong FS, Ayalon O, Millet I, Altieri M, Shintani S, Solimena M & Sherwin RS (1998) GAD-reactive CD4+ Th1 cells induce diabetes in NOD/SCID mice. J Clin Invest 101:68–73.

9

Fatty Acid Supply in Pregnant Women with Type 1 Diabetes Mellitus

Éva Szabó, Tamás Marosvölgyi and Tamás Decsi
University of Pécs, Department of Pediatrics, Pécs
Hungary

1. Introduction

Long-chain polyunsaturated fatty acids (LCPUFAs) play an important role in the human body in building up cell membranes and in regulating their fluidity. The most important fatty acids are the essential n-3 fatty acid, alpha-linolenic acid (C18:3n-3, ALA) and the essential n-6 fatty acid, linoleic acid (C18:2n-6, LA), and their most important metabolites, docosahexaenoic acid (C22:6n-3, DHA) and arachidonic acid (C20:4n-6, AA). LCPUFAs are precursors of different eicosanoids, and their availability may be disturbed in several diseases. As insulin is one of the most potent activators of $\triangle$-6 desaturase enzyme, type 1 diabetes mellitus (T1DM) is characterised by the diminished levels of n-3 LCPUFAs (Decsi et al., 2002, 2007; Szabó et al., 2010b).

2. Role of polyunsaturated fatty acids

Polyunsaturated fatty acids (PUFAs) are components of the lipid bilayer of cell membranes, where they also regulate membrane fluidity. Cell membranes containing more saturated fatty acids and cholesterol are more rigid, while PUFAs increase their fluidity as well as the number of receptors and their affinity to their substrates, like hormones and growth factors (Das, 2006).

PUFAs are also precursors of several second messengers. From the n-6 group, especially from AA proinflammatory eicosanoids are synthesized, while the n-3 fatty acids, especially eicosapentaenoic acid (C20:5n-3, EPA) are precursors of antiinflammatory eicosanoids.

The n-6 essential fatty acid (EFA), LA plays an important role in the maintenance of the epidermal water barrier (Koletzko & Rodriguez-Palmero, 1999), preventing thereby the transepidermal water loss and epidermal damage (Yen et al., 2008). There are data indicating that LA also lowers plasma total cholesterol levels (Nikkari et al., 1983). In an animal study the n-3 EFA, ALA lowered serum and liver triacylglycerol levels, while it increased serum HDL-cholesterol levels (Murano et al., 2007).

AA and DHA play an important role in the maturation of the developing nervous system: during the third trimester and in the first months of life there is an increased incorporation into the fetal/neonatal brain and retinal membranes (Farquharson et al., 1992; Martinez & Mougan, 1998).

Fish oil, containing EPA and DHA, may be beneficial not only during infancy, but also during adulthood. It may prevent the development of macula degeneration (Chua et al.,

2006), may lower the risk of developing dementia and Alzheimer-disease (Morris et al., 2003; Schaefer et al., 2006) and may be beneficial in bipolar depression (Noaghiul & Hibbeln, 2003). N-3 LCPUFAs play also an important role in the prevention of cardiovascular diseases: fish oil supplementation increased HDL-cholesterol levels, while decreased triacylglycerol levels (Laidlaw & Holub, 2003), reduced the progression of atherosclerosis (Erkkilä et al., 2004), the risk of coronary heart disease (Iso et al., 2006; Mozaffarian et al., 2005), fatal myocardial infarction (Yuan et al., 2001), sudden cardial death (Albert et al., 1998), incidence of atrial fibrillation (Mozaffarian et al., 2004) and the risk of stroke (Mozaffarian et al., 2005). In a longitudinal, observational study, fish oil supplementation reduced the risk of developing islet autoimmunity in children at increased genetic risk for T1DM (Norris et al, 2007).

Trans isomeric fatty acids increase serum lipoprotein(a), LDL-cholesterol, triacylglycerol (Katan et al., 1995) and total cholesterol levels (Louheranta et al., 1999), as well as significantly decrease the levels of HDL-cholesterol (Dyerberg et al., 2004; Louheranta et al., 1999; Sun et al., 2007); in summary, they increase the risk of cardiovascular diseases (Sun et al., 2007). In an animal study rats fed with *trans* fatty acid diet (similar to saturated fatty acid diet) had high levels of fasting plasma insulin and decreased adipocyte insulin sensitivity (Ibrahim et al., 2005). In contrast, in a human study *trans* fatty acid diet did not alter insulin sensitivity (Louheranta et al., 1999).

2.1 Biochemistry of fatty acids

The physiologically most important PUFAs contain 2-6 double bonds and have a chain length of 18, 20 or 22 carbon atom. The methyl end of the molecule is called the omega end. On the basis of the distance of the first double bond from the carbon atom at the omega end, three different groups of fatty acids can be distinguished: omega-3 (n-3), omega-6 (n-6) and omega-9 (n-9) fatty acids.

The human body is unable to establish double bond in the n-3 and n-6 position, so we have to ingest the EFAs, the n-3 ALA and n-6 LA with our diet. The most important dietary sources of these fatty acids are vegetables and vegetable oils.

From the essential n-6 LA, after $\triangle$-6 desaturation γ-linolenic acid (C18:3n-6, GLA) and after elongation dihomo-γ-linolenic acid (C20:3n-6, DHGLA) is synthesised. After a $\triangle$-6 desaturational step, the most important metabolite, AA is produced (Fig. 1).

The metabolism of the n-3 group is a longer, more complicated process. After elongation, $\triangle$-5 and $\triangle$-6 desaturation eicosapentaenoic acid (C20:5n-3, EPA) is formed. After chain elongation docosapentaenoic acid (C22:5n-3, DPA) is synthesised. The most important n-3 metabolite, DHA is produced after $\triangle$-6 desaturation and peroxisomal β-oxidation (Fig. 1).

Although the same enzymes are involved into the metabolism of the n-3 and n-6 group, these fatty acids cannot be transformed into each other, because the molecule can only be activated from the carboxyl end. In the metabolism, the elongation is a quicker, while desaturation is a slower step, so these desaturational steps determine the speed of metabolism (i.e. these are the rate-limiting steps).

In the nature, PUFAs can be found predominantly as cis isomers, while *trans* fatty acids are produced in the stomach of ruminants and during the partial hydrogenation of vegetable oils. Cis double bond bends the molecule, while *trans* double bond straightens the fatty acid, so it is similar to saturated fatty acids. From this difference arise their different physiological effects: *trans* isomers are similar to saturated fatty acids, while cis isomers have more beneficial effects. As cis and *trans* fatty acids use the same enzymes during their metabolism, several studies have indicated, that *trans* fatty acids may disturb the metabolism of the physiologically important n-3 and n-6 fatty acids (Szabó et al, 2007, 2010a; Vidgren et al., 1998).

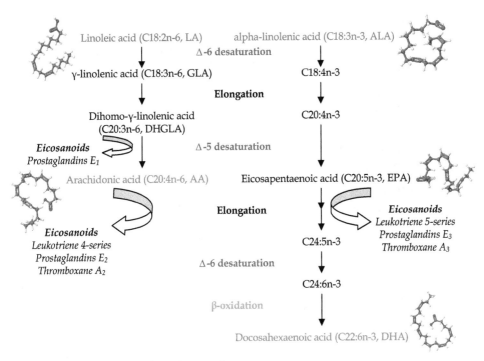

Fig. 1. Metabolism of n-6 and n-3 fatty acids
figure modified from http://www.lpi.oregonstate.edu; source of fatty acid figures:
http://www.3dchem.com/index.asp

2.2 Dietary sources of fatty acids

The n-3 EFA, ALA is found in the highest quantity in linseed oil, and considerable amounts are found in hempseed oil (20%) as well (Erasmus, 1993); however, from the dietary point of view its most important sources are walnut and rapeseed oils (Beare-Rogers et al., 2001). The n-6 EFA, LA can be found in the highest proportion in primrose (81%; Erasmus, 1993) and grapeseed oils, but its most important dietary sources are sunflower, corn and pumpkin seed oils (Table 1; Beare-Rogers et al., 2001). Compared to vegetable sources, animal lipid sources contain smaller quantities of ALA and LA (Table 2).

Flesh of herbivorous animals is very rich in the most important n-6 metabolite, AA (Table 2). On the other hand, haslets of terrestrial animals, like liver and kidney contains DHA also in relative high concentrations.

The most important n-3 LCPUFAs, EPA and DHA can be found in fatty sea fishes (Table 3). The DHA content of sea fishes may vary according to season, area of catching and to age and gender of the fish (Racine & Deckelbaum, 2007). Marine fish contains higher levels of n-3 PUFAs, EPA and DHA, while lower n-6 PUFAs, LA and AA compared to freshwater species. In a Chinese study, the edible meat of cultured freshwater fish contained more n-3

PUFAs, EPA and DHA, than the meat of wild freshwater fish (Li et al., 2011). Fatty acid composition of fishes living in the Mediterranean Sea showed seasonal variation (mackerel: lowest in winter-14.44%, highest in spring-38.27%; European eel: lowest in autumn-7.88%, highest in spring-9.46%; Soriguer et al., 1997).

	LA	ALA
Corn oil*	39.4-65.6	0.5-1.5
Grapeseed oil*	58-78	<1.0
Linseed oil*	17-30	47-55
Olive oil*	3.5-20.0	0.0-1.5
Palm kernel oil*	6.5-12	<0.5
Pumpkin seed oil#	42-57	0-15
Rapeseed oil*	11-23	5-13
Sesame oil*	41.5-47.9	0.3-0.4
Soya bean oil	49.8-57.1	5.5-9.5
Sunflower oil (high LA content)*	65.7	–
Walnut oil*	52.9	10.4

* data modified from Beare-Rogers et al., 2001
# data modified from Erasmus, 1993

Table 1. Fatty acid composition (g fatty acid/100 g fat) of selected vegetable sources, fats and oils

	LA	ALA	AA	DHA
Chicken flesh	26.5	1.1	1.7	0.6
Duck flesh	13.9	1.5	–	–
Heart (beef)	20.9	10.5	0.5	–
Kidney (lamb)	9.7	3.4	6.4	1.5
Kidney (veal)	13.4	1.7	7.8	0.7
Lamb	6.2	0.7	0.7	–
Liver (chicken)	14.0	4.2	0.3	2.0
Liver (pork)	13.6	17.2	1.3	1.0
Milk (cow)	2.6	1.6	–	–
Rabbit	20.2	5.2	–	–
Turkey flesh	24.2	1.3	2.3	0.5
Veal	9.4	0.6	2.3	–
Venison	14.6	3.3	4.7	–

Table 2. Fatty acid composition (g fatty acid/100 g fat) of selected terrestrial animal lipid sources (data modified from Beare-Rogers et al., 2001)

	LA	ALA	AA	DHA
*High fat fishes (>8%)**				
Blue fish, mature (31.3%)*	2.2	n.d.	4.2	13.8
Horse mackerel (12.8%) *	1.1	n.d.	1.4	6.6
Rainbow trout (9.0%)#	5.4	1.4	0.8	10.8
Sardine (11.3%)*	2.2	1.4	2.6	14.7
Striped mullet (11.0%)*	2.7	0.73	3.1	11.7
*Medium fat fishes (4-8%)**				
Anchovy (7.1%)*	2.8	1.4	2.4	16.2
Atlantic mackerel (6.1%)*	2.1	0.68	2.8	25.3
Crucian carp, wild (6.02%)$	11.4	4.0	3.6	5.0
Mackerel (7.45%)#	1.9	2.3	1.7	15.9
Silver carp (5.36%)$	2.4	4.4	4.9	15.5
White herring (6.88%)$	1.2	3.6	2.8	11.8
*Low fat fishes (2-4%)**				
Anchovy (3.49%)#	1.5	2.2	1.4	25.5
Crucian carp, cultured (3.60%)$	17.0	2.6	4.0	6.7
Swordfish (1.93%)#	0.7	1.0	1.1	9.3
Tuna (1.16%)#	2.3	1.3	1.8	16.9

data modified from: * Tanakol et al., 1999 [Black & Marmara Sea]; # Soriguer et al., 1997 [Atlantic Ocean & Mediterranean Sea]; $Li et al., 2011 [East China Sea & Quiantang River]

Table 3. Fat content and fatty acid composition (g fatty acid/100 g fat) of selected sea fishes

2.3 Fatty acids during pregnancy

LCPUFAs play an important role in the maturation of the developing nervous system. AA and DHA are accreted in large amounts into the fetal nervous system: into the cortex and retinal cell membranes during the third trimester of pregnancy and in the first months of life (Farquharson et al., 1992; Martinez & Mougan, 1998). DHA can be predominantly found in the grey matter and retina (Horrocks & Yeo, 1999), while the highest AA content is in the amygdala (Brenna & Diau, 2007). In a primate study (Diau et al., 2005), the highest DHA content was found in globus pallidus (15.8%), while the lowest in the optic nerve (4.5%). AA content was the highest in the amygdale (13.7%) and the lowest in the optic tract (6.8%). Grey matter was richer is both AA and DHA, but there was a discontinuity between grey and white matter DHA concentration, while this great difference wasn't seen in AA concentrations.

The human body has the enzymes needed to synthesise LCPUFAs from their parent essential fatty acids, but the synthesis is a very slow, limited process. In vivo human studies showed that from ALA only a little part is metabolised into EPA and DHA: when supplementing ALA in low dose (<100 mg) only 1.5-7.0% EPA and max. 0.3% DHA were synthesised, while supplementing ALA in high dose (>100 mg) resulted in the synthesis of 0.2-9.0% EPA and 3.8-10.4% DHA. Hence, rise of EPA by 20-100% can be seen in a dose-dependent manner after the administration of ALA. In contrast, the change in DHA values is rather negligible in healthy adults. Similarly, LA supplementation has little effect on AA supply, only ~0.1% of dietary LA is converted to AA in healthy adults (Plourde & Cunnane, 2007).

As AA and DHA play a key role in the fetal and neonatal brain and visual development, several authors investigated whether the fetus and/or the infant is capable to synthesise AA and DHA from LA and ALA, respectively. In an experimental study (Salem et al., 1996), in vivo conversion of EFAs in newborns was investigated. After the administration of deuterium-labeled LA and ALA, deuterium-labeled AA, EPA and DHA appeared in the neonatal blood. However, this capacity can hardly cover the LCPUFA requirement of the developing brain. Two groups of infants with sudden and unexpected death were studied (at the age of 2 to 48 weeks) and significantly higher AA and DHA values were found in erythrocyte and brain cortex lipids in breastfed infants than in infants fed formula that contained only LA and ALA, and the accretion of DHA was correlated with the length of breastfeeding (Makrides et al., 1994).

Since LCPUFA synthesis in the human organism is limited, the most important source of AA and DHA is diet. During pregnancy maternal diet covers the fetal requirements of these fatty acids, while after delivery either maternal diet (breastfeeding) or the independent diet of the infant (formula feeding). In an animal study (Diau et al., 2005), baboon neonates were fed either breastmilk or formula with or without AA and DHA. DHA supplementation restored the DHA supply in the grey matter to breastfed levels, while dietary AA had little effect on brain AA content. In other words: AA seems to be less sensitive to dietary manipulation than DHA.

Maternal diet and metabolism as well as maternal stores are the sources of fetal fatty acid supply. As the ability of the fetus to synthesise LCPUFAs is limited, placenta plays an important role in transferring AA and DHA from mother to the fetus. Several research groups (Berghaus et al., 1998; Gil-Sanchez et al., 2010; Ortega-Senovilla et al., 2009) investigated the differences in maternal and fetal (newborn) blood fatty acid composition and found a higher proportion of LCPUFAs, while lower proportion of the EFAs in the fetal circulation than in the mothers. This phenomenon is called "biomagnification" and may be related to the ability of the placenta to selectively transport LCPUFAs to the fetus. In an in vivo study (Larqué et al., 2003), pregnant women undergoing elective caesarean section received 4 h before delivery an oral dose of ^{13}C-labeled palmitic acid, oleic acid, LA and DHA. Venous blood was taken from the mothers every hour, and cord blood and placental tissues were also collected at delivery. All four fatty acids appeared in the placental tissues and cord blood triacylglycerol (TG) and non-esterified fatty acid (NEFA) lipids, and there was a preferential sequestration of DHA into the placenta. In a recent study (Gil-Sanchez et al., 2010), it was also shown that all labeled fatty acids were enriched in maternal plasma, as well as placental and cord blood lipids. This was the first study that showed a higher ratio of ^{13}C-labeled DHA in cord to maternal plasma. Unesterified fatty acids are transferred to the fetal circulation by both passive diffusion and through a complex, saturable, protein-mediated transport (Koletzko et al., 2007a). There are several fatty acid transfer proteins in the placenta, like fatty acid binding protein (FABP), that preferentially binds LCPUFAs, fatty acid translocase (FAT) and fatty acid transporter protein (FATP) located on both sides of trophoblast cells transporting fatty acids bidirectionally (Cetin et al., 2009). The plasma membrane FABP is located exclusively on the maternal side of membranes and might be involved in the preferential uptake of LCPUFAs by these cells (Koletzko et al., 2007a).

Fish or fish oil intake during pregnancy and lactation improves maternal fatty acid supply and, hence, may enhance fetal DHA concentrations. The increased DHA intake during pregnancy resulted in better visual and neural development in infants at the age of 18 months (Bouwstra et al., 2006), 3.5 years (Williams et al., 2001) and 4 years (Helland et al., 2003), while other studies failed to corroborate these findings (Bakker et al., 2003; Ghys et al., 2002). Because of the beneficial fetal/neonatal effects of n-3 LCPUFAs, for pregnant and lactating women, at least 200 mg/day DHA intake is recommended (Koletzko et al., 2007b).

3. Effect of type 1 diabetes mellitus on fatty acid supply

T1DM disturbs not only the carbohydrate, but also the lipid metabolism. The most extensively studied experimental animal model of T1DM is the alloxane or streptozotocin-induced diabetic rat or mouse. The results of animal studies are quite unequivocal: in diabetic animals significantly higher LA contents were found in liver, renal cortex and heart lipids (Ramsammy et al., 1993), in liver microsomes and erythrocyte membranes (Shin et al., 1995) as well as in plasma, liver and skeletal muscle phospholipids (Mohan & Das, 2001), while its most important metabolite, AA was significantly decreased in diabetic animals. These results can be explained with the diminished activity of $\triangle$-5 (Ramsammy et al., 1993) and $\triangle$-6 desaturase enzymes in T1DM (Ramsammy et al., 1993; Shin et al., 1995). On the basis of these animal studies, insulin is considered as the most potent activator of both $\triangle$-5 and $\triangle$-6 desaturase enzymes (Brenner, 2003).

Human studies are even less unambiguous than animal observations. Some studies found significantly higher LA values in diabetic patients (Decsi et al., 2002, 2007; Tilvis & Miettinen, 1985), while others found no significant differences (Ruiz-Gutierrez et al., 1993; Seigneur et al., 1994). On the other hand, most studies report significantly lower AA (Decsi et al., 2002; Ruiz-Gutierrez et al., 1993) and DHA values (Decsi et al., 2002; Ruiz-Gutierrez et al., 1993; Tilvis & Miettinen, 1985) in diabetic patients than in controls. In one study (Tilvis et al., 1986), diabetic patients treated with continuous insulin infusion therapy had significantly lower LA, and significantly higher AA and DHA values both in plasma and erythrocyte membrane lipids than patients with conventional insulin therapy. These results suggest that better diabetic control may improve the activity of $\triangle$-6 desaturase enzyme.

After a longer period, hyperglycaemia and hypoinsulinemia may lead to several complications in diabetic patients. Several studies investigated the relationship between disturbed fatty acid status in diabetic patients and a number of complications, like diabetic neuropathy, nephropathy and retinopathy. These relationships and the potential role of n-3 fatty acid supplementation in diabetic patients are reviewed elsewhere (Szabó et al., 2010b).

3.1 Fatty acid supply during pregnancy in women with type 1 diabetes mellitus: Maternal effects

T1DM disturbs the fatty acid supply, therefore maternal LCPUFA stores may be compromised compared to healthy pregnant women. Disturbed fatty acid supply and metabolism may influence the course of pregnancy and delivery and may lead both to maternal and fetal complications. Nevertheless, we found only two human studies investigating the fatty acid supply during pregnancy in women with T1DM and four studies investigating fatty acid supply in cord blood lipids of newborns born from mothers with T1DM (Table 4).

Ghebremeskel et al. (Ghebremeskel et al., 2002) induced diabetes with streptozotocin in pregnant rats and investigated the liver fatty acid composition. They found significantly higher essential fatty acid values (ALA and LA) as well as n-3 and n-6 LCPUFA values (AA, EPA, DPA and DHA) in the TG and NEFA fractions. In an earlier study (Chen CH et al.,

1965), only LA was determined and no significant differences were found in plasma NEFA fraction between diabetic and control mothers.

Author	Number	Change in EFAs	Change in LCPUFAs
T1DM: maternal effects			
Chen CH et al., 1965	n = 3	pl. NEFA: LA ↔	no data
Min et al., 2005a	n = 32	pl. TG, CPG: LA, ALA ↔ RBC PC, PE: LA, ALA ↔	pl. CPG: DHA ↓ RBC PC: DPA, DHA ↓ RBC PE: DHA ↓
T1DM: fetal effects			
Chen CH et al., 1965	n = 4	pl. NEFA: LA ↔	no data
Ghebremeskel et al., 2004	n = 31	pl. CPG: LA, ALA ↑ pl. TG: LA, ALA ↓ pl. STE: LA, ALA ↔	pl. CPG: AA, DPA, DHA ↓ pl. TG: DHGLA ↓ pl. STE: AA, DHA ↓
Min et al., 2005a	n = 26	pl. TG: ALA ↓ pl. CPG: LA, ALA ↔ RBC PC, PE: LA, ALA ↔	pl. TG: DHGLA, DPA, DHA ↓ pl. CPG: AA, DHA ↓ RBC PC: AA, DHA ↔ RBC PE: DHA ↓
Winkler et al., 2008*	a.) n = 23 b.) n = 25	a.) RBC PC, PE: LA, ALA ↔ b.) RBC PE: LA, ALA ↑ RBC PC: LA, ALA ↔	a.) RBC PC: DPA ↓ RBC PE: AA, DHA ↔ b.) RBC PE: DHA ↓ RBC PC: AA, DHA ↔

* a.) = age of 3 months; b.) = age of 12 months
Abbreviations: AA: arachidonic acid, ALA: alpha-linolenic acid, CPG: choline phosphoglycerol, DHA: docosahexaenoic acid, DHGLA: dihomo-gamma-linolenic acid, DPA: docosapentaenoic acid, EFAs: essential fatty acids, EPA: eicosapentaenoic acid, LA: linoleic acid, LCPUFAs: long-chain polyunsaturated fatty acids, NEFA: non-esterified fatty acid, PC: phosphatidylcholine, PE: phosphatidylethanolamine, pl.: plasma, PL: phospholipid, RBC: erythrocyte, SM: sphyngomyeline, STE: sterol esther, T1DM: type 1 diabetes mellitus, TG: triacylglycerol

Table 4. Change in essential fatty acid and long-chain polyunsaturated fatty acid values compared to controls in pregnant women with type 1 diabetes mellitus and newborns from mothers with type 1 diabetes mellitus

Plasma and erythrocyte membrane fatty acid composition was studied in women with and without T1DM at midgestation (Min et al., 2005a). In the maternal plasma only choline phosphoglyceride (CPG) DHA was found to be decreased in diabetic patients, while in the erythrocyte membrane lipids more pronounced differences were found. Both the phosphatidylcholine (PC) fraction and in the phosphatidylethanolamine (PE) fraction significantly lower DHA values were found in mothers with T1DM than in healthy pregnant women. The authors hypothesised that this difference might be due to the synergistic effect of diabetes and pregnancy.

3.2 Fatty acid supply in newborns of mothers with type 1 diabetes mellitus: Fetal effects

AA and DHA play an important role in the maturation of the fetal nervous system. Although the developing fetus can synthesise AA and DHA from their precursors, this synthesis is rather slow and can't meet the requirements of the fetus. As T1DM disturbs the fatty acid supply of pregnant women, newborns of mothers with diabetes may have inadequate in utero n-3 and n-6 LCPUFA supply. In contrast to the lack of data on maternal fatty acid supply, cord blood lipids in neonates of mothers with T1DM were published from several studies.

Chen CH et al. (Chen CH et al., 1965) found no differences between cord blood LA values between newborns of diabetic and control mothers. Cord blood of newborns from mothers with T1DM and healthy controls was analysed in detail in an English study (Ghebremeskel et al., 2004). In the plasma CPG fraction there were significantly higher LA and ALA values in cord blood of neonates from diabetic mothers, while their long-chain metabolites, AA and DHA were lower in both plasma CPG and sterin esther (STE) fractions, which may reflect impaired placental transfer of the n-3 and n-6 LCPUFAs. The authors speculated that the effect of T1DM and pregnancy-induced metabolic changes together with the Western diet might have resulted in decreased AA and DHA levels in pregnant women with T1DM.

In another study, cord blood samples of newborns of mothers with T1DM contained significantly lower ALA, DPA and DHA in the plasma TG fraction and significantly lower AA and DHA in the plasma CPG fraction (Min et al., 2005a). However, only DHA values were decreased in the erythrocyte PE fraction in the cord blood of the T1DM group.

In the BABYDIET study, newborns with increased genetic and familiar risk for T1DM were investigated (Winkler et al., 2008). Erythrocyte membrane PC and PE were determined in infants of mothers with and without T1DM at the age of 3 and 12 months. No differences were found in the values of the most important LCPUFAs, AA and DHA in the PC fraction, while significantly lower DPA values were found in the infants of diabetic mothers at the age of 3 months, than in those of the healthy controls. In contrast, comparing only the exclusively breastfed infants of mothers with and without T1DM, no differences were found in the values of n-3 and n-6 PUFAs. At the age of 12 months, infants from mothers with T1DM had significantly higher essential fatty acid (ALA and LA) values, but DHA values were decreased in the PE fraction.

As newborns of mothers with diabetes may have diminished AA and DHA supply, the neurodevelopment of these infants may also be affected. In an experimental animal study (Zhao et al., 2009), diabetes was induced in rats who were divided into two groups, one with good and one with poor diabetic control and were fed either with AA or control diet. After one week the animals were mated and the neurodevelopment of the pups was investigated. Maternal dietary AA supplementation through pregnancy and lactation resulted in improved sensorimotor and developmental performances of the offspring of both healthy controls and poorly controlled diabetic dams. Maternal AA supplementation also improved the AA supply of the offspring's liver, but not in the brain.

Maternal diabetes may disturb fetal fatty acid supply, however, from the epidemiological point of view the longer term effects are more important. Offspring of diabetic mothers may develop different malformations such as spina bifida, at birth they might be macrosomic and develop hypoglycaemia. The potential role of fatty acids in hyperglycaemia-induced teratogenesis was studied in an experimental animal model (Goldman et al., 1985). Diabetic pregnant rats without insulin treatment received subcutaneous AA injection during the period of organogenesis and although maternal glucose concentration didn't change, there was a significant decrease in the incidence of neural tube defects (from 11% to 3.8%), micrognathia (from 7% to 0.8%) and cleft palate (from 11% to 4%). These data suggest that beside good diabetes control also AA supplementation in diabetes might reduce the teratogenetic effect of hyperglycaemia.

4. Effect of gestational diabetes mellitus on fatty acid supply

Gestational diabetes mellitus (GDM) affecting 2-10% of pregnant women in the United States (National Diabetes Statistics, 2011) is associated with insulin resistance during pregnancy. Its prevalence is rising worldwide. Analysing the GDM screening results between 1994-2002 in Colorado state (Dabelea et al., 2005), the prevalence of GDM was increasing from 1994-1996 to 2000-2002 in all ethnic groups: Hispanic (2.8% to 5.1%), African American (2.5% to 4.6%), Asian (6.3% to 8.6%) and non-Hispanic white (1.9% to 3.4%). Women with GDM are at risk to develop type 2 diabetes mellitus either immediately after delivery (5-10%) or later, in 10-20 years (35-60%).

The risk factors of developing GDM during pregnancy are higher pre-pregnancy BMI, smoking, increasing maternal age and GDM during previous pregnancy. Western diet contains high fat intake with high n-6/n-3 fatty acid ratio, refined sugar, fried and snack foods with high *trans* fatty acid content; all these factors may play an important role in developing impaired glucose tolerance and, hence, GDM. Maternal high fat diet during pregnancy decreased EPA and DHA values in liver in newborn pups as well as in suckling pups born from both diabetic and control mothers (Ghebremeskel et al., 1999). In the Project Viva (Radesky et al., 2008), pregnant women with maternal age above 40 years (OR: 11.3), pre-pregnancy BMI above 30 kg/m² (OR: 3.44), GDM during prior pregnancy (OR: 58.3) and Hispanic ethnicity (OR: 3.19) had increased risk of developing GDM. However, dietary pattern during early pregnancy had no association with developing GDM.

4.1 Fatty acid supply during pregnancy in women with gestational diabetes mellitus: Maternal effects

As type 2 diabetes mellitus and obesity disturbs fatty acid supply, GDM may also have an effect on fatty acid metabolism in pregnant women. While only two studies were found investigating the effect of T1DM on maternal blood fatty acid composition, GDM was investigated in a number of studies. We found nine studies investigating the fatty acid supply during pregnancy in women with GDM and five studies investigating the fatty acid supply of newborns from mothers with GDM (Table 5).

In an early study (Chen CH et al., 1965), no difference was seen in LA values of mothers with GDM and controls at delivery. When in 2000 the diet and blood samples of pregnant women with GDM during the third trimester were analysed (Wijendran et al., 2000) women with GDM had significantly higher AA, EPA and DHA intakes than controls. Maternal erythrocyte PL contained more DHA, while other fatty acids didn't differ. The authors also determined the effect of fatty acid supply on plasma PL in these women at the 27-30th, 33-35th and 36-39th weeks of pregnancy (Wijendran et al., 1999). Although there were no significant differences in the LA and AA values between the two groups, values of DHGLA and C22:5n-6 were significantly lower at each investigated time points. In contrast, among the n-3 fatty acids, ALA and DPA were significantly lower, while DHA was significantly higher in women with GDM than in healthy controls. Wijendran et al. provided three possible explanations for the lower ALA and higher DHA values: 1. either increased desaturation and elongation of ALA to DHA may be responsible for these alterations, or 2. increased selective oxidation of ALA or 3. enhanced release of DHA into plasma PL. Both in controls and mothers with GDM, the n-3 and n-6 LCPUFAs decreased as the result of the physiologic adaptation in pregnant women to the increased fetal n-3 and n-6 LCPUFA requirement during the third trimester. The authors also investigated the correlations

Author	Number	Change in EFAs	Change in LCPUFAs
GDM: maternal effects			
Chen CH et al., 1965	n = 8	pl. NEFA: LA ↔	no data
Chen X et al., 2010	n = 49	pl.: LA, ALA ↑	pl.: AA, EPA, DHA ↑
Min et al., 2004	n = 53	pl. CPG: ALA ↓ RBC PC: ALA ↓ RBC PE: ALA ↑	pl. CPG: AA ↑ RBC PC: DHGLA, AA, EPA, DPA, DHA ↓ RBC PE: DHGLA, DPA, DHA ↓
Min et al., 2005b	n = 40	pl. TG: LA, ALA ↔ pl. CPG: ALA ↓ RBC PC, PE: LA, ALA ↔	pl. TG: AA, DHA ↔ pl. CPG: AA ↑ RBC PC: AA ↓ RBC PE: AA, DHA ↔
Min et al., 2006	n = 12	pl. TG: LA, ALA ↔ pl. PC: ALA ↓ pl. SM: LA ↔ RBC PC, PE: LA, ALA ↔ RBC SM: LA ↔	pl. TG: AA, DHA ↔ pl. PC: DHA ↑ pl. SM: AA, DHA ↔ RBC PC: AA ↓ RBC PE: AA ↓ RBC SM: AA, DHA ↔
Ortega-Senovilla et al., 2009	n = 15	pl.: LA, ALA ↔	pl.: AA, DHA ↔
Thomas et al., 2004	n = 44	pl. CPG: ALA ↓ pl. TG: LA ↑ pl. STE: ALA ↓	pl. CPG: AA ↑ pl. TG: DHA ↑ pl. STE: AA ↑
Wijendran et al., 1999	n = 15	pl. PL: ALA ↓	pl. PL: DHGLA, DPA ↓, DHA ↑
Wijendran et al., 2000	n = 13	RBC PL: ALA ↓	RBC PL: DHA ↑
GDM: fetal effects			
Chen CH et al., 1965	n = 9	pl. NEFA: LA ↔	no data
Min et al., 2005b	n = 40	pl. TG: LA, ALA ↓ pl. CPG: LA, ALA ↔ RBC PC, PE: LA, ALA ↔	pl. TG: AA, DHA ↔ pl. CPG: DHA ↓ RBC PC: DHA ↓ RBC PE: AA, DHA ↔
Ortega-Senovilla et al., 2009*	n = 15	a.) pl.: LA, ALA ↔ b.) pl.: LA, ALA ↔	a.) pl.: AA, DHA ↔ b.) pl.: AA, DHA ↓
Thomas et al., 2005	n = 37	pl. TG: ALA ↓ pl. CPG, STE: LA, ALA ↔	pl. CPG: DHGLA, DHA ↓ pl. STE: DHGLA ↓ pl. TG: AA, DHA ↔
Wijendran et al., 2000	n = 13	RBC PL: LA, ALA ↔	RBC PL: AA, DHA ↓

* a.) = umbilical vein; b.) = umbilical artery. Abbreviations: see Table 4.

Table 5. Change in essential fatty acid and long-chain polyunsaturated fatty acid values compared to controls in mothers with gestational diabetes mellitus and infants born from mothers with gestational diabetes mellitus (GDM)

between, on the one hand, maternal fatty acids and on the other hand, HbA$_{1c}$ and prepregnancy BMI. Though there was an inverse association between plasma HbA$_{1c}$ and plasma PL AA also in the controls, this association was more pronounced in women with GDM. Similarly, positive correlation was found between mean fasting plasma insulin and plasma PL AA values. These correlations may indicate impairment in the transport of AA to the fetus. Prepregnancy BMI was correlated inversely to maternal DHA and positively to maternal AA values in the diabetic group. These findings suggest that maternal alterations in plasma PL DHA values may be more pronounced in obese women with GDM.

An English research group (Thomas et al., 2006) investigated the diet of pregnant women with and without GDM during the third trimester, and reported several differences. Diabetic women ingested less fat than controls, and the ratios of fatty acids in the diet were also different: diabetic women had lower saturated, monounsaturated and *trans* fatty acid intake, but higher PUFA intake. Interestingly, the distribution of PUFAs was largely similar in the two groups, only one fatty acid differed between the two groups: mothers with GDM ingested more DHA. They also investigated the effect of ethnicity on dietary fatty acid intake. Afro-Caribbean mothers with GDM had lower total fat, saturated, monounsaturated, *trans* fatty acid and PUFA intake than Caucasian mothers. The diet of the Afro-Caribbean GDM group contained lower LA, AA, n-6 PUFA and ALA values, while higher EPA and DHA compared to Caucasian mothers with GDM.

The same authors also compared the plasma fatty acid supply of these women at diagnosis (Thomas et al., 2004). Women with GDM had significantly higher LA values in the plasma TG fraction, higher AA values in the plasma CPG and STE fraction and higher DHA values in the plasma TG fraction than healthy controls, while ALA was significantly lower in plasma STE in women with GDM. These alterations may be explained by the high glucose concentration that led to the mobilisation of LA, ALA, AA and DHA from adipose tissue and liver. When comparing the fatty acid supply of both plasma and erythrocyte membrane lipids in these women at diagnosis (Min et al., 2004), in plasma CPG higher AA and lower ALA values were found in the mothers with GDM, while values of DHGLA, AA, C22:4n-6 as well as ALA, EPA, DPA and DHA was significantly lower in erythrocyte CPG lipids in the diabetic than in the control group. This discrepancy between plasma and erythrocyte membrane lipid composition may arise as an effect of GDM causing reduction of incorporation of these fatty acids into red blood cells and other tissues. As erythrocyte membrane lipid composition is very similar to that of the vascular endothelium, these alterations in erythrocyte membrane lipids may indicate that endothelium may be also affected in GDM.

In another study carried out in London, significantly lower ALA and higher AA in plasma CPG fraction was found in diabetic mothers than in healthy controls at delivery (Min et al., 2005b). However, AA was significantly lower in erythrocyte membrane PC fraction.

Min et al. carried out a pilot study in Korea, where the habitual diet contains higher n-3 fatty acid and lower total fat intake than the typical Western-type diet (Min et al., 2006). Women with GDM had lower ALA and higher DHA in plasma PC fractions at delivery, while values of AA was lower in erythrocyte PC and PE fractions in women with GDM than in controls. Comparing the AA and DHA values in GDM patients and controls living in Korea or in the UK, in both study groups lower AA and DHA values were found in erythrocyte PC lipids of the GDM groups than in the controls. However, Korean women (both diabetic and control) had higher DHA values than British women. This finding suggests that the reduction of erythrocyte membrane AA and DHA values in women with GDM might be attributed to effects of the disease itself regardless of ethnicity, obesity or diet. In contrast, there were no significant differences in the fatty acid composition of plasma lipids between mothers with GDM and controls at delivery in an Italian study (Ortega-Senovilla et al., 2009).

As part of a prospective cohort study, a nested case-control study was carried out by Chen X et al. (Chen X et al., 2010) to investigate the differences in fatty acid status of women with impaired glucose tolerance, GDM and controls. In contrast to earlier studies (Wijendran et al., 2000; Thomas et al., 2006), this population had higher saturated fatty acid intake, while dietary LA, DHA and PUFA intakes were significantly lower in the diabetic group than in controls. At study entry (16th week) women who developed impaired glucose tolerance later, had higher plasma EPA absolute values; however, the percentage of PUFAs didn't differ significantly among the three groups. During the third trimester, mothers with GDM had higher AA, DHA and PUFA absolute concentrations, while women with impaired glucose tolerance had higher LA, ALA, EPA and DHA absolute values. Similarly to study entry, PUFA percents didn't differ among the groups. These data showed that not only GDM disturbs fatty acid supply of pregnant women, but impaired glucose tolerance as well. The authors also investigated the effect of BMI and found significantly higher concentrations of saturated and monounsaturated fatty acids and PUFAs in women with impaired glucose tolerance and BMI higher than 25 kg/m^2 at study entry than in normal weighted women with impaired glucose tolerance. During the third trimester, overweight and obese women with GDM had the highest fatty acid absolute concentration. These results indicate that the disturbance in the fatty acid metabolism is more pronounced when beyond the mild hyperglycaemia obesity is also present. Results of this study raised the possibility that reducing pregravid weight and modifying diet (increasing PUFAs and reducing saturated fatty acids) may reduce circulating free fatty acids, therefore decreasing insulin resistance and inflammation and lower future maternal risk of type 2 diabetes mellitus.

4.2 Fatty acid supply in newborns of mothers with gestational diabetes mellitus: Fetal effects

Macrosomia and lipid abnormalities are common complications associated with maternal diabetes during pregnancy. Offspring of diabetic mothers are prone to develop obesity, type 2 diabetes mellitus and cardiovascular diseases during adulthood. In an animal study (Soulimane-Mokhtari et al., 2008), diabetic and control rats were fed a control diet or diet rich in EPA and DHA. During pregnancy of the diabetic rats, VLDL- and LDL-cholesterol were significantly decreased in the intervention group. Moreover, similar changes were seen in the macrosomic offspring: maternal fish oil diet significantly decreased VLDL- and LDL-cholesterol. As n-3 LCPUFA supplementation during pregnancy restored tissue lipase activities to normal range and ameliorated long-term prognosis of macrosomia, n-3 fatty acid supplementation may be beneficial for mothers with GDM.

Maternal diabetes during pregnancy (characterised by hyperglycaemia, hyperlipidaemia, hyperlipoproteinaemia and altered T-cell function) may result in metabolic programming of the offspring causing obesity, impaired glucose tolerance, hyperlipidaemia and hyperlipoproteinaemia during adulthood (Khan, 2007). In Chinese children of mothers with GDM, significantly higher systolic and diastolic blood pressures and lower HDL-cholesterol levels were seen than in controls at the age of 8 years. High umbilical cord insulin was an independent risk factor of both abnormal glucose tolerance and obesity; hence, in utero hyperinsulinaemia and hyperglycaemia may have long-term effects on developing type 2 diabetes and metabolic syndrome (Tam et al., 2008). Type 2 diabetes was diagnosed at younger ages if the patients were exposed to maternal diabetes intrauterine, whereas this difference wasn't seen in the onset of type 1 diabetes (Pettitt et al., 2008). This finding suggests, that intrauterine hyperglycaemia predisposes to an earlier onset of type 2 diabetes, while type 1 diabetes is little influenced by the intrauterine milieu.

In the pioneer study published in 1965 by Chen CH et al. (Chen CH et al., 1965) newborns of mothers with GDM were also analysed and no differences were found in LA values between the diabetic and control groups. Wijendran et al. analysed not only the maternal diet and fatty acid composition of maternal erythrocyte PL, but also the fatty acid composition of cord blood erythrocyte membrane lipids (Wijendran et al., 2000). Though in the maternal blood only DHA differed between mothers with GDM and controls, in the cord blood several differences were found. Values of AA and n-6 PUFAs as well as DHA and n-3 PUFAs were significantly lower in the GDM group than in controls. The DHA sufficiency index calculated from DHA divided with C22:5n-6 was also decreased. This impaired AA and DHA supply in cord blood suggested the impaired fetal accretion of these LCPUFAs in pregnancy with GDM. The authors also correlated maternal and fetal fatty acids both in the GDM group and controls. Though in controls significant positive correlations were found between maternal plasma PL AA and DHA and cord blood plasma PL AA and DHA, these correlations were lost in the GDM group. In controls also an enrichment of AA and DHA in fetal erythrocyte was found, while in the GDM group fetal DHA was lower than maternal, and no difference in AA values were found. These alterations raised the possibility that placental transfer of maternal LCPUFAs during the third trimester may be altered in GDM. Maternal HbA$_{1c}$ was also significantly and inversely correlated to fetal AA and DHA values. Although mothers had their HbA$_{1c}$ values between 4-6%, these values were significantly higher than in controls suggesting a moderate impairment of glucose control. This altered glucose control may also have a negative impact on fetal LCPUFA accretion.

Min et al. (Min et al., 2005b) investigated cord blood samples of newborns from mothers with and without GDM in London and found significantly decreased ALA, LA, DHA and AA values in the plasma TG fraction. In contrast, in the plasma CPG fraction only DHA values were significantly lower in the diabetic group. Similarly, in the PC fraction of erythrocyte membrane lipids significantly decreased DHA values were found. This altered cord blood fatty acid supply may suggest the compromised placental fatty acid transport and/or fetal lipid metabolism.

In another English study (Thomas et al., 2005) also significantly lower DHA values were found in the cord blood plasma CPG lipids in the diabetic group. DHGLA was also decreased in plasma CPG and STE fractions. Values of LA, ALA and AA were not significantly different between the two groups in the plasma TG, CPG and STE fractions, but values of AA were reduced. Although mothers with GDM consumed more DHA, their neonates had reduced levels of both DHA and AA, suggesting that mothers with GDM have impaired placental transfer of LCPUFAs. Mead acid, which is considered as an indicator of shortage of EFAs, was increased in the plasma CPG and TG fractions. The elevated Mead acid values in the cord plasma TG and CPG fraction suggested fetal EFA deficiency.

In a recent study (Ortega-Senovilla et al., 2009) umbilical arterial and venous plasma fatty acid composition was analysed in women with GDM and controls who underwent elective caesarean section. While there were no significant differences in umbilical venous blood fatty acids between the two groups, in the umbilical arterial blood significantly lower AA, n-6 PUFA, DHA and n-3 PUFA values were found. Umbilical arterial and venous blood of both

GDM and control groups had lower LA and higher AA and DHA than their mothers. As umbilical venous blood comes from placental capillaries, these higher proportions of AA and DHA in umbilical venous than in maternal blood may indicate that the placental transfer remained unimpaired. However, the decreased n-3 and n-6 LCPUFA values might indicate enhanced utilization of these fatty acids.

4.3 Differences between fatty acid supply in pregnant women with type 1 diabetes mellitus and with gestational diabetes

We found ten studies about fatty acid supply of pregnant women with either T1DM or GDM. Five different research groups performed human investigations: Chen CH et al. from Cleveland, Chen X et al. from New Jersey, Min et al. from London (Min, Thomas), Ortega-Senovilla et al. from Madrid, finally Wijendran et al. from Hartford.

To the best of our knowledge, only one study investigated the LCPUFA supply in pregnant women with T1DM. In this study no differences were found in n-3 and n-6 EFA values, while the most important n-3 metabolite, DHA was lower in all lipid fractions. In GDM most of the studies found decreased or unchanged ALA values, while LA values remained in most cases stable. In case of LCPUFAs, the results are less unambiguous and there was a difference between plasma and erythrocyte LCPUFA values. In general we can say, that plasma LCPUFAs in most cases were higher in mothers with GDM than in controls or it remained unchanged. In contrast, in erythrocyte membrane lipids LCPUFAs were either lower or unchanged in women with GDM compared to healthy controls except for one study (Wijendran et al., 2000).

Although we found only one study about fatty acid supply of pregnant women with T1DM, it seems, that diabetes had no influence on the EFA supply in mothers. In contrast, GDM may diminish EFA supply during pregnancy. T1DM significantly lowered the LCPUFA values in both plasma and erythrocyte membrane lipids, while there was a discrepancy in the effect of GDM: in plasma lipids it rather increased while in erythrocyte membrane lipids decreased the availability of LCPUFAs.

4.4 Differences between fatty acid supply in neonates from mothers with type 1 diabetes mellitus and with gestational diabetes

There were seven human studies investigating the fatty acid supply in cord blood or blood from infants born from mother with either T1DM or GDM. Four different research groups have data about blood lipid fatty acid composition of these offspring: Min et al. from London (Ghebremeskel, Min, Thomas), Ortega-Senovilla et al. from Madrid, Wijendran et al. from Hartford, finally Winkler et al., from Munich.

In contrast to maternal data, four studies investigated the fatty acid composition of newborns or infants of mothers with T1DM. Findings of EFA values are rather unequivocal: values of LA and ALA are either higher or lower or remained unchanged in the T1DM group. However, result are more clear in the case of LCPUFAs, all three studies found significantly lower AA and/or DHA values in plasma lipids, while erythrocyte membrane DHA values were either lower or similar to AA values, they remained unchanged in the offspring of T1DM mothers.

Looking at the results about the effect of GDM, in most cases EFA values remained stable, while LCPUFAs, predominantly DHA was significantly lower in the GDM group. In cord blood there was no deviation between plasma and erythrocyte LCPUFA values: AA and

DHA were either lower or no significantly different in the offspring of GDM mothers than in controls.

To sum it up: T1DM has no clear effect on EFA status of the offspring, while GDM might lower it. In contrast, both T1DM and GDM lowered the availability of LCPUFAs in newborns and infants of diabetic mothers.

5. Conclusion

Data reviewed here indicate that both T1DM and GDM disturb the fatty acid supply in pregnant women and their offspring. Both types of diabetes during pregnancy may result in lower values of n-3 and n-6 LCPUFA in maternal erythrocyte lipids as well as in cord blood plasma and erythrocyte lipids. Therefore incorporation of fatty sea fishes rich in n-3 fatty acids into the diet (e.g. in the form of two 200 g pieces weekly) or other ways of n-3 LCPUFA supplementation during pregnancy may be beneficial.

6. References

Albert, CM., Hennekens, CH., O'Donnell, CJ., Ajani, UA., Carey, VJ., Willett, WC., Ruskin, JN. & Manson, JE. (1998). Fish consumption and risk of sudden cardiac death. *JAMA: The Journal of the American Medical Association*, Vol.279, No.1, (January 1998), pp. 23-28, ISSN 0098-7484

Bakker, EC., Ghys, AJ., Kester, AD., Vles, JS., Dubas, JS., Blanco, CE. & Hornstra, G. (2003). Long-chain polyunsaturated fatty acids at birth and cognitive function at 7 y of age. *European Journal of Clinical Nutrition*, Vol.57, No.1, (January 2003), pp. 89-95, ISSN 0954-3007

Beare-Rogers, J., Dieffenbacher, A. & Holm, JV. (2001). Lexicon of lipid nutrition (IUPAC Technical Report). *Pure and Applied Chemistry*, Vol.73, No.4, (April 2001), pp. 685-744, ISSN 0033-4545

Berghaus, TM., Demmelmair, H. & Koletzko, B. (1998). Fatty acid composition of lipid classes in maternal and cord plasma at birth. *European Journal of Pediatrics*, Vol.157, No.9, (September 1998), pp. 763-768, ISSN 0340-6199

Bouwstra, H., Dijck-Brouwer, J., Decsi, T., Boehm, G., Boersma, ER., Muskiet, FA. & Hadders-Algra, M. (2006). Neurologic condition of healthy term infants at 18 months: positive association with venous umbilical DHA status and negative association with umbilical trans-fatty acids. *Pediatric Research*, Vol.60, No.3, (September 2006), pp. 334-339, ISSN 0031-3998

Brenna, JT. & Diau, GY. (2007). The influence of dietary docosahexaenoic acid and arachidonic acid on central nervous system polyunsaturated fatty acid composition. *Prostaglandins, Leukotrienes, and Essential Fatty Acids*, Vol.77, No.5-6, (November-December 2007), pp. 247-250, ISSN 0952-3278

Brenner, RR. (2003). Hormonal modulation of delta6 and delta5 desaturases: case of diabetes. *Prostaglandins, Leukotrienes, and Essential Fatty Acids*, Vol.68, No.2, (February 2003), pp. 151-162, ISSN 0952-3278

Cetin, I., Alvino, G. & Cardellicchio, M. (2009). Long chain fatty acids and dietary fats in fetal nutrition. *The Journal of Physiology*, Vol.587, No.14, (July 2009), pp. 3441-3451, ISSN 0022-3751

Chen, CH., Adam, PA., Laskowski, DE., McCann, ML. & Schwartz, R. (1965). The plasma free fatty acid composition and blood glucose of normal and diabetic pregnant women and of their newborns. *Pediatrics*, Vol.36, No.6, (December 1965), pp. 843-855, ISSN 0031-4005

Chen, X., Scholl, TO., Leskiw, M., Savaille, J. & Stein, TP. (2010). Differences in maternal circulating fatty acid composition and dietary fat intake in women with gestational diabetes mellitus or mild gestational hyperglycemia. *Diabetes Care*, Vol.33, No.9, (September 2010), pp. 2049-2054, ISSN 0149-5992

Chua, B., Flood, V., Rochtchina, E., Wang, JJ., Smith, W. & Mitchell P. (2006). Dietary fatty acids and the 5-year incidence of age-related maculopathy. *Archives of Ophthalmology*, Vol.124, No.7, (July 2006), pp. 981-986, ISSN 0003-9950

Dabelea, D., Snell-Bergeon, JK., Hartsfield, CL., Bischoff, KJ., Hamman, RF., McDuffie, RS. & Kaiser Permanente of Colorado GDM Screening Program. (2005). Increasing prevalence of gestational diabetes mellitus (GDM) over time and by birth cohort: Kaiser Permanente of Colorado GDM Screening Program. *Diabetes Care*, Vol.28, No.3, (March 2005), pp. 579-584, ISSN 0149-5992

Das, UN. (2006). Essential Fatty acids - a review. *Current Pharmaceutical Biotechnology*, Vol.7, No.6, (December 2006), pp. 467-482, ISSN 1389-2010

Decsi, T., Minda, H., Hermann, R., Kozári, A., Erhardt, E., Burus, I., Molnár, S. & Soltész, G. (2002). Polyunsaturated fatty acids in plasma and erythrocyte membrane lipids of diabetic children. *Prostaglandins, Leukotrienes, and Essential Fatty Acids*, Vol.67, No.4, (October 2002), pp. 203-210, ISSN 0952-3278

Decsi, T., Szabó, É., Burus, I., Marosvölgyi, T., Kozári, A., Erhardt, É. & Soltész, G. (2007). Low contribution of n-3 polyunsaturated fatty acids to plasma and erythrocyte membrane lipids in diabetic young adults. *Prostaglandins, Leukotrienes, and Essential Fatty Acids*, Vol.76, No.3, (March 2007), pp. 159-164, ISSN 0952-3278

Diau, GY., Hsieh, AT., Sarkadi-Nagy, EA., Wijendran, V., Nathanielsz, PW. & Brenna, JT. (2005). The influence of long chain polyunsaturate supplementation on docosahexaenoic acid and arachidonic acid in baboon neonate central nervous system. *BMC Medicine*, Vol.23, No.3, (June 2005), pp. 11-22, ISSN 1741-7015

Dyerberg, J., Eskesen, DC., Andersen, PW., Astrup, A., Buemann, B., Christensen, JH., Clausen, P., Rasmussen, BF., Schmidt, EB., Tholstrup, T., Toft, E., Toubro, S. & Stender, S. (2004). Effects of trans- and n-3 unsaturated fatty acids on cardiovascular risk markers in healthy males. An 8 weeks dietary intervention study. *European Journal of Clinical Nutrition*, Vol.58, No.7, (July 2004), pp. 1062-1070, ISSN 0954-3007

Erasmus, U. (1993). *Fats that Heal, Fats that Kill*, (1st Edition) Alive Books, ISBN 978-0-920470-38-1, Vancouver, Canada

Erkkilä, AT., Lichtenstein, AH., Mozaffarian, D. & Herrington, DM. (2004). Fish intake is associated with a reduced progression of coronary artery atherosclerosis in postmenopausal women with coronary artery disease. *The American Journal of Clinical Nutrition*, Vol.80, No.3, (December 2004), pp. 626-632, ISSN 0002-9165

Farquharson, J., Cockburn, F., Patrick, WA., Jamieson, EC. & Logan, RW. (1992). Infant cerebral cortex phospholipid fatty-acid composition and diet. *Lancet*, Vol.340, No.8823, (October 1992), pp. 810-813, ISSN 0140-6736

Ghebremeskel, K., Bitsanis, D., Koukkou, E., Lowy, C., Poston, L. & Crawford, MA. (1999). Maternal diet high in fat reduces docosahexaenoic acid in liver lipids of newborn and sucking rat pups. *The British Journal of Nutrition*, Vol.81, No.5, (May 1999), pp. 395-404, ISSN 0007-1145

Ghebremeskel, K., Bitsanis, D., Koukkou, E., Lowy, C., Poston, L. & Crawford, MA. (2002). Liver triacylglycerols and free fatty acids in streptozotocin-induced diabetic rats have atypical n-6 and n-3 pattern. *Comparative Biochemistry and Physiology, Toxicology & Pharmacology*, Vol.132, No.3, (July 2002), pp. 349-354, ISSN 1532-0456

Ghebremeskel, K., Thomas, B., Lowy, C., Min, Y. & Crawford, MA. (2004). Type 1 diabetes compromises plasma arachidonic and docosahexaenoic acids in newborn babies. *Lipids*, Vol.39, No.4, (April 2004), pp. 335-342, ISSN 0024-4201

Ghys, A., Bakker, E., Hornstra, G. & van den Hout, M. (2002). Red blood cell and plasma phospholipid arachidonic and docosahexaenoic acid levels at birth and cognitive development at 4 years of age. *Early Human Development*, Vol.69, No.1-2, (October 2002), pp. 83-90, ISSN 0378-3782

Gil-Sánchez, A., Larqué, E., Demmelmair, H., Acien, MI., Faber, FL., Parrilla, JJ. & Koletzko, B. (2010). Maternal-fetal in vivo transfer of [13C]docosahexaenoic and other fatty acids across the human placenta 12 h after maternal oral intake. *The American Journal of Clinical Nutrition*, Vol.92, No.1, (July 2010), pp. 115-122, ISSN 0002-9165

Goldman, AS., Baker, L., Piddington, R., Marx, B., Herold, R. & Egler, J. (1985). Hyperglycemia-induced teratogenesis is mediated by a functional deficiency of arachidonic acid. *Proceedings of the National Academy of Sciences of the United States of America*, Vol.82, No.23, (December 1985), pp. 8227-8231, ISSN 0027-8424

Helland, IB., Smith, L., Saarem, K., Saugstad, OD. & Drevon, CA. (2003). Maternal supplementation with very-long-chain n-3 fatty acids during pregnancy and lactation augments children's IQ at 4 years of age. *Pediatrics*, Vol.111, No.1, (January 2003), pp. e39-44, ISSN 0031-4005

Horrocks, LA. & Yeo, YK. (1999). Health benefits of docosahexaenoic acid (DHA). *Pharmacological Research: the Official Journal of the Italian Pharmacological Society*, Vol.40, No.3, (September 1999), pp. 211-225, ISSN 1043-6618

Ibrahim, A., Natrajan, S. & Ghafoorunissa, R. (2005). Dietary trans-fatty acids alter adipocyte plasma membrane fatty acid composition and insulin sensitivity in rats. *Metabolism: Clinical and Experimental*, Vol.54, No.2, (February 2005), pp. 240-246, ISSN 0026-0495

Iso, H., Kobayashi, M., Ishihara, J., Sasaki, S., Okada, K., Kita, Y., Kokubo, Y., Tsugane, S. & JPHC Study Group. (2006). Intake of fish and n3 fatty acids and risk of coronary heart disease among Japanese: the Japan Public Health Center-Based (JPHC) Study Cohort I. *Circulation*, Vol.113, No.2, (January 2006), pp. 195-202, ISSN 0009-7322

Katan, MB., Zock, PL. & Mensink, RP. (1995). Trans fatty acids and their effects on lipoproteins in humans. *Annual Review of Nutrition*, Vol.15, (July 1995), pp. 473-493, ISSN 0199-9885

Khan, NA. (2007). Role of lipids and fatty acids in macrosomic offspring of diabetic pregnancy. *Cell Biochemistry and Biophysics*, Vol.48, No.2-3, (July 2007), pp. 79-88, ISSN 1085-9195

Koletzko, B. & Rodriguez-Palmero, M. (1999). Polyunsaturated fatty acids in human milk and their role in early infant development. *Journal of Mammary Gland Biology and Neoplasia*, Vol.4, No.3, (July 1999), pp. 269-284, ISSN 1083-3021

Koletzko, B., Larqué, E. & Demmelmair, H. (2007a). Placental transfer of long-chain polyunsaturated fatty acids (LC-PUFA). *Journal of Perinatal Medicine*, Vol.35, No.Suppl 1, (February 2007), pp. S5-11, ISSN 0300-5577

Koletzko, B., Cetin, I., Brenna, JT., Perinatal Lipid Intake Working Group; Child Health Foundation; Diabetic Pregnancy Study Group; European Association of Perinatal Medicine; European Society for Clinical Nutrition and Metabolism; European Society for Paediatric Gastroenterology, Hepatology and Nutrition, Committee on Nutrition; International Federation of Placenta Associations; & International Society for the Study of Fatty Acids and Lipids. (2007b). Dietary fat intakes for pregnant and lactating women. *The British Journal of Nutrition*, Vol.98, No.5, (November 2007), pp. 873-877, ISSN 0007-1145

Laidlaw, M. & Holub, BJ. (2003). Effects of supplementation with fish oil-derived n-3 fatty acids and gamma-linolenic acid on circulating plasma lipids and fatty acid profiles in women. *The American Journal of Clinical Nutrition*, Vol.77, No.1, (January 2003), pp. 37-42, ISSN 0002-9165

Larqué, E., Demmelmair, H., Berger, B., Hasbargen, U. & Koletzko, B. (2003). In vivo investigation of the placental transfer of (13)C-labeled fatty acids in humans. *Journal of Lipid Research*, Vol.44, No.1, (January 2003), pp. 49-55, ISSN 0022-2275

Li, G., Sinclair, AJ. & Li, D. (2011). Comparison of lipid content and fatty acid composition in the edible meat of wild and cultured freshwater and marine fish and shrimps from China. *Journal of Agricultural and Food Chemistry*, Vol.59, No.5, (March 2011), pp. 1871-1881, ISSN 0021-8561

Louheranta, AM., Turpeinen, AK., Vidgren, HM., Schwab, US. & Uusitupa, MI. (1999). A high-trans fatty acid diet and insulin sensitivity in young healthy women. *Metabolism: Clinical and Experimental*, Vol.48, No.7, (July 1999), pp. 870-875, ISSN 0026-0495

Makrides, M., Neumann, MA., Byard, RW., Simmer, K. & Gibson, RA. (1994). Fatty acid composition of brain, retina, and erythrocytes in breast- and formula-fed infants. *The American Journal of Clinical Nutrition*, Vol.60, No.2, (August 1994), pp. 189-194, ISSN 0002-9165

Martínez, M. & Mougan, I. (1998). Fatty acid composition of human brain phospholipids during normal development. *Journal of Neurochemistry*, Vol.71, No.6, (December 1998), pp. 2528- 2533, ISSN 0022-3042

Min, Y., Ghebremeskel, K., Lowy, C., Thomas, B. & Crawford, MA. (2004). Adverse effect of obesity on red cell membrane arachidonic and docosahexaenoic acids in gestational diabetes. *Diabetologia*, Vol.47, No.1, (January 2004), pp. 75-81, ISSN 0012-186X

Min, Y., Lowy, C., Ghebremeskel, K., Thomas, B., Offley-Shore, B. & Crawford, M. (2005a). Unfavorable effect of type 1 and type 2 diabetes on maternal and fetal essential fatty acid status: a potential marker of fetal insulin resistance. *The American Journal of Clinical Nutrition*, Vol.82, No.6, (December 2005), pp. 1162-1168, ISSN 0002-9165

Min, Y., Lowy, C., Ghebremeskel, K., Thomas, B., Bitsanis, D. & Crawford, MA. (2005b). Fetal erythrocyte membrane lipids modification: preliminary observation of an early sign of compromised insulin sensitivity in offspring of gestational diabetic women. *Diabetic Medicine: a Journal of the British Diabetic Association*, Vol.22, No.7, (July 2005), pp. 914-920, ISSN 0742-3071

Min, Y., Nam, JH., Ghebremeskel, K., Kim, A. & Crawford, M. (2006). A distinctive fatty acid profile in circulating lipids of Korean gestational diabetics: a pilot study. *Diabetes Research and Clinical Practice*, Vol.73, No.2, (August 2006), pp. 178-183, ISSN 0168-8227

Mohan, IK. & Das, UN. (2001). Prevention of chemically induced diabetes mellitus in experimental animals by polyunsaturated fatty acids. *Nutrition*, Vol.17, No.2, (February 2001), pp. 126-151, ISSN 0899-9007

Morris, MC., Evans, DA., Bienias, JL., Tangney, CC., Bennett, DA., Wilson, RS., Aggarwal, N. & Schneider, J. (2003). Consumption of fish and n-3 fatty acids and risk of incident Alzheimer disease. *Archives of Neurology*, Vol.60, No.7, (July 2003), pp. 940-946, ISSN 0003-9942

Mozaffarian, D., Psaty, BM., Rimm, EB., Lemaitre, RN., Burke, GL., Lyles, MF., Lefkowitz, D. & Siscovick, DS. (2004). Fish intake and risk of incident atrial fibrillation. *Circulation*, Vol.110, No.4, (July 2004), pp. 368-373, ISSN 0009-7322

Mozaffarian, D., Ascherio, A., Hu, FB., Stampfer, MJ., Willett, WC., Siscovick, DS. & Rimm, EB. (2005). Interplay between different polyunsaturated fatty acids and risk of coronary heart disease in men. *Circulation*, Vol.111, No.2, (January 2005), pp. 157-164, ISSN 0009-7322

Murano, Y., Funabashi, T., Sekine, S., Aoyama, T. & Takeuchi, H. (2007). Effect of dietary lard containing higher alpha-linolenic acid on plasma triacylglycerol in rats. *Journal of Oleo Science*, Vol.56, No.7, (July 2007), pp. 361-367, ISSN 1345-8957

National Diabetes Statistics, 2011, Available from http://diabetes.niddk.nih.gov/dm/pubs/statistics/

Nikkari, T., Räsänen, L., Viikari, J., Akerblom, HK., Vuori, I., Pyörälä, K., Uhari, M., Dahl, M., Lähde, PL., Pesonen, E. & Suoninen, P. (1983). Serum fatty acids in 8-year-old Finnish boys: correlations with qualitative dietary data and other serum lipids. *The American Journal of Clinical Nutrition*, Vol.37, No.5, (May 1983), pp. 848-854, ISSN 0002-9165

Noaghiul, S. & Hibbeln, JR. (2003). Cross-national comparisons of seafood consumption and rates of bipolar disorders. *The American Journal of Psychiatry*, Vol.160, No.12, (December 2003), pp. 2222-2227, ISSN 0002-953X

Norris, JM., Yin, X., Lamb, MM., Barriga, K., Seifert, J., Hoffman, M., Orton, HD., Barón, AE., Clare-Salzler, M., Chase, HP., Szabo, NJ., Erlich, H., Eisenbarth, GS. & Rewers, M. (2007). Omega-3 polyunsaturated fatty acid intake and islet autoimmunity in children at increased risk for type 1 diabetes. *JAMA : the Journal of the American Medical Association*, Vol.298, No.12, (September 2007), pp. 1420-1428, ISSN 0098-7484

Ortega-Senovilla, H., Alvino, G., Taricco, E., Cetin, I. & Herrera, E. (2009). Gestational diabetes mellitus upsets the proportion of fatty acids in umbilical arterial but not venous plasma. *Diabetes Care*, Vol.32, No.1, (January 2009), pp. 120-122, ISSN 0149-5992

Pettitt, DJ., Lawrence, JM., Beyer, J., Hillier, TA., Liese, AD., Mayer-Davis, B., Loots, B., Imperatore, G., Liu, L., Dolan, LM., Linder, B. & Dabelea, D. (2008). Association between maternal diabetes in utero and age at offspring's diagnosis of type 2 diabetes. *Diabetes Care*, Vol.31, No.11, (November 2008), pp. 2126-2130, ISSN 0149-5992

Plourde, M. & Cunnane, SC. (2007). Extremely limited synthesis of long chain polyunsaturates in adults: implications for their dietary essentiality and use as supplements. *Applied Physiology, Nutrition, and Metabolism*, Vol.32, No.4, (August 2007), pp. 619-634, ISSN 1715-5312

Racine, RA. & Deckelbaum, RJ. (2007). Sources of the very-long-chain unsaturated omega-3 fatty acids: eicosapentaenoic acid and docosahexaenoic acid. *Current Opinion in Clinical Nutrition & Metabolic Care*, Vol.10, No.2, (March 2007), pp. 123-128, ISSN 1363-1950

Radesky, JS., Oken, E., Rifas-Shiman, SL., Kleinman, KP., Rich-Edwards, JW. & Gillman, MW. (2008). Diet during early pregnancy and development of gestational diabetes. *Paediatric and Perinatal Epidemiology*, Vol.22, No.1, (January 2008), pp. 47-59, ISSN 0269-5022

Ramsammy, LS., Haynes, B., Josepovitz, C. & Kaloyanides, GJ. (1993). Mechanism of decreased arachidonic acid in the renal cortex of rats with diabetes mellitus. *Lipids*, Vol.28, No.5, (May 1993), pp. 433-439, ISSN 0024-4201

Ruiz-Gutierrez, V., Stiefel, P., Villar, J., García-Donas, MA., Acosta, D. & Carneado, J. (1993). Cell membrane fatty acid composition in type 1 (insulin-dependent) diabetic patients: relationship with sodium transport abnormalities and metabolic control. *Diabetologia*, Vol. 36, No.9, (September 1993), pp. 850-856, ISSN 0012-186X

Salem, N. Jr., Wegher, B., Mena P. & Uauy, R. (1996). Arachidonic and docosahexaenoic acids are biosynthesized from their 18-carbon precursors in human infants. *Proceedings of the National Academy of Sciences of the United States of America*, Vol.93, No.1, (January 1996), pp. 49-54, ISSN 0027-8424

Schaefer, EJ., Bongard, V., Beiser, AS., Lamon-Fava, S., Robins, SJ., Au, R., Tucker, KL., Kyle, DJ., Wilson, PW. & Wolf, PA. (2006). Plasma phosphatidylcholine docosahexaenoic acid content and risk of dementia and Alzheimer disease: the Framingham Heart Study. *Archives of Neurology*, Vol.63, No.11, (November 2006), pp. 1545-1550, ISSN 0003-9942

Seigneur, M., Freyburger, G., Gin, H., Claverie, M., Lardeau, D., Lacape, G., Le Moigne, F., Crockett, R. & Boisseau, MR. (1994). Serum fatty acid profiles in type I and type II diabetes: metabolic alterations of fatty acids of the main serum lipids. *Diabetes Research and Clinical Practice*, Vol.23, No.3, (April 1994), pp. 169-177, ISSN 0168-8227

Shin, CS., Lee, MK., Park, KS., Kim, SY., Cho, BY., Lee, HK., Koh, CS. & Min, HK. (1995). Insulin restores fatty acid composition earlier in liver microsomes than erythrocyte membranes in streptozotocin-induced diabetic rats. *Diabetes Research and Clinical Practice*, Vol.29, No.2, (August 1995), pp. 93-98, ISSN 0168-8227

Soriguer, F., Serna, S., Valverde, E., Hernando, J., Martín-Reyes, A., Soriguer, M., Pareja, A., Tinahones, F. & Esteva, I. (1997). Lipid, protein, and calorie content of different Atlantic and Mediterranean fish, shellfish, and molluscs commonly eaten in the south of Spain. *European Journal of Epidemiology*, Vol.13, No.4, (June 1997), pp. 451-563, ISSN 0393-2990

Soulimane-Mokhtari, NA., Guermouche, B., Saker, M., Merzouk, S., Merzouk, H., Hichami, A., Madani, S., Khan, NA. & Prost, J. (2008). Serum lipoprotein composition, lecithin cholesterol acyltransferase and tissue lipase activities in pregnant diabetic rats and their offspring receiving enriched n-3 PUFA diet. *General Physiology and Biophysics*, Vol.27, No.1, (March 2008), pp. 3-11, ISSN 0231-5882

Sun, Q., Ma, J., Campos, H., Hankinson, SE., Manson, JE., Stampfer, MJ., Rexrode, KM., Willett, WC. & Hu, FB. (2007). A prospective study of trans fatty acids in erythrocytes and risk of coronary heart disease. *Circulation*, Vol.115, No.14, (April 2007), pp. 1858-1865, ISSN 0009-7322

Szabó, É., Boehm, G., Beermann, C., Weyermann, M., Brenner, H., Rothenbacher, D. & Decsi, T. (2007). trans Octadecenoic acid and trans octadecadienoic acid are inversely related to long-chain polyunsaturates in human milk: results of a large birth cohort study. *The American Journal of Clinical Nutrition*, Vol.85, No.5, (May 2007), pp. 1320-1326, ISSN 0002-9165

Szabó, É., Boehm, G., Beermann, C., Weyermann, M., Brenner, H., Rothenbacher, D. & Decsi, T. (2010a). Fatty acid profile comparisons in human milk sampled from the same mothers at the sixth week and the sixth month of lactation. *Journal of Pediatric Gastroenterology and Nutrition*, Vol.50, No.3, (March 2010), pp. 316-320. ISSN 0277-2116

Szabó, É., Soltész, Gy. & Decsi, T. (2010b). Long-chain polyunsaturated fatty acid supply in diabetes mellitus, In: *Handbook of Type 1 Diabetes Mellitus*, L. Aucoin, T. Prideux (Ed.), pp. 265-295, Nova Science Publishers Inc., ISBN: 978-1-60741-311-0, New York, USA

Tam, WH., Ma, RC., Yang, X., Ko, GT., Tong, PC., Cockram, CS., Sahota, DS., Rogers, MS. & Chan, JC. (2008). Glucose intolerance and cardiometabolic risk in children exposed to maternal gestational diabetes mellitus in utero. *Pediatrics*, Vol.122, No.6, (December 2008), pp. 1229-1234, ISSN 0031-4005

Tanakol, R., Yazici, Z., Sener, E. & Sencer, E. (1999). Fatty acid composition of 19 species of fish from the Black Sea and the Marmara Sea. *Lipids*, Vol.34, No.3, (March 1999), pp. 291-297, ISSN 0024-4201

Thomas, B., Ghebremeskel, K., Lowy, C., Min, Y. & Crawford, MA. (2004). Plasma AA and DHA levels are not compromised in newly diagnosed gestational diabetic women. *European Journal of Clinical Nutrition*, Vol.58, No.11, (November 2004), pp. 1492-1497, ISSN 0954-3007

Thomas, B., Ghebremeskel, K., Lowy, C., Offley-Shore, B. & Crawford, MA. (2005). Plasma fatty acids of neonates born to mothers with and without gestational diabetes. *Prostaglandins, Leukotrienes, and Essential Fatty Acids*, Vol.72, No.5, (May 2005), pp. 335-341, ISSN 0952-3278

Thomas, B., Ghebremeskel, K., Lowy, C., Crawford, M. & Offley-Shore, B. (2006). Nutrient intake of women with and without gestational diabetes with a specific focus on fatty acids. *Nutrition*, Vol.22, No.3, (March 2006), pp. 230-236, ISSN 0899-9007

Tilvis, RS. & Miettinen, TA. (1985). Fatty acid compositions of serum lipids, erythrocytes, and platelets in insulin-dependent diabetic women. *The Journal of Clinical Endocrinology and Metabolism*, Vol.61, No.4, (October 1985), pp. 741-745, ISSN 0021-972X

Tilvis, RS., Helve, E. & Miettinen, TA. (1986). Improvement of diabetic control by continuous subcutaneous insulin infusion therapy changes fatty acid composition of serum lipids and erythrocytes in type 1 (insulin-dependent) diabetes. *Diabetologia*, Vol.29, No.10, (October 1986), pp. 690-694, ISSN 0012-186X

Vidgren, HM., Louheranta, AM., Agren, JJ., Schwab, US. & Uusitupa, MI. (1998). Divergent incorporation of dietary trans fatty acids in different serum lipid fractions. *Lipids*, Vol.33, No.10, (October 1998), pp. 955-962, ISSN 0024-4201

Wijendran, V., Bendel, RB., Couch, SC., Philipson, EH., Thomsen, K., Zhang, X. & Lammi-Keefe, CJ. (1999). Maternal plasma phospholipid polyunsaturated fatty acids in pregnancy with and without gestational diabetes mellitus: relations with maternal factors. *The American Journal of Clinical Nutrition*, Vol.70, No.1, (July 1999), pp. 53-61, ISSN 0002-9165

Wijendran, V., Bendel, RB., Couch, SC., Philipson, EH., Cheruku, S. & Lammi-Keefe, CJ. (2000). Fetal erythrocyte phospholipid polyunsaturated fatty acids are altered in pregnancy complicated with gestational diabetes mellitus. *Lipids*, Vol.35, No.8, (August 2000), pp. 927-931, ISSN 0024-4201

Williams, C., Birch, EE., Emmett, PM., Northstone, K. & Avon Longitudinal Study of Pregnancy and Childhood Study Team. (2001). Stereoacuity at age 3.5 y in children born full-term is associated with prenatal and postnatal dietary factors: a report from a population-based cohort study. *The American Journal of Clinical Nutrition*, Vol.73, No.2, (February 2001), pp. 316-322, ISSN 0002-9165

Winkler, C., Hummel, S., Pflüger, M., Ziegler, AG., Geppert, J., Demmelmair, H. & Koletzko, B. (2008). The effect of maternal T1DM on the fatty acid composition of erythrocyte phosphatidylcholine and phosphatidylethanolamine in infants during early life. *European Journal of Nutrition*, Vol.47, No.3, (April 2008), pp. 145-152, ISSN 1436-6207

Yen, CH., Dai, YS., Yang, YH., Wang, LC., Lee, JH. & Chiang, BL. (2008). Linoleic acid metabolite levels and transepidermal water loss in children with atopic dermatitis. *Annals of Allergy, Asthma & Immunology : Official Publication of the American College of*

Allergy, Asthma, & Immunology, Vol.100, No.1, (January 2008), pp. 66-73, ISSN 1081-1206

Yuan, JM., Ross, RK., Gao, YT. & Yu, MC. (2001). Fish and shellfish consumption in relation to death from myocardial infarction among men in Shanghai, China. *American Journal of Epidemiology*, Vol.154, No.9, (November 2001), pp. 809-816, ISSN 0002-9262

Zhao, J., Del Bigio, MR. & Weiler, HA. (2009). Maternal arachidonic acid supplementation improves neurodevelopment of offspring from healthy and diabetic rats. *Prostaglandins, Leukotrienes, and Essential Fatty Acids*, Vol.81, No.5-6, (November-December 2009), pp. 349-356, ISSN 0952-3278

10

Therapeutic Modelling of Type 1 Diabetes

Nilam Nilam[1], Seyed M. Moghadas[2] and Pappur N. Shivakumar[3]

[1]Department of Mathematics, Delhi Technological University, Delhi
[2]Centre for Disease Modelling, York University, Toronto, Ontario
[3]Department of Mathematics, University of Manitoba, Winnipeg, Manitoba
[1]India
[2,3]Canada

1. Introduction

In this Chapter, we are mainly concerned with mathematical modelling (using differential equations) of controlled continuous subcutaneous infusion of insulin in Type 1 diabetes using pumps. It occurs mainly in children where controlling levels of sugar is entirely dependent on external infusion of insulin. Type I diabetes is a result of loss of beta-cell functions in the body due to an autoimmune reaction There is vast literature concerning continuous infusion of insulin where feedback is intermittent and the dosage is adhoc. Other ways of combating Type I diabetes include transplantation of insulin producing tissues or introducing artificial beta cells. We mathematically model the sugar concentration in the body and use it to dovetail a previously medically prescribed sugar concentration curve. The modelling, for the first time, aids the continuous infusion of insulin based upon individuals requirements in terms of the curve of decay of sugar concentration in a prescribed time. For each individual, depending on many personal factors like obesity, age, kidney functions, etc., a prescription is made of the desirable curve of sugar concentration from its highest level to the desired lowest level in a given period of time. This fine tunes the delivery of insulin as it takes away much guesswork of amounts of insulin given intermittently or continuously. Devices attached to continuous monitoring device will infuse insulin continuously and as per prescribed curve of reduction of sugar concentration. Thus, the pumps delivery takes into consideration the time profile of the insulin release, with the release stopping after the prescribed values are attained. The amount released in a dual wave shaped insulin bolus combining [8] both the usual normal and square wave methods. The therapy described will be the forerunner of intense clinical research work.Mathematical models with numerical simulations and analysis based on experimental data can be more effective in terms of costs and an extraordinary amount of time dealing with diverse physiological situations. This is particularly so in view of the complexities of the functions in the human body and incomplete existing knowledge.

This chapter provides an overview of mathematical modelling of type 1 diabetes, with particular focus on pump therapy as a management strategy for continuous subcutaneous insulin infusion. Previous models describing the mechanism of glucose metabolism have mostly focused on type 2 diabetes, most notably the classical minimal model for explaining the profile of glucose concentration over time.[4,5] Here we summarize the conclusions of these studies for management of diabetes, and attempt to lay out a framework for further development of these models to include pump therapy. These models are often formulated as a system of differential equations that describes the profile of insulin release and the dynamics of glucose concentration over specified period of time. In addition to providing background on existing modelling frameworks, the practical implications of their outputs are discussed.

The main goals are (a) formulation of the model using the pump mechanism (b) defining the parameters (c) profiling the insulin release (d) simulating using estimated parameter values and (e) modelling extensions to include obesity as it had been well established that obesity promotes insulin resistance through the inappropriate inactivation of a process called gluconeogenesis, where the liver creates glucose for fuel. The model consists of blood glucose concentration, remote insulin action and amount of insulin. The model predictions include insulin secreted, if any, in pancreas, role of other organs, tissue uptake etc. This chapter closes with future direction in mathematical modelling of type 1 diabetes for optimal usage of external insulin and measuring insulin dependency with an insight into the role of obesity in developing diabetes.

2. Diabetes

2.1 What is diabetes?

Diabetes is a global problem with devastating human, social and economic impact. Diabetes is a growing epidemic threatening to overwhelm global healthcare services, wipe out some indigenous populations and undermine economies worldwide, especially in developing countries. Today more than 250 million people worldwide are living with diabetes and by 2025, this total is expected to increase to over 380 million people. Approximately 24 million people are diabetics in United States which is about 8 percent of the total population. The number of people with diabetes is increasing due to population growth, aging, urbanization, and increasing prevalence of obesity and physical inactivity. Diabetes is a highly prevalent disease in India where more than 35 million people suffer from diabetes. Alarmingly, as much as 13 million cases remains undiagnosed which leads to long term complications. The prevalence of diabetes is greater amongst the urban South Asian population (12-15%) compared to urban population in the West (6%).[9] That is why Diabetes has been one of the most important subjects for biomedical research for many years.

Diabetes Mellitus, commonly referred to as Diabetes, means sweet urine. Consistently elevated levels of blood glucose lead to spillage to glucose into urine, hence the term sweet urine. When the blood sugar level consistently runs too high in our blood stream, the condition is named as Diabetes. In patients with Diabetes Mellitus, the absence or insufficient production of insulin by the liver causes hyperglycemia. Diabetes Mellitus is a syndrome characterized by chronic hyperglycemia resulting from absence or relative impairment in insulin secretion and/or insulin action. It can also be referred to as a condition characterized by the disturbances of carbohydrate, protein and fat metabolism, the way our bodies use digested food for growth and energy. The chronic hyperglycemia of diabetes is associated with long term damage, dysfunction and failure of various organs, especially the eyes, kidneys, nerves, heart and blood vessels.[7] Diabetes is the most common endocrine disorder. It is a chronic medical condition meaning it can last a lifetime which can be controlled but can not be cured completely.

Human body functions best at a certain level of sugar in the blood stream. Blood sugar levels are tightly controlled by insulin, the principal hormone that makes it possible for many cells (primarily muscle and fat cells) to use glucose from the blood. It is manufactured by the beta cells of the pancreatic islets of Langerhans, a small section of the pancreas. Secretion of insulin primarily occurs in response to increased concentration of glucose in the blood. Insulin helps the glucose from food get into the body cells. If body does not make enough insulin or if the insulin does not work the way it should, glucose can not get into the cells. It stays in the blood instead and blood glucose level gets too high causing to have Diabetes. Deficiency of insulin or its action plays a central role in all forms of diabetes. There are three major forms of diabetes:[18]

2.1.1 Type 1 diabetes

Type 1 diabetes is one of the most challenging medical disorder because of the demands it imposes on day-to-day life. It was formerly known as insulin dependent diabetes mellitus (IDDM) or juvenile onset diabetes mellitus.

In this type of diabetes, the pancreas undergoes an autoimmune attack by the body itself and is rendered incapable of making insulin. It is an autoimmune disorder, in which body's own immune system attacks the beta cells in the islets of Langerhans of the pancreas destroying them or damaging them sufficiently to reduce insulin production. The pancreas then produces little or no insulin. At present, scientists do not know exactly what causes the body's immune system to attack the beta cells, but it is believed that autoimmune, genetic, and environmental factors, possibly viruses, are involved. It develops most often in children and young adults, but can appear at any age.Type 1 diabetes, which predominately affects youth, is rising alarmingly worldwide, at a rate of 3% per year. Some 70,000 children worldwide are expected to develop type 1 diabetes annually. If not diagnosed and treated with insulin, a person with type 1 diabetes can lapse into a life-threatening diabetic coma, also known as diabetic ketoacidosis.

2.1.2 Type 2 diabetes

Type 2 diabetes, formerly called adult-onset diabetes or non-insulin- dependent diabetes mellitus (NIDDM), is the most common form of diabetes. Type 2 diabetes is responsible for 90 -95% of diabetes cases and is increasing at alarming rates globally as a result of increased urbanization, high rates of obesity, sedentary lifestyles and stress. Type 2 diabetes is increasingly being diagnosed in children and adolescents though it can occur at any age. Millions of people don't even know they have it because it can arise with minimal outward signs or symptoms. It is diagnosed with insulin resistance in which the pancreas is producing enough insulin but for unknown reasons, the body can not use the insulin effectively. This leads to a situation similar to type 1 diabetes in which the pancreas can't secrete enough insulin because of which glucose builds up in the blood and the body cannot make efficient use of its main source of fuel. This form of diabetes is associated with obesity, older age, a family history of diabetes, a history of gestational diabetes, certain medications, impaired glucose metabolism, psychological factors, and physical inactivity. Type 2 diabetes can be controlled with exercise, diet and lifestyle modifications.[6] This type of diabetes may develop microvascular complications, which may lead to retinopathy, nephropathy and peripheral and autonomic nephropathies, and macrovascular complications include atherosclerotic coronary and peripheral arterial disease.

2.1.3 Gestational diabetes

This type of diabetes develops just before or during the pregnancy. Though the patient may have diabetes before the onset of the pregnancy, it is termed gestational only if it is first identified after the pregnancy has occurred. Gestational diabetes is caused by the hormones of pregnancy which is produced when the placenta supports the growing fetus. These hormones may interfere with the mother's ability to produce and use her own insulin. Usually this form of diabetes goes away after the delivery but women who have had gestational diabetes have a 20 to 50 percent chance of developing type 2 diabetes within 5 to 10 years especially those who require insulin during pregnancy and those who are overweight. Untreated Gestational Diabetes Mellitus (GDM) can lead to fetal macrosomia, hypoglycemia, hypocalcemia and hyperbilirubinemia. Also chances of cesarean delivery and chronic hypertension increases in women with GDM.

2.2 History and causes of diabetes

Diabetes is not a newly born disease, it has been with human race from long back but, we came to knew about it in 1552 B.C. Since after than, many of Greek as well French **physicians** had worked on it and threw some light on the nature of disease, organs responsible for it etc. Diabetes was recognized and categorized with complete details and its types, Type 1and Type 2 in 1959. In 1870s, a French physician had discovered a link between Diabetes and diet intake, and then diabetic diet was formulated with inclusion of milk, oats and other fiber containing foods in 1900-1915. Dr. Frederick Banting, Prof. Macleod and Dr. Collip discovered the function of **insulin**, its nature, along with its use started at the University of Toronto from 1920 -1923, who were awarded a Noble prize. In 1922, 14 year old Leonard Thompson becomes the first human to receive insulin. In the decade of 1940, it has been discovered that different organs like kidney and skin are also affected if diabetes is creeping from a long term. A major turn in this **research** was in 1955, when the oral hypogycemic drugs had been manufactured. Paul E. Lacy, a JDRF – funded researcher at Washington University School of Medicine performs the first successful islets transplantation in diabetic animal models in 1976. The first experimental insulin pump was developed in 1979 which leads to further refined pumps to provide the infusion of insulin in a way which closely mimics the glucose response of human islets. Since then, scientists are trying their best to produce results with the most impact.

Diabetes and its complications occur among Americans of all ages and ethnicities but the elderly and certain racial/ethnic groups are more commonly affected. In comparison of non – Hispanic whites, African Americans and Hispanics/Latino Americans are about two times more likely to be affected by the disease. It has been found that one tribe in Arizona has the highest rate of diabetes in the world, with about 50 percent of the adults between the ages of 30 and 64 with the disease. Population of type 2 diabetes sufferers has officially reached epidemic proportions.

Diabetes mellitus is developed when pancreatic tissue responsible for the production of insulin is absent because it is destroyed by disease such as chronic pancreatitis, trauma or surgical removal of pancreas. It can also result from other hormonal disturbances such as excessive growth hormone production (acromegaly, in which a pituitary gland tumor at the base of the brain causes excessive production of growth hormone leading to hyperglycemia) and Cushing's syndrome, in which the adrenal glands produce an excess of cortisol which promotes blood sugar elevation. Several other factors that make it more likely that a person develop diabetes are as follows:

- Age-older than 45 years
- Obesity
- Family history of diabetes in a first degree relative (parent or sibling)
- History with gestational diabetes mellitus
- Hispanic, Native American, African American, Asian American or Pacific Islander descent
- Hypertension (>140/90 mm Hg) or dyslipidemia (high-density lipoprotein HDL cholesterol <35mg/dl or triglyceride level >250mg/dl)

2.3 Symptoms and diagnosis of diabetes mellitus

Diabetes mellitus (DM) has diverse intial presentations. The early symptoms of diabetes are related to elevated blood sugar levels in the body and loss of glucose in the urine. It usually presents with symptomatic hyperglycemia. Common sign and symptoms may include any of the following:

- Being very thirsty
- Urinating often
- Feeling very hungry or tired
- Losing weight without trying
- Repeated or slow healing infections
- Having dry, itchy skin
- Extreme fatigue
- Blurred vision
- Tingling or loss of feeling in the hands or feet

2.4 Biological terms commonly used in diabetes

Insulin: An anabolic hormone, produced by the beta cells of the islets of Langerhans of pancreas in response of elevated blood sugar level in the body. It helps to control the blood sugar level in the desirable range.

Glucose: Glucose is a simple sugar present in everyone's body. It is an essential nutrient that provides energy for the proper functioning of the body cells. After meals, food is digested in the stomach and intestines. The glucose in digested food is absorbed by the intestinal cells into the blood stream and is carried by the blood to all the cells in the body. Glucose needs insulin to enter into the body as it can not get into the cells alone.

Glucagon: Glucagon is a hormone synthesized and secreted from alpha cells of the pancreatic islets used for carbohydrate metabolism. Its secretion increases rapidly when the sugar level is too low in the body. It maintains the level of glucose in the blood by binding to specific receptors on hepatocytes causing the liver to release its intracellular stores of glucose. As these stores become depleted, glucagon then encourages the liver to synthesize glucose by gluconeogenesis which will be released to prevent the development of hypoglycemia, low sugar level.

Insulin Resistance: Sometimes the cells throughout the body become resistant to the insulin produced by the pancreas due to which it becomes difficult for the sugar to enter the cells. This condition is known as insulin resistance.

Diabetic Ketoacidosis: It is a condition in which the cells of muscle, liver and other body parts are unable to take up glucose for producing energy due to the absence of insulin. It is a state of absolute or relative **insulin deficiency** aggravated by hyperglycemia, dehydration, and acidosis-producing derangements in intermediary metabolism. To avoid starvation the body begins to break down fat for energy. Fatty acids and ketone bodies are released due to the break down of fat causing chemical imbalance (metabolic imbalance) called Diabetic Ketoacidosis. Moderate or large amounts of **ketones** in urine are dangerous. They upset the chemical balance of the blood.

Chronic hyperglycemia: Chronic hyperglycemia means elevated blood sugar level in the blood.

2.5 Treatment therapies for diabetes

Type 1 Diabetes is very serious, with a sudden and dramatic onset, usually in youth. Type 1 diabetes is an autoimmune condition, where the body attacks its own insulin producing cells. The body's immune cells, or white blood cells, include B cells and T cells. B cells make antibodies and present 'antigens' to T cells, allowing them to recognize, and kill invaders. People with Type 1 diabetes must maintain an insulin-monitoring and insulin-injecting regimen for the rest of their lives as the islets of Langerhans are destroyed in this type of diabetes. Treatment for type 1 diabetes includes taking insulin shots or insulin pump to deliver insulin in the body, making wise food choices, exercising regularly and controlling blood pressure and cholesterol.

Type 2 diabetes can be treated successfully with diet, physical activity and medication, if necessary.[23] Physical activity can help to control blood sugar levels and increases body's sensitivity to insulin.[6] Also, it helps delays or stop heart diseases, a leading complication of diabetes. Diet plays an extremely important role in controlling this type of diabetes. Being overweight can increase the chances of developing type 2 diabetes. Usually GDM in pregnant women disappears itself after delivery.

2.6 Mathematical model

The first approach to measure the insulin sensitivity *in vivo* was introduced by Himsworth and Ker [24] and the first mathematical model to estimate the glucose disappearance and insulin sensitivity was proposed by Bolie. In this model, he assumed that glucose disappearance is a linear function of both glucose and insulin. The insulin secretion and disappearance is proportional to glucose and plasma insulin concentration respectively.

The main objective here is to prescribe a more accurate, but less simple, method of arranging the palatable composition of a diabetic diet.

The modified coupled differential equations for the plasma glucose and insulin concentration [1-14, 16-22], when the normal fasting level of plasma glucose is 70 - 120 mg/dl, are given as follows

$$\frac{dg}{dt} = -l_1 h \bar{g} + l_2 \left(g_0 - g \right) U \left(g_0 - g \right) + l_3 F(t) \tag{1}$$

$$\frac{dh}{dt} = l_4 \left(g - g_0 \right) U \left(g - g_0 \right) - l_5 h_0 + l_6 I(t) \tag{2}$$

where, g(t) - plasma glucose concentration, h(t) - insulin concentration, l_i - sensitivity constants, i = 1,2,3,4,5,6, F(t) - food source input for plasma glucose, I(t) – insulin input and $U(g_0 - g)$ is unit step function.

The insulin input I(t) will be given through injection at subcutaneous level at periodic intervals, which leaks its contents into the system over a period of time. Therefore, I(t) may be defined as

$$I(t) = \frac{\rho t}{t - t_0} + b$$

At t = t_0, I(t) = 0

$$\Rightarrow b = -\frac{\rho t_0}{t - t_0} \qquad \therefore I(t) = \frac{\rho(t - t_0)}{t - t_0} \qquad = \lambda + \mu t \qquad (3)$$

where, $\lambda = -\frac{\rho t_0}{t - t_0}$, $\mu = \frac{\rho}{t - t_0}$, ρ - quantity of injection, t_0 – time of injection, $\bar{t}$ -time lag to

maximum.

Food input source term, F(t), is the source for food input to the plasma glucose level, the contents of which are reduced in a simple exponential manner. Therefore, F(t) may be modeled as

$$F(t) = \begin{cases} Se^{-\alpha(t - t_0)}, & t > t_0 \\ 0, & t \le t_0 \end{cases} \qquad (4)$$

where, S - quantity constant of meal, α - delay parameter.

For $t \ge t_0$, in non – diabetic case, $F(t) \ne 0$ and $I(t) = 0$ and for diabetic case, $F(t) \ne 0$, $I(t) \ne 0$.

A mathematical model for the dynamics of glucose concentration in patients with type 1 diabetes using CSII [15] therapy as an external source of insulin has been developed by us. We attempt to model the effect of an external source of insulin release, as a prescribed function of time, on glucose levels. The model is then used to assess the optimal insulin release profile, and the threshold amount required to bring the level of glucose to within a normal physiological range.

To model the pump's delivery of insulin, we take into account three major factors: (i) the total amount of insulin released over a specific period; (ii) the time profile of insulin release, f(t); and (iii) the glucose threshold concentration Gc, below which the pump stops releasing insulin. The amount of insulin (TDD) is proportional to the total amount of glucose, whose concentration is assessed by the sensor in the pump's controller. This amount is released by the pump in a dual wave shaped insulin bolus which allows the patient to combine both normal and square wave techniques. The body characteristics of the patient determine how much insulin is needed to maintain the glucose level within the normal physiological range after each meal. The dual wave shape also provides a rapid increase in insulin plasma concentration, and sustained high circulating insulin levels while a meal is being consumed. Here, we extend the minimal model to incorporate the above factors, which leads to the following differential equations:

$$\frac{dG}{dt} = -XG + l_1(G_b - G)^+, \qquad (5)$$

$$\frac{dX}{dt} = -p_1 X + p_2 (I - I_b),\tag{6}$$

$$\frac{dI}{dt} = -l_2 (G - G_c)^+ f(t) - l_3 (I - I_b),\tag{7}$$

where G is the blood glucose concentration, X is an auxiliary function representing remote insulin action, and I is the insulin plasma concentration. A description of the model parameters and their values are given in Table 1.

The important part of this extension is the first term of (7) which models all three factors mentioned above. This term contributes to the insulin plasma when the glucose concentration exceeds the threshold Gc, and is defined as

$$l_2 (G - G_c)^+ = \begin{cases} l_2 (G(t) - G_c) f(t) & if\ G(t) > G_c \\ 0 & if\ G(t) < G_c \end{cases}\tag{8}$$

The function models the profile of insulin release from the pump, and the coefficient represents a scaling factor determining TDD of insulin released by the pump. In the next section, we discuss different profiles of insulin release and compare their effects on the optimal control of glucose concentration. The newer generation of pumps can be programmed to release insulin using three different bolus techniques.

A normal bolus can be used if small amounts of carbohydrates are consumed or if a correction to the blood glucose level outside the physiological range needs to be made. A square wave profile is helpful when eating foods that are high in both fat/protein and carbohydrate (fat and protein delay the absorption of carbohydrates). If a normal bolus is given for a meal high in protein and fat concentrations, circulating insulin levels rise rapidly and may peak before the carbohydrates are absorbed. This mismatch in insulin and blood glucose levels can result in postprandial hypoglycemia. Therefore, a dual wave bolus, as a combination of the normal and square wave bolus techniques, can be introduced. Using this technique, half of the insulin dose is given (over a short period of time) at the onset of the meal, and the remainder over a 2–4 h period. The profile of a dual wave bolus is modeled as a function of time, f(t), in Eq. (4) over a period of 3 h (Fig. 1(a)–(c)).

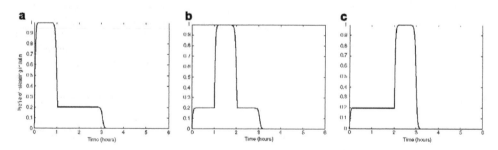

Fig. 1. Profile of insulin release by the pump $f(t)$, for 3h: HLL release; (b)LHL release; (c) LLH release, where H stands for high amount release of insulin and L stands for its low amount per hour $f(t)$ is normalized so that $H=L$

S No	Parameter	Description	Value	Unit
1	G_b	Base line value of glucose concentration in plasma	118	mg dl^{-1}
2	G_c	Glucose threshold concentration in plasma	100-107	mg dl^{-1}
3	I_b	Baseline value of insulin concentration in plasma	7	μU ml^{-1}
4	I_1	The insulin dependent rate of tissue glucose uptake	10	Min^{-1}
5	I_2	Scaling factor determining TDD of insulin	Variable	min^{-1} μU mg^{-1}
6	I_{3}	The rate of decay for insulin in plasma	0.264	min^{-1}
7	p_1	The rate of spontaneous decrease of glucose uptake	0.0107	min^{-1}
8	p_2	The rate of insulin – dependent increase in tissue glucose uptake due to insulin concentration excess over its baseline	0.007	min^{-2} μU ml^{-1}

Table 1. Description and values of the model parameters obtained from the published literature

This particular work is published in Applied Mathematics and computation, 2007, pages 1476 – 1483 and has been cited by Kato, R, Munkhjargal, M and Takahashi, D "An autonomous drug release system based on chemo- mechanical energy conversion "Organic Engine" for feedback control of blood glucose", Biosensors and Bioelecetronics in 2010 Vol 26(4), pages 1455 - 1459.

2.7 Future work
More advanced mathematical models can be formulated to explain the effects of obesity on diabetes, effects of exercise on management of type 2 diabetes. Parameters involving glucose sensors can be added to the insulin pump model for a better programmed insulin delivery by insulin pump.

3. References

[1] D. Araujo-Vilar, C.A. Rega-Liste, D.A. Garcia-Estevez, F. Sarmiento-Escalona, V. Mosquera-Tallon, J. Cabezas-Cerrato, Minimal model of glucose metabolism: modified equations and its application in the study of insulin sensitivity in obese subject, Diabetes Res. Clin. Pract. 39 (1998) 129–141.

[2] R.N. Bergman, L.S. Phillips, C. Cobelli, Physiologic evaluation of factors controlling glucose tolerance in man, J. Clin. Invest. 68 (1981) 1456–1467.

[3] B.W. Bode, R.D. Steed, P.C. Davidson, Reduction in severe hypoglycemia with long term continuous subcutaneous insulin infusion in type 1 diabetes, Diabetes Care 19 (1996) 324–327.

[4] A. Boutayeb, E.H. Twizell, K. Achouayb, A. Chetouani, A mathematical model for the burden of diabetes and its complications, BioMed. Eng. (2004), doi:10.1186/1475-925X-3-20, Online.

[5] A. De Gaetano, O. Arino, Mathematical modelling of the intravenous glucose tolerance test, J. Math. Biol. 40 (2000) 136–168.

[6] M. Derouich, A. Boutayeb, The effect of physical exercise on the dynamics of glucose and insulin, J. Biomech. 35 (2002) 911–917.

[7] Diabetes Control and Complications Trial Research Group, The effect of intensive treatment of diabetes on the development and progression of long-term complications in insulin-dependent diabetes mellitus, New. Engl. J. Med. 329 (1993) 977–985.

[8] T.M. Gross, D. Kayne, A. King, C. Rother, S. Juth, A bolus calculator is an effective means of controlling postprandial glycemia in patients on insulin pump therapy, Diabetes Technol. Ther. 5 (2003) 365–369.

[9] A.P. Harmel, R. Mathur, Davidson's Diabetes Mellitus: Diagnosis and Treatment, fifth ed., 2004.

[10] W.B. Saunders, A.E. Kitabchi, J.N. Fisher, G.A. Burghen, M.S. Gaylord, N.M. Blank, Evaluation of a portable insulin infusion pump for outpatient management of brittle diabetes, Diabetes Care 2 (1979) 421–424.

[11] R. Linkeschova, M. Raoul, U. Bott, M. Berger, M. Spraul, Less Severe hypoglycemia, better metabolic control and improved quality of life in type 1 diabetes mellitus with continuous subcutaneous insulin infusion (CSII) therapy; an observational study of 100 consecutive patients followed for a mean of 2 years, Diabetes Med. 19 (2002) 746–751.

[12] R.S. Parker, F.J. Doyle, N.A. Peppas, A model-based algorithm for blood glucose control in type I diabetic patients, IEEE Trans. BioMed. Eng. 46 (1999) 148–157.

[13] L. Perko, Differential Equations and Dynamical Systems, Springer-Verlag, New York, 1996.

[14] J.C. Pickup, M.C. White, H. Keen, J.A. Parsons, K.G. Alberti, Long-term continuous subcutaneous insulin infusion in diabetics at home, Lancet 2 (1979) 870–873.

[15] J. Pickup, H. Keen, Continuous subcutaneous insulin infusion at 25 years: evidence base for the expanding use of insulin pump therapy in type 1 diabetes, Diabetes Care 25 (2002) 593–598.

[16] G. Pillonetto, G. Sparacino, C. Cobelli, Numerical non-identifiability regions of the minimal model of glucose kinetics: superiority of Bayesian estimation, Math. Biosci. 184 (2003) 53–67.

[17] W. Regittnig, Z. Trajanoski, H.J. Leis, M. Ellmerer, A. Wutte, G. Sendlhofer, L. Schaupp, G.A. Brunner, P. Wach, T.R. Pieber, Plasma and interstitial glucose dynamics after intravenous glucose injection, Diabetes 48 (1999) 1070–1081.

[18] Report of the expert committee on the diagnosis and classification of diabetes mellitus, Diabetes Care 20 (1997) 1183–1197.

[19] The UK Prospective Diabetes Study (UKPDS) Group, Intensive blood glucose control with sulphonylureas or insulin compared withconventional treatment and risk of complications in patients with type 2 diabetes (UKPDS33), Lancet 352 (1998) 837–853.

[20] G. Toffolo, E. Breda, M.K. Cavaghan, D.A. Ehrmann, K.S. Polonsky, C. Cobelli, Quantitative indexes of b-cell function duringgraded up and down glucose infusion from C-peptide models, Am. J. Physiol. Endocrinol. Metab. 280 (2001) E2–E10.

[21] I.M. Tolic´, E. Mosekilde, J. Sturis, Modelling the insulin–glucose feedback system: the significance of pulsatile insulin secretion, J. Theor. Biol. 207 (2000) 361–375.

[22] J. Unger, A primary care approach to continuous subcutaneous insulin infusion, Clin. Diabetes 17 (1999) 113–127.

[23] Management of Type 2 Diabetes, N ENGL J MED 358;3, 2008.

[24] Himsworth/ H. 1. and 5er/ R. B./ Insulin sensiti<e and insulin insensiti<e types of diabetes mellitus/ Clinical Science/ 4 D1F3FH 11F.

Permissions

The contributors of this book come from diverse backgrounds, making this book a truly international effort. This book will bring forth new frontiers with its revolutionizing research information and detailed analysis of the nascent developments around the world.

We would like to thank Dr. Chih-Pin Liu, for lending his expertise to make the book truly unique. He has played a crucial role in the development of this book. Without his invaluable contribution this book wouldn't have been possible. He has made vital efforts to compile up to date information on the varied aspects of this subject to make this book a valuable addition to the collection of many professionals and students.

This book was conceptualized with the vision of imparting up-to-date information and advanced data in this field. To ensure the same, a matchless editorial board was set up. Every individual on the board went through rigorous rounds of assessment to prove their worth. After which they invested a large part of their time researching and compiling the most relevant data for our readers. Conferences and sessions were held from time to time between the editorial board and the contributing authors to present the data in the most comprehensible form. The editorial team has worked tirelessly to provide valuable and valid information to help people across the globe.

Every chapter published in this book has been scrutinized by our experts. Their significance has been extensively debated. The topics covered herein carry significant findings which will fuel the growth of the discipline. They may even be implemented as practical applications or may be referred to as a beginning point for another development. Chapters in this book were first published by InTech; hereby published with permission under the Creative Commons Attribution License or equivalent.

The editorial board has been involved in producing this book since its inception. They have spent rigorous hours researching and exploring the diverse topics which have resulted in the successful publishing of this book. They have passed on their knowledge of decades through this book. To expedite this challenging task, the publisher supported the team at every step. A small team of assistant editors was also appointed to further simplify the editing procedure and attain best results for the readers.

Our editorial team has been hand-picked from every corner of the world. Their multi-ethnicity adds dynamic inputs to the discussions which result in innovative outcomes. These outcomes are then further discussed with the researchers and contributors who give their valuable feedback and opinion regarding the same. The feedback is then collaborated with the researches and they are edited in a comprehensive manner to aid the understanding of the subject.

Apart from the editorial board, the designing team has also invested a significant amount of their time in understanding the subject and creating the most relevant covers. They scrutinized every image to scout for the most suitable representation of the subject and create an appropriate cover for the book.

The publishing team has been involved in this book since its early stages. They were actively engaged in every process, be it collecting the data, connecting with the contributors or procuring relevant information. The team has been an ardent support to the editorial, designing and production team. Their endless efforts to recruit the best for this project, has resulted in the accomplishment of this book. They are a veteran in the field of academics and their pool of knowledge is as vast as their experience in printing. Their expertise and guidance has proved useful at every step. Their uncompromising quality standards have made this book an exceptional effort. Their encouragement from time to time has been an inspiration for everyone.

The publisher and the editorial board hope that this book will prove to be a valuable piece of knowledge for researchers, students, practitioners and scholars across the globe.

List of Contributors

Paulo Ivo Homem de Bittencourt Jr.
Department of Physiology, Institute of Basic Health Sciences, Federal University of Rio Grande do Sul, Brazil
Federal University of Rio Grande do Sul School of Physical Education, Porto Alegre, RS, Brazil
National Institute of Hormones and Women's Health, Brazil

Philip Newsholme
School of Biomolecular and Biomedical Science and Institute for Sport and Health, UCD Dublin, Belfield, Dublin 4, Ireland

Elisavet Efstathiou and Nicos Skordis
Paediatric Endocrine Unit, Department of Paediatrics, Makarios Hospital, Nicosia, Cyprus

Elena Matteucci and Ottavio Giampietro
Department of Internal Medicine, University of Pisa, Italy

Adriana Mimbacas
Instituto de Investigaciones Biológicas Clemente Estable, Department of Genetics, Human Genetic Group, Uruguay

Gerardo Javiel
ASSE-Ministry of Health, Hospital Pasteur, Uruguay
IAMPP-Centro de Asistencia del Sindicato Médico del Uruguay,(CASMU), Diabetologic Service, Uruguay

Kjersti S. Rønningen
Department of Pediatric Research, Oslo University Hospital, Rikshospitalet, Oslo, Norway

Mamdouh Abdulrhman, Rasha Ali and Ahmad Abou El-Goud
Pediatric Department, Faculty of Medicine, Ain Shams University, Abbasia – Cairo, Egypt

Mohamed El Hefnawy
National Institute of Diabetes, Cairo, Egypt

Momir Mikov and Svetlana Golocorbin-Kon
Department of Pharmacology, Toxicology and Clinical Pharmacology, Medical Faculty, Univeristy of Novi Sad, Serbia
Pharmacy Faculty, University of Montenegro, Podgorica, Montenegro

Hani Al-Salami
Senior Lecturer, School of Pharmacy, Curtin University, Perth, Australia

Agustin Busta, Bianca Alfonso and Leonid Poretsky
Albert Einstein College of Medicine, Beth Israel, Medical Center New York, U.S.A.

Éva Szabó, Tamás Marosvölgyi and Tamás Decsi
University of Pécs, Department of Pediatrics, Pécs, Hungary

Nilam Nilam
Department of Mathematics, Delhi Technological University, Delhi, India

Seyed M. Moghadas
Centre for Disease Modelling, York University, Toronto, Ontario, Canada

Pappur N. Shivakumar
Department of Mathematics, University of Manitoba, Winnipeg, Manitoba, Canada

Printed in the USA
CPSIA information can be obtained
at www.ICGtesting.com
JSHW011426221024
72173JS00004B/684